Medicine, Sport and the Body

Medicine, Sport and the Body
A Historical Perspective

Neil Carter

B L O O M S B U R Y

LONDON · NEW DELHI · NEW YORK · SYDNEY

Bloomsbury Academic
An imprint of Bloomsbury Publishing Plc

50 Bedford Square
London
WC1B 3DP
UK

1385 Broadway
New York
NY 10018
USA

www.bloomsbury.com

Bloomsbury is a registered trade mark of Bloomsbury Publishing Plc

First published in 2012
Paperback edition first published 2014

British Library Cataloguing-in-Publication Data
A catalogue record for this book is available from the British Library.

ISBN: HB: 978-1-8496-6067-9
       PB: 978-1-4725-5854-1
       ePDF: 978-1-8496-6681-7
       ePUB: 978-1-8496-6680-0

Library of Congress Cataloging-in-Publication Data
A catalog record for this book is available from the Library of Congress.

Printed and bound in Great Britain

Contents

Acknowledgements

My first debt of gratitude is to Emily Drewe, Rhodri Mogford and Jenny Dodd at Bloomsbury Academic for both their professionalism and patience.

My biggest debt of gratitude is to Mike Cronin who was the joint-grant holder for a Wellcome Trust-funded history of sports medicine, jointly run between De Montfort University and the University of Manchester. I was a research fellow for this project and this book is a product of that collaboration. I would like to thank Ian Burney and Michael Worboys for their help and I am especially grateful to Vanessa Heggie for her contribution throughout.

During the research for this book many people have generously given their time, particularly John Lloyd Parry, John Rowlands, and Robin Harland as well as my interviewees. Patrick Milroy also kindly passed on the archives of the British Association of Sport and Exercise Medicine (now deposited in the Wellcome Archives).

Richard Holt and Tony Mason kindly read drafts and made typically sensible suggestions while my colleagues – Matt Taylor, Tony Collins, Jean Williams, Jeff Hill and Dil Porter – also provided advice and support in equal measure.

Introduction

Published in 1962, *Sports Medicine* was the first English language book with the phrase 'sports medicine' in the title.[1] Edited by John G.P. Williams, a pioneering figure in British sports medicine, this collection of essays, aimed mainly at general practitioners but also coaches and trainers, was a landmark study. In the preface it was claimed that the book was necessary because of the intensity of modern competitive sport, which had resulted in the emergence of a new type of person – the trained athlete; hence the need for a book, which could cater for the special demands of this lifestyle. There are chapters on both the physiological and psychological aspects of sport, training methods as well as the treatment of injuries. 'The Athlete's Life' is the final chapter. Written by Williams, it touches upon aspects of physical hygiene and includes advice on cleanliness and oral health. There is also a section that gives guidance on an athlete's sexual habits. It was recommended that a 'married couple should maintain the normal pattern of sexual relationship during the training and competition season'. So far, so good. The advice then gradually takes on a decidedly moral tone. Single athletes are advised 'most strongly against extramarital intercourse'. Athletes are advised against masturbation on moral grounds but if he – and there is no mention of she – feels he must then he should go ahead. Nocturnal emissions, i.e., wet dreams, are explained as 'a natural and normal part of adolescence', and there is no need, as one male athlete did, to tie a soft-drink bottle around his waist to prevent himself lying on his back. Homosexuality is regarded as a perversion. This 'problem', it is stated, 'must be handled with sympathy and delicacy', which includes the seeking of psychiatric advice. Williams cautioned that if 'cases' appear – like an outbreak of the measles – among members of a touring team they may have to be sent home and classified as 'sick'. Interestingly, in a later book, published in 1965, Williams makes no reference to homosexuality, although he repeats his other advice on 'sexual hygiene'. It perhaps indicates how even within three years the Sixties were having an impact on social discourse.[2] The aim here is not to criticize Williams' attitudes towards sex. Instead it is to demonstrate the increasing role doctors were now playing in the lives of athletes and how far this extended, as well as how their views on the bodies of athletes were shaped by wider social and cultural forces.

The actions of the body have become part of the sporting language. Whether through the pushing of an athlete's body to the limit of its capabilities or the breaking down of a particular part of this 'machine' through injury, sport has been expressed in medical terms. In his study of American sporting autobiographies, James Pipkin has identified how athletes base their identity on their bodies and have an obsession with body image. However, while their 'super fitness' and athletic prowess engenders a feeling of indomitability, there is also the constant pressure of competing and the fear of injury and that this indomitability will be taken away from them with the loss of identity that this would entail.[3]

In her autobiography, Paula Radcliffe makes the reader fully aware of the importance she places on her relationship with medicine. It reads in part like a medical logbook due to the numerous visits she makes to various practitioners. However, she puts more faith in one form of therapy than the others – and this 'faith' is a recurrent theme throughout. Moreover, another important part of the life of the modern athlete that comes through in the book is the time spent coping with and recuperating from injury.[4] The obsession with medicine, therefore, is unsurprising. An athlete's body is his or hers only resource. How this resource has been studied and managed through the prisms of sport and medicine is the focus of this book.

Sport and medicine have been two of the major cultural and scientific growth areas of the twentieth century. Medicine has become 'increasingly central to changing expectations of life and death' and has 'pervasively and profoundly influenced the ways in which people come to maintain their bodies, to mind their minds and to interact with the world around them'.[5] Sport similarly exerts powerful but largely unseen influences on much of the world's population. It has not only influenced leisure and consumption patterns, moral values, aesthetics, conceptions of time and space, work and play, individual and society but also ideas about race and gender, and the body.[6]

The aim here is to write a history of the relationship between sport and medicine in its widest possible context. In many ways sport and medicine are natural bedfellows because of the emphasis on bodily experiences. As Richard Holt has observed, 'Sport is cultural as well as physical, and what we do with our bodies is very much a product of what we think we ought to do with them'.[7] Similarly, while much of medicine is based on knowledge about the body in sickness and health, these 'ideas and practices do not develop through their own inexorable logic'.[8] Instead, as Cooter and Pickstone argue, medical knowledge is subject to the social, political and cultural contexts in which it is produced and used.[9] These 'bodily experiences', therefore, have not been politically or socially neutral because both sport and medicine also act as cultural agencies. In linking the two together, Patricia Vertinsky has identified how the expanding power of medical knowledge in the production and regulation of sporting bodies has been one of the most significant developments in sport over the second half of the twentieth century.[10] Sport has also been an expression of twentieth century modernity in which the rational, scientific measurement of the performer as well as the performance has been an integral part. As athletes have come to see the benefits of medicine so scientists have become interested in investigating the possibilities and potential of the athletic body.

However, we can also identify elements within sport that makes its relationship with medicine seem peculiar to other areas of society. In particular, although the idea of regular exercise has long been thought of as a pathway to good health, sport at the elite level (and even at recreational level to a certain extent) is about excess and it can be considered unhealthy – maybe pathological – due to the general wear and tear on the body and the injuries sustained. Whereas the function of medicine has generally been to act as a rational response to ill health, elite sports, especially those that involve physical contact, have produced different responses from doctors. As a consequence, it can lead to dilemmas for practitioners, patients and medical organizations alike that are alien to the 'normal' response.

Sports medicine or sport and medicine?

The breadth of the relationship between sport and medicine is wide as well as complex. One means of simplifying the relationship has been to just call it 'sports medicine'. However, like 'medicine' itself, the phrase sports medicine is protean. Cooter and Pickstone have stated that medicine can range from what we take or receive 'for our own good' from a bottle, as pills or products from multi-national companies. It can also mean the professional practices of healers as well as refer to institutions of research and education, hospitals or the local GP's surgery. Medicine is often equated to the provision nation-states make for the fitness of their populations through national health schemes.[11]

The term 'sports medicine' had not been coined by 1914 and as a specialism sports medicine has been a relatively late modern innovation. It was only in 1932 that the first book to use the term was probably written: Dr Hermann Herxheimer's *Grundriss im Sportsmedizin* (*Foundations of Sports Medicine*) was published in Germany. An international organization, the Fédération Internationale de Médecine Sportive (FIMS), was founded in 1928.[12] However, sports medicine was not used regularly in the English language until the formation of the American College of Sports Medicine in 1954. Medical specialisms have tended not to have had fixed definitions. Instead they have evolved, making any definition problematic. Defining sports medicine is further complicated because it is a holistic practice, covering a wide range of interests, such as the treatment of injuries and performance enhancement.[13]

At the heart of sports medicine's identity have been debates over whether it should be directed more towards elite athletes or the general population. In the late 1950s, for example, the Canadian doctor, Doris Plewes argued that sports medicine was about 'the physical efficiency of normal people' not with athletes *per se*. Any experiments on elite athletes, therefore, should be for the benefit of the population as a whole.[14] In 1999 the British Association of Sport and Medicine (BASM), which had been formed in 1952, changed its name to the British Association of Sport and Exercise Medicine (BASEM).

This was to accommodate a shift towards a greater emphasis on exercise medicine by the state, partly due to concern over rising obesity levels. In 2005 the UK government bestowed specialty status on sport and exercise medicine despite no consensus amongst sports medicine practitioners in the United Kingdom (nor in many other countries) over what actually constituted a sports medicine specialist.[15] In 2006 Paul McCrory, the editor of the *British Journal of Sports Medicine* could still state:

> There is no universally accepted definition of sports and exercise medicine (SEM). The nature of the discipline has changed over time and continues to do so as SEM begins to clarify its scope more clearly and delineates itself from the traditional medical specialities.[16]

As McCrory also pointed out, the British government now set the parameters of the discipline whereas previously an unregulated sports medicine landscape allowed for much flexibility in its definition.

Because it has held different meanings at different periods throughout recent history, there is a danger of seeing sports medicine solely in terms of the medical profession and how it has developed as a medical specialty. The development of sports medicine as a specialty is an important element in the story of the relationship between sport and medicine but it is only one part. Because of this elasticity, therefore, rather than make claims about writing a hermetically-sealed history of sports medicine, this book is more concerned with the relationship between sport and medicine and how this has developed over time and place.

Histories of sport and medicine

The histories of medicine and sport have followed similar trajectories, although medical history was being written from the nineteenth century – by doctors to mainly illuminate scientific or professional issues – whereas academic histories of sport emerged only in the 1970s.[17] Each benefited from not only the expansion of higher education and with this the growth in academics and newly researched subjects but also both drew upon the new social history from the Sixties. Initially, the history of medicine placed an emphasis on medical knowledge whereas labour history provided a framework for the history of sport. Both sub-disciplines later came under the influence of cultural history and the linguistic turn. As a consequence, the history of medicine has seen a growth of cultural and historical studies of the body and its diseases and a shift away from the history of science and technology, health services and demographics. Within the history of sport there has been a quest to locate its meanings, especially identities, whether local or national, or increasingly the self.[18]

What attempts have been made to merge these two branches of history? Unsurprisingly the shifting debates over definition have also been mirrored in the scope of the academic work on sports medicine. In their edited collection, Berryman and Park make a similar observation about the difficulties in nailing down a definition, and indeed, their ground-breaking book is perhaps confusingly titled, *Sport and Exercise Science: Essays in the History of Sports Medicine*.[19] Some early histories of sports medicine and sports science were written by practitioners and had teleological tendencies.[20] There continues to be a sense in some of the literature that emphasizes the idea of the 'progress' of both sport and medicine; possibly a product of sport being judged by the stop-watch and tape. Even the otherwise excellent doctoral thesis of Nicholas Bourne on a history of sports science tends to look upon the subject uncritically and with an inevitable sense of improvement.[21] But just as improvements in health have resulted in people living longer and has shifted debates towards issues such as Alzheimer's, so with sport, improvements in human athletic performance has provoked debate over topics such as drugs. This book is concerned with the historical context in which these 'improvements' have taken place.

Pioneered amongst others by Roberta Park, much of the early academic literature focused on the fusion of ideas that liked health and wellbeing through the pursuit of physical activity as well as the development of physical education in North America.[22] Patricia Vertinsky, another pioneer, has analysed how prevailing medical discourses concerning women's exercise since the nineteenth century have shaped gender power relations[23] while some of Park's work has also overlapped with the history of sports science.[24] Other work here has tended to focus on the idea of performance enhancement within specific contexts.[25] The area that has attracted most academic attention though has been on drugs in sport, a subject not only tightly linked to athletic performance but also tied to ethical and moral debates around cheating, which has led to a focus on the anti-doping regulations of sporting authorities in their attempts to eradicate cheating.[26] More recently there has been a shift towards seeing drugs in sport in a wider historical context and the questioning of some past assumptions.[27]

In 2007 Mike Cronin noted that there had been a gap in the historiography of sports medicine as 'a practice that treats injury'. While there is now some work in this area stressing continuities and discontinuities[28] there is also a large sociological literature, which has mainly focussed on the notion of pain and the professional credentials of sports medicine practitioners.[29] Linked to debates on the culture of risk, a considerable literature on the working lives of physiotherapists and doctors – and their professional status – in football and rugby has been produced.[30] Ken Sheard has similarly examined how injuries in boxing have been managed as well as the moral implications for the sport.[31]

In her recent book, Vanessa Heggie has written persuasively on how in Britain the history of sport and exercise medicine as a formal medical specialty can be explained through a biomedical understanding of the athletic body: 'It is only when the athlete becomes "not normal" – that is, both supernormal as well as abnormal – that one can have sports medicine as distinct area of expertise'.[32] While the emergence of a distinct athletic body is not denied, this book takes a slightly different direction. Because sports medicine has traditionally been a space occupied by a variety of practitioners – medical and non-medical – the objective here is to explore the multi-faceted relationship between sport and medicine through a number of the constituent elements that have emerged such as fitness, injuries, performance enhancement and ethics as well as a specialty. In the heart of every athletic body beats a strong competitive impulse but this book also gives a nod to the different types of athletic bodies, which have been inscribed with different meanings. While sport – through its rules – has been an artificial construction, it has also been a cultural agent that has had a power to work on its participants and consumers ideologically,[33] and as the meaning of sport has mutated there has been a subsequent shift in the demand for medicine.

Through sport, for example, meanings of gender have been produced and re-produced. Sport has been a largely masculine affair with an emphasis on the values of courage, loyalty and hardness as well as an ability to withstand pain that have been traditionally associated with men. However, in their attempts to claim some of the cultural space filled by men, female athletes have also appropriated some of these qualities. Moreover, sports with physical contact have also engendered attitudes that they are about the giving and taking of hard knocks. As a consequence, playing with injury has become an acceptable part of the sporting sub-culture. Some sports created their own individual meanings. Cricket was seen as a gentlemanly game while prize-fighting became a metaphor for British patriotism. The Tour de France, through the media, developed a heroic ethos and a cult of suffering and survival.[34]

In addition, sport has created its own ideologies. In the early twentieth century, sporting values had been seen as a preparation for war, for example.[35] The amateur ideology was the most persistent. Amateurism is a slippery concept but it carried heavy moral and ethical overtones. It was essentially a state of mind in which social status was all important. British 'gentleman amateur' administrators ran sports for themselves in order to transmit the values of *esprit de corps*, the character building nature of sport, fair play and sportsmanship, as well as to *de facto* exclude the working classes and to keep the professionals in their place. Tensions between amateurs and professionals reverberated throughout the twentieth century. Amateurs loathed the association of sport with money, especially through gambling. There was also a dislike of winning through any form of 'specialization'. Yet for many amateurs winning was important. This was partly the reason why in 1882 the Amateur Rowing Association had excluded manual workers because amateur oarsmen could not hope to compete with the watermen of the Thames and Tyne. Also in 1882, the formation of the Corinthians, that bastion of amateurism, had been underpinned by competition. The club's founder 'Pa' Jackson, fed up with Scotland regularly defeating England in the annual football international, wanted to build a team that comprised the best English (amateur) players so that they would become familiar with each other's play.[36] Amateurism ran deep into British society. It was also an aspect of the Victorian obsession with health and the idea of *mens sana in corpore sano*. Sporting administrators emphasized active participation and there were attempts to regulate violent play: the amateur body had to be protected as well as developed. As a consequence, moderation in exercise became the watchword.[37]

Moreover, given their middle-class backgrounds many doctors were instilled with these notions and a number of them played an important role in running British sport during the twentieth century. Amateur values were also present in professional sports like football, which was largely resistant to coaching. The amateur hegemony within British sport ran into the 1960s, although amateurism was not applied uniformly by each sport and the nature and meanings of amateurism itself shifted in light of changes in the sporting world. However, these attitudes coloured the sport-medicine relationship and can be summed up by Geoff Dyson, who was the first chief coach of the Amateur Athletic Association from 1947 to 1961,

> the British attitude, particularly in Oxford and Cambridge, the Fighting Services perhaps a little less so but at public schools, would go something like this – if you do well in sport and you train, 'Good show', but if you do well in sport and you don't train, 'Bloody good show'.[38]

Similar views about the 'amateur nature' of British sport would be aired frequently throughout the twentieth century. International sport had begun to emerge from the early 1900s due to the founding of organizations like the International Olympic Committee (1894) and football's world governing body FIFA (1904) and the values of amateurism later became embedded in the administration of these bodies. Yet this did not mean notions of fair play and competition were incompatible. Out of his admiration for the English sporting model, Pierre de Coubertin, the founder of the IOC, advocated an (elitist) ideology of Olympic universalism. While invoking Greek classicism, 'Olympism' also promoted notions of athletic excellence because de Coubertin felt that men should strive to their physical limits in order to aspire to heroism; an ideal that has much resonance in the twenty-first century.

While amateurism was not absent in American sport either, it was defined more in monetary than moral terms. Amateur athletes did not get paid but that did not prevent them from adopting a 'professional' attitude. American sport was mainly based on its collegiate system, and this was very competitive. In particular, college football had become *de facto* professionalized by the 1920s. Moreover, American culture promoted a more competitive society than Britain, certainly in sport, which had consequences for the demands put on athletes. This ultra competitiveness is illustrated in Philip Roth's *The Great American Novel*:

'I am talking about winning, Roland, winning – what made this country what it is today. Who in his right mind can be against that?'

Who, indeed. Winning! Oh, you really can't say enough good things about it. There is nothing quite like it ... Winning is the tops. Winning is the name of the game. Winning is what it's all about. Winning is the be-all and the end-all, and don't let anybody tell you otherwise. All the world loves a winner.

Show me a good loser, said Leo Durocher, and I'll show you a loser ... Losing is tedious ... Losing makes for headaches, muscle tension, skin eruptions, ulcers, indigestion and for mental disorders of every kind. Losing is bad for confidence, pride, business, peace of mind, family harmony, love, sexual potency, concentration ... Losing makes the benign malicious, the generous stingy, the brave fearful, the healthy ill and the kindly bitter. Losing is universally despised, as well it should be. The sooner we get rid of losing, the happier everyone will be.

'But winning. To win! It was everything Roland remembered.'[39]

Following the establishment of international sporting competition, nationalism came to the fore, starting at the 1908 Olympics and the rivalry between Britain and America. Other nations not only began to take a greater interest in sporting success but also the fitness of their populations. During the twentieth century many countries, especially new ones, appropriated sport for the construction of national identity. The Olympic Games and the football World Cup were particularly important in providing a forum for these national rivalries to be played out. This process was further intensified after 1945 with the onset of the Cold War and the rivalry between East and West. Greater resources were devoted to sport as topping the medal table for those leaders of countries in Eastern Europe gave justification for their political system. It was during this period that the relationship between science and sport became closer. The Cold War had ended by 1990 and global sport entered a phase of intense commercialization with television as the paymaster. With greater rewards available, there was an analogous increase in the quest of athletes and coaches for the extra edge that could make the difference between winning and losing. Even in Britain, the mantra of winning would become all-important and hence the need of sportsmen and women to train hard and have access to the best medical and scientific resources.

The role of the state, another theme of this book, has been evident on a number of levels. Public health became an increasing concern for national governments from the nineteenth century and resulted in a drift to increasingly welfarist policies. Through physical education, sport became part of the state. In addition, sport was later used as a tool to boost national prestige. However, this was an uneven process, which was contingent on national political cultures. In America, for example, there was no national health service similar to the one in Britain, nor was there any wish that the state would interfere in sporting matters. At the other end of the spectrum, communist states controlled all aspects of society through central planning. They were particularly keen on using physical culture to improve the health of their populations as well as exploit sport for matters of politics and prestige.

Britain fell somewhere in-between these two extremes.[40] While concern and spending for welfare grew throughout the twentieth century, especially with the establishment of the National Health Service in 1948, the mark of British civil society was its voluntary tradition. Associational life continued to be strong throughout the twentieth century. Many nineteenth century charities, for example, had acted as social services but their role was later taken over by the state. But gaps that were left continued to be filled by the voluntary sector. However, there was a great reluctance for the British state to interfere in sporting affairs. Sport was seen as a voluntary activity by a political class, most of whom were imbued with the amateur ethic. Even when a Sports Council was formed in the 1960s, intervention was still constrained. Nevertheless, from the 1990s the British government had begun to see and use sport in the same way as other Western countries like Canada and Australia.

The history of sport and medicine has also been a history of power, especially power in the hands of the medical profession, patients and institutions. In addition, the history of sports medicine – as a medical specialty – has been bound up with tensions between orthodox and alternative medicine. The medical profession has sought to exclude certain practitioners in order to defend their place in the medical marketplace and this has been reflected in sports medicine.

Structure

The book's main focus is on elite sport but developments here are also aligned with the issue of fitness amongst the masses. The British (mostly English) experience is the primary focus but international examples (mainly Western countries) are used to illuminate general points about the relationship between sport and medicine. One justification for this preference is that Britain, America and Europe were the pioneers of modern sport and hence it developed a longer relationship with medicine. Moreover, developments here have tended to be copied elsewhere although more research on the subject, especially in Asia, would be welcome. The book has a thematic structure with each chapter based on a chronological framework, covering both the nineteenth and twentieth centuries. A variety of sources have been employed. These include archival material, newspapers and medical journals as well as secondary sources. A number of interviews have been conducted with doctors, physiotherapists and players from English association football in conjunction with a questionnaire survey (for qualitative purposes) regarding their medical experiences. In a subject as wide as this one book cannot cover all the ground but some omissions requires acknowledgement. In particular, there is little on sport and disability and sport and race although there is a growing literature on both subjects.[41]

The opening chapter places the relationship between sport and medicine in the wider context of health. It explores how, since the nineteenth century, sport, exercise and physical culture were incorporated into cultural and scientific ideas about health, wellbeing and the body. In particular, it examines the impact of eugenics on ideas of national degeneration and the role of the state in its increasing promotion of public health. Sport and exercise were seen as vital in increasing the 'fitness of the nation' throughout the twentieth century. From the late twentieth century, the relationship between exercise and wellbeing became increasingly consumerist. There was a boom in the recreational sport and leisure market more generally that reflected greater individual concerns and solutions over health.

Chapter 2 looks at the occupational culture of athletes and how this shaped the nature of medical provision in its social, cultural and legal context. Attitudes to sporting injuries have been forged by an amalgam of ideas concerning masculinity as well as an intensification in competition and later sport's exponential commercialization, at least in Britain and America. Moreover, because sport was seen as a voluntary activity separate from the state, national sporting bodies acted as quasi-legal organizations that made the rules and had a *de facto* duty of care to athletes. The ever-present threat of injury to professionals, who relied on staying healthy for their ability to earn, was a factor in a gradual shift towards a greater emphasis on the health and safety of athletes.

The third chapter is concerned with the rise of sports medicine as a medical specialty. Initially, a doctor's interest in sport was often personal, reflected by the role – and case study here – of the football club doctor. However, it is also a story about medical politics as the medical profession attempted to bring sports medicine under its umbrella in a professional and institutional sense. Germany had been an early pioneer while an international federation for sports medicine was established in the 1930s. A case study of the British Association of Sport and Medicine, which was founded in 1952, charts how the aims of sports medicine – as a specialty – evolved in the context of medical politics. As a consequence, in 2005 sports medicine was recognized by the government as a medical specialty and became available on the NHS.

Because of the escalating stress placed on their bodies during training and competition it is unsurprising that athletes increasingly sought the expertise of medical practitioners. The fourth chapter is essentially a history of sports science, thus reflecting the wide-ranging nature of sport and medicine's relationship. But this was a bottom-up process and is reflected in an on-going tension between coaches, who were from a practical tradition, and emerging scientific theories and their application to sport, particularly track and field athletics, the main case study here. At first, athletes' training methods were based on empirical notions but by the twentieth century, modern science played a more influential role and a paradigm shift took place. However, it was not a smooth transition. Not only does the chapter map the evolution in training techniques but it also highlights how they have been shaped by prevailing discourses, both medical and sporting.

Chapter 5 is an extension of the previous one due to its implications for the enhancement of sporting performance. However, the subject is deserving of a chapter on its own because there has been no more emotive subject in sport over the last few decades than the use of drugs. The aim here, similar to the approach adopted by Paul Dimeo,[42] is to cut across this emotion and see the topic in its wider historical context. In particular, it examines how discourses have been constructed around the topic in light of sporting ideologies of fair play as well as how the issue was inflamed through the sporting Cold War and how doping controls emerged. While much of the literature has focussed on athletics and cycling, the sport of snooker is used as a case study to show how the tentacles of this issue reached into every corner of the sporting world.

For many people, the popular perception of sports medicine's *raison d' étre* has been to treat the injuries of athletes and to ensure that they return to the sporting arena as soon as possible. Chapter 6 charts how the treatment of injuries has developed from the application of the 'magic sponge' to more modern sophisticated techniques and a case study of the football trainer plots the professionalization of this role. Moreover, this chapter also highlights how the sporting arena places peculiar demands and provides ethical challenges for medical practitioners due to the not always identical objectives of athletes and coaches.

Chapter 7 is an example of the wider social implications of sport's relationship with medicine. Whilst not the only reason, medicine has been a key factor in shaping the development of women's sport. Importantly, it shaped perceptions of female athletes and reinforced gender stereotypes that were projected through the media and everyday discourse. Starting in the nineteenth century, this chapter will show how notions of 'eternally wounded' women and their perceived role as mothers, persisted along with other medical theories to constrain women's involvement in sport. From medical pronouncements on what exercise was deemed suitable for women to issues such as gender testing by international sporting authorities, the medical profession has played a significant role in shaping the growth in the participation of females in sport and physical activity generally.

Finally, in his review on the historiography of boxing, John Welshman expressed surprise that 'there has been almost no interest in the links between boxing and the medical establishment'.[43] The final chapter attempts to fill this lacuna. In medical terms, boxing has been one of the most controversial sports and this chapter shows how from an early stage doctors began to take an interest in it. Rather than injuries being incidental to the sport, it is the specific aim of boxers to injure and harm their opponents, and has seen high profile incidents of medical intervention, as in the Michael Watson case. This chapter charts how the boxing debate, mainly in Britain, has evolved over the twentieth century, especially in light of a welfarist ethos and growing medical evidence that boxing caused brain damage, leading to a vociferous lobby that wanted the sport banned. It also highlights how the rhetoric of the medical profession came to shape the story of boxing during the twentieth century and how through growing safety measures the sport was increasingly subject to medical control.

1

Sport as Medicine

Ideas of Health, Sport and Exercise

Health Fanatic
John Cooper Clarke (1978)

… Shadow boxing – punch the wall
One-a-side football… what's the score… one-all
Could have been a copper… too small
Could have been a jockey… too tall
Knees up, knees up… head the ball
Nervous energy makes him tick
He's a health fanatic… he makes you sick

This poem, written by the 'punk poet' John Cooper Clarke, the bard of Salford, encapsulated the reaction in some quarters to the health and fitness boom, and its increasing visibility, in the post-war period. However, concern with personal health and wellbeing has not been a new phenomenon. Moreover, the use of sport and physical activity as a form of preventive medicine has been a cornerstone regarding ideas over the attainment of health. In 1929 the New Health Society proposed ten 'Health Rules' and, at number ten, after advice on topics such as diet, internal and external cleanliness and sunlight, was exercise in which the individual was encouraged to, 'Take out-of-door exercise every day. Also practice daily exercises for a few minutes every morning or evening, especially such as will bring into play the abdominal muscles'.[1] This chapter is mainly concerned with how sport and exercise has been incorporated into ideas and debates over health from around 1800 in Western countries, but mainly in Britain. While attention is also given to voluntary activity and commercial entrepreneurs, the central focus is on how the state has played an ever more interventionist role in looking after the 'fitness of the nation'. In charting the link between health and exercise, it aims to provide a broader political and cultural context for the relationship between sport and medicine. In addition, it highlights how ideas, such as eugenics, have not only shaped notions of health but also provided a basis for how medicine influenced sport.

By starting in 1800 the chapter provides a sense of how contemporary notions over health and exercise have paralleled wider developments in the origins and growth of state welfare provision and social policy more generally. The beginnings of industrialization – first in Britain and later in other Western countries – prompted a response by government and other sections of society to the economic, social and practical problems this posed.[2] While the charting of this process maybe seen as having teleological overtones, the response by government needs to be understood in terms of its adaptation to prevailing circumstances. Each country developed its own distinctive pattern of welfare provision subject to that country's particular political and cultural traditions as well as through the acceptance or rejection of competing ideologies. National governments also adapted their own responses to the use of sport.

Early ideas of health and physical activity

Before looking more closely at the relationship between the state and fitness, it would be beneficial to ask what do we mean by 'health'? There has never been a fixed definition for health and the term and the concept of health has constantly changed subject to its particular historical context. While health in the twenty-first century is bound up with science, in ancient Greece, for example, it was tied up with religious traditions. Klaus Bergoldt has argued that any definition is problematic and that health is not measurable. There is also the question of where health finishes and sickness starts, something which the World Health Organisaton's rather simplistic definition of health – 'complete physical, mental and social wellbeing' – fails to take into account as it only applies to a minority of relatively wealthy Europeans. Lugwig Borne was quoted as saying that, 'There are a thousand illnesses, but only one health'.[3] Not only is the idea of health subjective and dependent on an individual's perceptions of his or her own health, it is a social and cultural construction in which these perceptions are subject to a multiplicity of political influences and fluctuations. Defining health, therefore, can have important implications for the relationship between sport and medicine, especially in the twentieth century when the medical profession became a more powerful group and had the capacity to proclaim what was healthy and what was not. Before looking at the 'modern' era it would be useful to reflect on how earlier notions of health emerged and how sport and exercise were incorporated into them.

An early Graeco-Roman hygiene ideal was *mens sana in coropore sano* – a healthy mind in a healthy body – which was revived during the Victorian era and still has resonance today. An important part of this principle was, and continues to be, the promotion of the benefits of exercise and forms of physical activity. Plato, for example, while advocating moderate forms of exercise, was critical of extreme forms of gymnastics and dietetics, something that echoed modern medical concerns over competitive sport.[4] Ideas of health were conditioned by both prevailing medical theories and notions of the body

football and gymnastics. During the nineteenth century, to crudely summarize, a struggle within physical culture emerged between modern sport and gymnastics.[23] In Britain, and later America, physical exercise was expressed mainly through modern sport and especially team sports. In continental Europe indigenous gymnastics movements were deeply entrenched. However, by 1900 the British version had gained a foothold in Europe.

The nature of physical culture had been shaped by contemporary ideas concerning medicine and the body. These ideas included a revival of a forgotten body aesthetic: the muscular, symmetrical example of Ancient Greece, which was part of the emergence of classicism within Britain from the late eighteenth century. Greek statues in museums came to be viewed as 'living examples of the perfection which the human form is capable of attaining'.[24] The power of classical Greece continued to run strong in the imagination of the Western world deep into the twentieth century. This was not only evident in the architecture of state buildings but also through many of the staff of Western governments who were products of a classical education.[25] A number of European physical training instructors, such as Johann Friedrich Simon, GusMuths and Gotliff Salzman, were similarly impressed, and their programmes were imbued with notions of the classical world, especially in Germany where the 'Philanthropic Education' movement emerged.[26]

While the application of sport and exercise to improve the health of populations was partly a response to concerns over a country's preparedness for war, the nature of physical culture itself was determined by national characteristics. In Prussia, gymnastics, or Turnen, had been born out of its defeat to the French at Jena in 1806. It was essentially a movement that was begun by Friedrich Ludwig Jahn who had proclaimed the benefits of Turnen for military readiness and the strengthening of the Germanic race. He saw the 'Turner' as the core of the army to drive out the French and in 1811 he constructed a Turnplatz with towers, platforms, ropes and rings. Inspired by his example and publications, Turnen spread throughout Germany. Jahn had been part of a movement that emerged in the late eighteenth century, which included both writers on physical exercise as well as philosophers, such as Friederich Schiller and Wilhelm von Humboldt, in which ideas of physical exercise and the healthy body were formed in the image of physical culture in Ancient Greece.[27] Following years of suspicion by the political establishment, Turnen was institutionalized within German schools, and the Deutsche Turnerschaft (DT), founded in 1868, became a chauvinistic supporter of the German empire following the Franco-Prussian War.[28] As a popular system of exercise, Turnen promoted a German philosophy of health, vigour and patriotic ethnic identity. By 1914 the DT had 1.4 million members, seven times as many who participated in modern sports.[29]

The Scandinavian gymnastics movement was based on the Ling system. In 1805 Per Henrik Ling, a Swede, had launched a system of exercise routines that were based on anatomical and physiological principles. Whereas Turnen placed a greater emphasis on athleticism, strength and agility through the use of parallel bars, Ling used movements to provide enhanced military dexterity for fencing or bayonet fighting. Ling's ideas formed the basis of Swedish remedial exercises (later called medical or remedial gymnastics), which would become part of the work of masseurs and physiotherapists.[30] Both Turnen and Ling would be influential in the development of physical education in Britain and America.

The struggle for ascendancy between the physical education of the Germans and Swedes against the influence of modern sports like football invented by the British was most apparent in France. Initially, gymnastic societies flourished following France's defeat in 1871 as it was felt that physical training would contribute to national preparedness for any future war. Educational reformers were also patriots. In 1880 a law made gymnastic training – two hours of physical training and military exercises – compulsory in all public boys' schools. In the 1880s, however, the young Baron Pierre de Coubertin became a convert to English sports. According to him, and perhaps contrary to evidence, French secondary schools had become too scholastic while the pupils of private schools were 'narrow-chested, round-shouldered aesthetes'.[31] He looked to the games culture of English public schools like Eton and the emphasis placed on manliness to rectify this situation.[32] De Coubertin was imbued with both a keen sense of classicism and the potential physical and moral benefits of sport. These ideas would be the basis for his vision of 'Olympism' as a secular faith and the foundations for the formation of the International Olympic Committee in 1894.

British physical culture and the rise of public health

In the late eighteenth century British physical culture was built on sports such as pugilism and pedestrianism. Pedestrians, such as Foster Powell and Captain Barclay, won fame for their feats of endurance. Although physical culture was more commercial in its nature – mainly gambling – it highlighted contemporary fascination with the athletic body of Ancient Greece. Jackson's Rooms in Regency London, for example, was at the centre of British sport and were frequented by the nobility as well as members of the Cabinet and the Prince of Wales. Here they received a course of lessons from Gentleman John Jackson that included fencing and boxing. Jackson had been a champion of the prize ring and despite his lowly social status the elite of society admired his physical appearance. So much so that in 1797 and 1800 the Royal Academy commissioned portraits of him. This helped to fuel a growing pre-occupation with the physical appearance of the male body by the sporting elite, the Fancy, who began to dress in tight-fitting breeches to show their manliness and flaunt their well-muscled arms.[33]

While Britain was demilitarized compared to its Continental neighbours and did not have a standing army between 1815 and 1914, the army developed new attitudes towards physical training. Here the influence of Captain Phokion Heinrich Clias (1782–1854) was important. An American by birth, Clias had trained soldiers in Switzerland before becoming a captain in the British Army in 1822. Influenced by GusMuths and admired for his muscular physique, he was made superintendant of physical training at a number of military academies including Sandhurst. Clias placed an emphasis on medical gymnastics as well as remedial and hygienic exercises, and he wrote a number of exercise manuals for women.[34] Archibald Maclaren was a successor to Clias. He had built gymnasiums and was also widely acknowledged as a written authority on 'the scientific study of physical education'. In 1861 an army training school and a gymnasium were established at Aldershot and the following year his system was adopted in all military gymnasia. Maclaren's methods and writings popularized the use of dumb-bells, bar-bells, climbing ropes, horizontal bars, vaulting horses, and climbing walls, as well as running and free-standing exercises.[35] Later, many of the physical training instructors in public schools had been in the army and had trained under the system developed by Maclaren.[36]

While British physical culture developed differently compared to Europe, health also became an obsession in Victorian Britain. Bruce Haley has claimed, that 'No topic more occupied the Victorian mind than Health – not religion, or politics, or Improvement, or Darwinism'.[37] The dominant idea, reflecting new attitudes towards mental wellbeing, was 'total health or wholeness'.[38] New attitudes to bodily discipline found receptive audiences in all areas of Victorian society and its institutions. Religion, for example, was an important source of recreation with churches playing an important part in setting up football and cricket clubs. In a new interpretation on the ideal of 'muscular Christianity', Daniel Erdozain has argued that in Victorian Britain evangelicalism itself was to be expressed through 'active participation' in sport and recreational activities as opposed to churches just being seen as sites of recreation.[39]

At public schools a cult of athleticism emerged around team games such as football and cricket. In 1864 the Clarendon Commission had commended the public schools, especially Rugby, for 'their love of healthy sports and exercise'.[40] It was felt that sport inculcated character formation and moral discipline as well as trying to root out the 'problems' of homosexuality and masturbation.[41] Football played at Rugby school was ascribed a set of moral values through Thomas Hughes's semi-autobiographical *Tom Brown's Schooldays* (1857). Schoolboy sport and literature generally during this era reflected wider Victorian culture in which ideas of health were transmitted through a radical conceptualization of the adolescent body.[42] Following the Clarendon Commission, Rugby, under its headmaster, Thomas Arnold, became the model for the mid-Victorian public school and so its moral philosophy stretched far beyond the school. Not only were middle-class expectations of public school life shaped in part by Hughes's book but the sport of rugby itself became an ideology. These attitudes, combined with notions of muscular Christianity, were exported throughout the world where the game was played, especially in the British Empire, which adopted the Arnoldian model of public school life. In addition, the Rugby-style game flourished in an environment where sport at Ivy League universities was closely interwoven with the North American form of muscular Christianity.[43]

Public school values were also associated with patriotism imperialism, and war was regularly referred to as a form of sport.[44] A 'hegemonic masculinity' emerged in which manliness was felt to imbue the ideal of a moral and civilized man. Victorian reformers like Charles Kingsley believed that games created 'hardy, quick-thinking men' who could run the Empire.[45] Importantly, the attitudes of those who attended the public schools, such as doctors, were carried on into other areas of public life, including that of health.

In wider British society Holt has argued that the spread of amateurism within sport not only complemented the inculcation of the values of muscular Christianity but an amateur cult of the active body emerged that was shaped to a greater extent by the bodily requirement of work and health. The values of work inspired the idea of competition while those who advocated amateur values were influenced by medical and public opinion concerning health. As a result, amateurs advocated active participation over professional sport. Outdoors activities also combated changing work patterns, where growing numbers of middle class men spent their working lives sitting at a desk as well as the spread of the suburbs, which led to a reliance on the commuter train.[46]

Moreover, through a growing raft of public health legislation, the state took a greater interest in the health and fitness of the British people. The initial focus had been on sanitary reform but the state regularly intervened in areas such as food, drugs and the workplace, highlighted by the 1864 Factory Act.[47] State interest also began to stretch to the application of physical activity to improve the health of the population. At the municipal level a host of parliamentary legislation, such as the 1846 Baths and Wash Houses Act, had allowed local authorities to use permissive powers that were aimed at ensuring basic standards of health by developing leisure amenities.[48] Later, the 1878 Baths and Wash Houses Act enabled local authorities to build covered swimming pools, which now became places for physical recreation and sport.[49]

While sport was an important aspect of life for pupils at the public schools, physical culture spread only slowly into Britain's new mass education system. In 1866 there had been just over one million children attending schools in England but through the 1870 and 1880 Education Acts this had risen to 4.5 million in 1886. The passing of these acts gave a – potentially – more formal structure to physical training programmes in schools. By the late 1880s physical exercises, mainly in the form of gymnastic-based military drill, had become an established part of the timetable in many voluntary and government controlled board schools, although it was not compulsory at this stage.[50] The main emphasis was on Swedish gymnastics but in 1900 the Board of Education had permitted organized games as a substitute for Ling-type drill or physical exercises, although it was not until 1906 that games were officially allowed in elementary schools.[51] With the appointment of the first Chief Medical Officer, George Newman, in 1907, physical education was given a higher priority. Under that year's Education Act, a system of medical inspections was established and Newman saw PE as a cheap form of preventive medicine.[52] In his annual report of 1909, Newman wrote that 'physical exercises are now recognized to be a desirable and indeed a necessary part of the school curriculum'.[53]

The motivations behind these initiatives were both utilitarian and moral. Leisure was seen as part of a grander mission to build a new humane society of cultivated individuals.[54] It was an example of the middle class paternalism that would be a constant theme in the politics of health and would continue through the twentieth century. This 'grander mission' was to be found within the voluntary sector in the shape of 'rational recreation'. Alongside the provision of parks and baths, bourgeois reformers aimed to create a healthy, moral and orderly workforce through sport.[55] Although Victorian reformers didn't succeed, the idea of using sport as a tool for health purposes as well as a social service has continued to persist into the twenty-first century. In the mid-1880s a National Physical Recreation Society had been founded to promote physical recreation, especially gymnastics, among the working classes.[56] Youth movements, like the Boys Brigade, established in 1883, the Church Lads' Brigade (1892), the Boy Scouts (1908) and the Girl Guides (1910) all provided boys and girls with opportunities for outdoor activities.[57] Similarly, schools' football (soccer) developed through voluntary associations and in 1904 the English Schools Football Association was founded.[58] Interestingly, reflecting the influence of classical Greece, some amateur football leagues in London were called the Isthmian League, the Spartan League and the Hellenic League while the premier amateur club was the Corinthians. In addition, from the second half of the nineteenth century, sports provision became a common aspect of welfare capitalism amongst some employers such as Cadbury's and Rowntree's, albeit with mixed motivations.[59]

Underpinning much of the debate concerning physical fitness were contemporary anxieties over the health of national populations, caused by the population boom that had accompanied industrialization, and ultimately fears about racial degeneration. Debates around public health and health generally – including exercise – became increasingly informed through the widespread reception, if not wholesale acceptance, of eugenicist ideals.[60] Eugenics, first coined by Francis Galton in 1883, was based on ideas about heredity and evolution and aimed to address these fears over 'race suicide'. A statistical as much as a biological and social science, eugenics had a broad appeal across all political classes. Although eugenics was applied in various contexts, the language of 'struggle' and 'fitness' and superior and inferior 'types' relating to both people and nations permeated social and political discourse.[61] There were two strands. Positive eugenics aimed to achieve racial improvement through encouraging the fit to breed, and this thinking was behind initiatives such as ante-natal and baby clinics, while preventing breeding among the unfit was the goal of negative eugenics. Here it was argued that for the race to survive social amelioration should be abandoned in favour of selective breeding and the elimination of those who were eugenically deficient such as the sickly, the deformed and the demented. Policies were applied differently in different countries. Negative eugenics was taken to its most extreme form in Germany with the Final Solution while American states and even Sweden adopted compulsory sterilization laws.[62]

Latent fears amongst the upper and middle classes over national efficiency, race degeneration and ultimately Britain's imperial ambitions had crystallized during the Boer War. Not only were British forces defeated in its early stages by mostly volunteer farmers but when conscription was introduced (for the first time) over thirty-five per cent of male recruits, mainly from the masses, were found to be physically unfit for service.[63] Eugenic fears had important implications for policies regarding the health of schoolchildren.[64] The Inter-departmental Committee on Physical Deterioration had been set up after the conflict, although its recommendations in 1904 favoured environmental reforms rather than an overtly eugenicist solution. The reforms were mainly aimed at improving the physique of schoolchildren and included the medical inspection of schoolchildren, the feeding of children in elementary schools and physical exercise for all schoolchildren because of its 'character-building qualities'. It also recommended that local education authorities should provide playgrounds and other indoor facilities. Ultimately, all policy initiatives were designed with the aim of 'building an imperial race of healthy, fit workers and soldiers to defend the nation and empire'.[65]

Health and physical culture in the United States

Whereas in Western Europe there was a trend towards the bureaucratization and centralization of public health, in America the response was different. In the early nineteenth century a 'rugged individualism' prevailed and the persistence of Jacksonian democracy kept government to a minimum. Instead, any reform was dominated by local voluntary and philanthropic efforts and promoted by Puritan morality. In particular, it was felt that social cleanliness was next to godliness:[66] 'to follow the rules of hygiene was a moral act and a religious duty, and sanitary regeneration was a crusade to improve the poor'.[67] In ante-bellum America there had been great concern for the physical degeneracy of the population, especially in the expanding towns and cities. Developments were built on the American self-help tradition with health being seen as a personal responsibility while concerns over the health of the population became part of a general reform movement. This was reflected by a growth in the popularity of prevention literature and hygiene instruction amongst medical practitioners.[68] The American medical market also provided opportunities for entrepreneurs like the 'botanic' physician Samuel Thomson (1769–1843) whose herbal remedies were very popular in rural America.[69]

In America there had initially been a boom in physical training in the early years of the nineteenth century. However, due to a cholera epidemic in the early 1830s, the focus shifted to matters of nutrition, sanitation and public health.[70] Migrants later introduced Turnen into America, although it would undergo a process of 'Americanization'.[71] The Civil War gave further impetus to matters of health by provoking an interest in calisthenics, gymnastics, physical training, outdoor activities and competitive sports. As well as the emergence of PE in colleges and high schools, a number of organizations were founded, such as the American Association for the Advancement of Physical Education in 1885, which devoted their attention to promoting health through exercise regimens and gymnastics.[72] The idea that underpinned these movements resonated with that of muscular Christianity in England; that perfection of the body was an essential part of Christian morality and should, therefore, be kept free from disease.[73] In the late 1800s physical education had begun to emerge as a professional field. Its development was assisted through the staging of various international expositions and world fairs, many of which hosted congresses and meetings on aspects of PE, bodily hygiene and physical training. At the 1876 Philadelphia Centennial Exhibition there was a section on the 'Physical, Social and Moral Condition of Man while two years later there was a special section on gymnastics at Paris's International Exposition.[74]

During the Progressive era (1890–1920) public health became more national in its outlook. It was now supported by qualified public health workers who promoted an ethic of scientific management within social and political reform, which had coincided with the development of the bacteriological theory of disease.[75] Anxieties over the health of the nation persisted, however, and were increasingly based on fears in America of 'race suicide' because of the perception of a dwindling in the Puritan stock. One response, from the mid-nineteenth century, was for schoolgirls to participate in calisthenic exercises, and from the 1890s their athletic opportunities increased. Physical educators justified the need for exercise and sport as a way to better develop women for the struggle for race survival (see Chapter 7).[76]

Through his own lifestyle, President Theodore Roosevelt embodied and popularized the philosophy of 'strenuous life'. Roosevelt's outlook had been shaped by his experience as a frail and sickly young man who earned his 'manliness' from hunting and athletic sports. He later advocated the popular idea of sport as a form of rejuvenation for the neurasthenic and dyspeptic American male. Sports, especially team games such as football, rowing and baseball, and strength sports like boxing and wrestling became the preferred activities of the middle-class American male. Borrowing the ideals of English public schools, as well as developing young men physically, sport, it was said, developed character. Football was particularly important to Roosevelt. He placed the game at the heart of a young man's training for life, believing that this 'manly game' inculcated them with 'virile virtues' and acted as a preparation for the 'rough work of the world'. However, his pursuit of the strenuous life was directed more towards his own class, in particular the Ivy League, than the nation as a whole.[77] Through the craze for sport and physical culture in the American higher education system, and the success of American sportsmen at the first Olympic games, a change in the ideal body shape took place. The image of the svelte Greek athlete that had characterized the somatic ideal from antiquity through the Renaissance and up to the early nineteenth century was now being challenged. Instead, the Olympian examples of 'American muscle and brawn, began to redefine the image of the well-developed male body'.[78]

The commercialization of physical culture

The creation of healthy citizenry was not limited to government action. From the late nineteenth century, commercial interests 'turned the construction of the healthy body into a moral crusade and a vastly profitable industry'.[79] Ina Zweiniger-Bargielowska has argued that the emergence of a commercial physical culture reflected changing notions and meanings of 'bodily discipline'. Not only were health and fitness important but because new ideas about body management were set in a modern urban industrial society, the pursuit of beauty was also part of wider discourses that were framed around patriotism, degeneration, eugenics and modernity.[80]

Commercial physical culture also highlighted a shift in emphasis in the responsibility from the state to the individual to pursue health and fitness. Chief amongst physical cultural entrepreneurs was the bodybuilder Eugen Sandow. Initially a fairground entertainer due to his physical strength, he built up a highly successful business through his world tours and publications from the 1890s.[81] In advocating exercise, which included weight-training, Sandow invoked the rhetoric of deterioration and national efficiency: 'Physical decadence or physical degeneracy will be almost invariably accompanied by mental and moral deterioration, for as Herbert Spencer said, "we must never forget that there is such a thing as physical morality."'[82]

While Sandow represented a new distinctive Herculean body other physical culturalists advocated different lifestyles. Eustace Miles, a tennis player, rejected the Sandow ideal. Instead, he promoted a 'hygienic regimen' that was directed at the middle classes. It 'combined mental health practices and vegetarianism – he had his own vegetarian restaurant – with exercises based on movement such as swimming, golf and tennis and activities like gardening.[83] Similarly, I.P. Muller rejected the use of apparatus and the pursuit of an overly muscular body. Instead, with '15 minutes exercise a day', he placed an emphasis on the pursuit of general health 'in all the vital organic functions' through a regimen that included daily exposure to fresh air and 'brisk' exercise.[84]

Another entrepreneur in this field was the American Bernarr Macfadden who advertised his own brand of physical culture through his magazine, *Physical Culture*, founded in 1899. He established several 'healthoriums' where he outlined his theories of 'physcultopahy'. His aim was to allow people to develop 'absolute purity of their blood through a regimen of exercise, fresh air, bland diet and no medicines'. Despite his reputation as an apostle of strength and fitness, he later earned notoriety for his unconventional attitudes towards sex. He was also an advocate of eugenics and as such national racism in which the aim of marriage was to produce healthy offspring for the sake of the nation.[85]

In addition to gymnastics and weight-training, swimming and its accompanying lifestyle became a feature of physical culture, especially in America and Australia. In fact, through the image and body of the champion Olympic swimmer Johnny Weissmuller, the American government attempted to export American culture in the form of sports goods. It also highlighted a growth in beach culture in Europe that the Americans strove to exploit.[86] These developments contributed to the era of the 'Body Beautiful' and was further highlighted through the building of outdoor modernist lidos in Britain.[87]

Physical culture both complemented and was part of a wider international health and life reform movement that advocated exercise along with dietary reform such as vegetarianism, sun- and air-bathing plus personal cleanliness and temperance.[88] In 1906 the Health and Strength League was formed in Britain, and its journal, *Health and Strength*, had a circulation of about 75,000 in 1909. The inter-war years were also marked by health and hygiene pressure groups, the most influential of which was the New Health Society.[89] Launched by Sir William Arbuthnot Lane in 1925, its members included prominent politicians and industrialists such as Ramsay MacDonald and Alfred Mond. The society aimed to convert 'a rapidly degenerating community' from a C3 nation into an A1 nation. It generally eschewed environmental causes of degeneration and rather than a redistribution of wealth as the key to improve individual and racial health, the society emphasized Victorian moral character and self-discipline instead.[90]

Sport, fitness and the state in inter-war Europe

The fall-out from the Great War loomed large in European inter-war health policies. Fears of national decline continued and were reinforced by a long-term fall in birth-rates. 'A new organic vision of society emerged' within Europe based on a collective responsibility for welfare. The mixed economy of welfare that featured in this era provided the foundation for the establishment of classic welfare states after 1945.[91] Interestingly, although perhaps unsurprisingly, the motivations of different states, whether totalitarian or liberal democracies, for promoting sport and exercise were remarkably similar: hygiene, preparedness for war and industrial production. Increasingly, however, totalitarian states began to appropriate sport for national prestige, which marked a demarcation from sport's previous function as an aid to national fitness.

In Fascist Italy the government imbued physical education with a military utility in which young people were understood as soldier-citizens. Physical education and sport was largely controlled through the establishment of the *Opera Nazionale Dopolavoro* (OND). Set up in 1926, it coordinated the after-work recreational activities of Italians. In addition, Mussolini himself was the personification of the fascist body. He was often depicted in the press riding horses, fencing, skiing and flying or even driving a racing car. 'He was never afraid to display his body … he believed that a healthy and strong body was testimony to great effort.' He also gave instructions that all fascist chiefs should keep fit through physical activity.[92]

It was during this period that modern sport displaced traditional gymnastics and workers' sport as the leading form of physical culture in Europe. With the growth of international competition, sport provided a means of mediating between national and international identities and acting as a forum for nationalist rivalry.[93] Yet this had not been an inevitable process. Following the revolution, Western sport had been rejected by the Soviet Union because of its bourgeois links. Initially the Bolsheviks attempted to build on the Russian legacy of *fizkul'tura*. Alongside Turnen and Sokol, *fizkul'tura* represented a third variation of the pre-1914 PE movement in Central and Eastern Europe. *Fizkul'tura* was proletarianized by the Soviets some of whom rejected competitive sport completely due to its association with capitalism while others felt that certain sports could be used in moderation to encourage the masses into a regimen of health and exercise. All agreed that 'individualism, record-seeking and competitive habits were vices to be discouraged'. However, Soviet physical culture failed to take a grip amongst not only the domestic population but also communists worldwide. The Red Sport International (Sportintern) had been formed in 1921 to oversee an international proletarian sports culture as an alternative to both the workers' sports system run by the Socialist Workers' Sport International and Western sports bodies such as the International Olympic Committee. But Sportintern remained a marginal organization throughout its 16-year existence. Instead, the Supreme Council for Physical Culture, the main Soviet government body for sport, took a greater interest in Western sport because it offered greater opportunities for prestige on an international scale. Prefacing the Soviet Union's Olympic bow in 1952 was the council's decision in 1933 to sanction competition between Soviet athletes and those from non-workers' clubs, which essentially meant an acceptance of the Western model of competitive, achievement-oriented sport. Back at home football became the national sport as Soviet attempts to develop a domestic and international system of physical culture lost out to a capitalist and elite-centred transnational sports culture.[94]

Nazi Germany similarly embraced a form of physical culture in modern sport that it had initially opposed. On the face of it, modern sport was inimical to Nazism because of its foreign origins and the threat of internationalism which it posed. Moreover, Turnen with its strong völkisch tradition continued to be an important strand of German physical culture and because the Nazis sought to control culture for the purposes of mass mobilization it offered the Nazis an opportunity to build 'an autarkic cultural alternative'. Nevertheless, as Keys has pointed out, under Hitler Germany became a full member of the international sport community, highlighted by its staging of and the success of German athletes at the 1936 Olympics.[95] Success at international sport was seen as an opportunity to vindicate the superiority of the Aryan race and the pursuit of success was woven into notions of racial hygiene that were a central part of the Nazi public health agenda. These ideas had been built on the promotion of social hygiene policies during Weimar with a focus on eugenic and racial issues pre-1933.[96] Moreover, German attitudes to health and fitness were also highlighted through an emphasis on the natural body.[97] It was in this context of racial hygiene that the Nazis developed a sports system, based on Italy's OND, through its policy of *Gleichschaltung*: the coordination and centralization of sports clubs and societies into a central programme, Kraft durch Freude (Strength through Joy) under the control of the Reichssportführer, Hans von Tschammer.[98] Even the Deutsche Turnerschaft had to be incorporated into the centralized system. Gymnastics still heavily influenced PE but organized physical activities at all levels, including gender, were now defined in terms of service to the state and its drive towards militarization.[99]

The British state and national fitness

A British response to continental developments came in the form of the 1937 Physical Training and Recreation Act.[100] Zweiniger-Bargielowska has argued that the National Fitness Campaign, which was a product of the act, was important 'because the cultivation of health and fitness, which had been advocated by physical culture promoters, life reform campaigners, public health professionals, and leaders of voluntary associations for decades, was finally elevated to the status of a major government policy'.[101] The horrors of the First World War had proved a catalyst more generally for health initiatives by commercial and voluntary groups. In addition, central government played an increasing role in the administration of health policies. There was an extension of welfare reforms generally and in 1919 a Ministry of Health was established. It promised health policies on an integrated and national basis but due to the permissive nature of these policies much of the provision was a patchwork of un-coordinated services.[102]

Nevertheless, both central and local government had begun to devote more resources to sport and physical recreation to promote the virtues of healthy living. There was also a clearer demarcation between work and leisure, highlighted by legislation like the 1938 Holidays with Pay Act.[103] A greater concern for open spaces at the municipal level led to an expansion of sporting facilities such as football and cricket pitches.[104] Physical education continued to be seen as a form of preventive medicine as well as a cheap and effective way of promoting better health amongst schoolchildren. As a result, through the School Medical Service there was an – albeit uneven – expansion in the teaching of PE, the provision of improved recreational facilities for all age groups and installing gymnasium equipment in board schools.[105] A closer relationship between central government and independent voluntary organizations developed in order to facilitate the public's greater access to recreational facilities. In 1925, for example, the National Playing Fields Association (NPFA) was founded as a charity to protect the UK's sports fields, recreation grounds and public open spaces. In 1935 it was given responsibility for nearly 500 fields that were presented to the nation by George V to mark his Silver Jubilee.[106] Of greater significance was the formation of the Central Council of Physical Recreation (CCPR) through the prompting of the Board of Education in 1935.[107] In 1936 the British Medical Association's Physical Education committee published a report that preached the message of a 'healthy body means a healthy mind', and was particularly concerned with the physical, mental and moral welfare of young people in an era of mass unemployment.[108]

The Physical Training Act had initially been a reaction to Britain's relatively poor performance and the strong showing by the host nation at the Berlin Olympics. There was also awareness that organizations such as Strength Through Joy were having a beneficial impact on the health of the German population. A National Fitness Council (NFC) was established but rather than a portent of militarism it needs to be seen in British context. As Zweiniger-Bargielowska has pointed out, 'the concept was understood in a wider sense of good citizenship which depended on voluntary participation'.[109] Essentially the NFC was tapping into the growth of sporting and outdoor activities during the thirties. The campaign had a mixture of activities. It included mass displays of physical culture such as one at the Festival of Youth in 1937 and annual ones by the Women's League of Health and Beauty as well as hundreds of local and regional demonstrations and festivals. Grants were also made available for the construction of sporting facilities and various other schemes, which were attractive to governing bodies of sports. The Amateur Athletic Association, for example, used Council funds to appoint a national coach. While historians have argued over its merits and success, the philosophy behind the NFC not only provided continuities regarding the relationship between sport and exercise and fitness this idea continued to have salience, albeit in a changing health and medical landscape.

Welfarism, individual health and the fitness boom

Dorothy Porter has argued that in post-war Europe a new universal vision of society emerged with the establishment of the 'classic welfare state', highlighting a larger role for the state in undertaking collective responsibility of welfare.[110] There was a shift in the nature of health care provision from an emphasis on voluntarism towards compulsory state insurance and universal welfare provision. This process, however, in national terms was uneven. In France a comprehensive social security system was introduced in 1945, although voluntarism maintained a significant role in health care delivery due to the persistence of liberal values. The concept of universal comprehensive welfare policy was applied most vigorously in Sweden following the introduction of state insurance in 1955.[111]

The shift in provision was most pronounced in Britain. Here the balance of the mixed economy of voluntary and state welfare swung away from the liberal collectivism of the Edwardian period to a new philosophy of universalism by the Second World War, highlighted by the publication of the *Beveridge Report* (1942) and then the establishment of the National Health Service in 1948. In addition, these ideological shifts redefined the boundaries of citizenship. 'The citizenship of voluntary service was replaced by a citizenship of rights to statutory relief in times of need'.[112] Bernard Harris has pointed out that, despite many disagreements between the main British political parties over the development of social policy after 1945, 'there was still an underlying consensus concerning the role that the state might justifiably play in meeting social needs'.[113] Following the Second World War the medical profession became more interested in the scientific link between health and physical activity. In 1953, in a landmark study, Jerry White *et al* established a positive link between exercise and health through a study of bus drivers and bus conductors. It found that the more active conductors had far less heart attacks than sedentary drivers. Similar conclusions were reached when comparing postal workers with civil servants.[114] These findings provided a launch pad for further state intervention regarding the health of the nation.

While public health services grew, from the 1960s, there was also a greater pre-occupation with personal health; what Crawford has termed 'healthism'.[115] This drift towards individual lifestyles complemented what Berridge has identified as a new ideology in public health which stressed 'individual responsibility for good health, lifestyle and behaviour.'[116] In addition, this shift in the public health agenda was reinforced through publicity campaigns and a much greater visibility of doctors within the media giving expert opinion on medical and health matters. This approach, in combination with the growing use of evidence-based medicine, first came to public attention with the 1962 report of the Royal College of Physicians on smoking and the subsequent campaign to ban tobacco advertising.[117] The 'individualisation of health issues' continued during the Thatcher administrations of the 1980s.[118] As Zweiniger-Bargielowska has shown, however, the new emphasis on the individual drew on long-standing beliefs about health, stressing the value of a healthy lifestyle of diet, exercise and moderate living.[119]

Growing concerns with personal health had both reflected and shaped a rise in demand for alternative medicine. From the 1960s a counter culture emerged that challenged the ascendancy of orthodox medicine. It formed part of a general challenge to mainstream materialistic values in the Western world as well as a decline in deference throughout society. Importantly, the notion of 'progress', based on a scientific world, was demythologized. As a result, alternative lifestyles, such as meditation and mysticism, gained in popularity as a reaction to the perceived moral bankruptcy of Western material values.[120] In addition to the greater demand for more 'natural' forms of health care like homeopathy, acupuncture, osteopathy and alternative practitioners such as herbalists, the holistic approach that underlies these therapies has challenged the very essence of orthodox medicine. One such alternative activity/therapy that enjoyed popularity was yoga. A 'yogi's' true concern with his/her body was a spiritual one with the ultimate objective the liberation of the soul with the universe. It originated in India and was popular amongst middle-class housewives, although yoga had actually gone through a process of modernization from around 1900.[121]

The popular health consciousness that pervaded Western culture in the 1970s was also accompanied by a fitness boom. In addition, an aggressive anti-smoking lobby emerged along with an expansion of popular health magazines as well as a proliferation of articles on health in newspapers and advertisements for health-related products. There was also a sharp increase in demand for health food items. The most emblematic activity from this period was jogging, something that was parodied in the film *Forrest Gump* (1994), and also portrayed more sensitively in the 1983 biopic of the Canadian charity runner Terry Fox (1958–81). The jogging boom was highlighted further by the inception of the London Marathon in 1981, and then by its growth in runners from 7,747 to 22,000 from 70,000 applications in 1985. In addition, the numbers playing football had increased.[122] Elite sport itself was on television more often, acting as an advertisement for itself as well as health and fitness.

By 2000 consumer spending on sporting goods in the UK was £4 billion. During the 1990s the number of health and fitness clubs expanded by nearly a quarter and catered for a membership of 8.6 million people, generating an estimated £1.25 billion for the UK economy. Similarly, in Italy a keep fit culture emerged in which, like elsewhere, lifestyle as much as physical activity was being sold. From the late 1980s fitness clubs were advertised on television as 'fashionable, modern places full of interesting people'. By 2000 nearly 4 million Italians frequented around 4,000 gyms and spent $1.4 billion a year on sports clothing. However, the USA remains the largest health and fitness market. In 1976 Americans spent $147 million on running shoes, rising to $471 million in 1982. Spending on sporting goods was worth $47.3 billion in 2002 and the US had over 22,000 commercial health clubs, more than in Germany, Italy, Spain, France and the UK combined.[123] This Western capitalist fashion also began to penetrate the Iron Curtain from the 1970s. In the German Democratic Republic there was an emergence of *Trendsport* (fashionable sports) that included windsurfing, bodybuilding and jogging as well as increased gym membership. These activities had been imported partly through West German television and were part of wider international movements that included youth culture and a bourgeoning football fan culture.[124] Even in communist East Germany, wellbeing was increasingly seen in individualistic terms.

Since the late twentieth century a fetishization of health has taken place, argues Dorothy Porter. First, body-building, which traces its roots back to Sandow and Macfadden, became more freakish as the aim of body-builders was to look 'alien'. In addition to their bulk, they need to look 'cut' through a low fat diet. The taking of steroids and human growth hormones has been an important part of this sub-culture. Moreover, changes in body shape and the shift to a bulkier physique can also been seen through the changing covers of *Marvel* comics in which Superman has got bigger in order to reflect, and maintain, his status against mortal men. Second, an offspring of body-building was the goal of a 'designer body' with an emphasis on 'shape' rather than bulk and whose defining characteristic is sexual desirability; a central goal of the healthy body from the beginning of the twentieth century.[125]

International sport and the state

The post-1945 period was marked by a closer relationship between sport and the state amongst virtually all countries. The nature of this process though was reflected both by individual national political cultures and sporting rivalries created by the Cold War. Sport was now seen not just in terms of health by governments but it also became more closely linked with national prestige, especially after the Soviet Union's entry into the Olympics in 1952. In the Eastern Bloc mass physical cultural displays, which promoted an all-round physical and mental education, were swept away – in 1948 Sokol gymnastics were banned in Czechoslovakia and Poland – to be replaced by an emphasis on sporting excellence.

Anxieties over the health of populations, which were increasingly being shaped by the Cold War, still remained the main priority in the West but there was also a greater awareness of the sporting threat posed by communist nations. In 1961 the Canadian Federal Government's, 'An Act to Encourage Fitness and Amateur Sport' had been stimulated by both poor levels of physical fitness and Canadian failure in international ice-hockey.[126] America's post-war sport policy initially revolved around the ideas of national physical fitness and mass participation. This policy was also linked to pre-war concerns over the problem of youth and anxieties over the fitness, both physical and mental, of boys and girls. The construction of adolescence as a life-stage had been partly established through the work of the American psychologist G. Stanley Hall. By the 1920s adolescence as a specific psychological and biological stage in the development of the child to adult had become firmly established in psychology.[127] Physical education in American schools received greater prominence as did outdoor recreations such as summer camps. The playground movement also continued to expand and there was also a growth in other municipal activities and facilities where alongside better health, training children to become good citizens was also deemed important. In addition, throughout the Depression the value of sport and recreation for the psycho-social health of adolescents, especially boys, was continually repeated, something that reflected growing concerns over the perceived threat of juvenile delinquency.[128] Following a report in 1953, which concluded that European children were fitter than their American counterparts, a President's Council on Youth Fitness was established three years later and further promoted under the Kennedy administration. However, national sporting prestige, in light of the rivalry with the Soviet Union, became a more pressing issue. There was a turn away from the use of sport as an instrument to promote national fitness, a process that culminated in the Amateur Sports Act of 1978.[129]

More generally in the West there was now a greater investment in sport for reasons of national prestige. In Western Europe France led its neighbours in its commitment to elite sport and was the first to establish a strong state-sport relationship. From the 1960s to the 1980s French sport adopted what Phil Dine has called a 'middle way' between the 'big state' Soviet model and the 'small state' model of Britain and America.[130] Following the creation of the Fifth Republic in 1958 de Gaulle placed a greater emphasis on a stronger state.[131] No longer a superpower, sport for de Gaulle offered an opportunity for France to regain international prestige. To rejuvenate the nation it relied on 'rationalized athletic development to produce elite athletes'.

Following France's poor showing at the 1960 Olympics the desire for success was given greater priority. In 1963 Maurice Herzog was appointed Secretary of State for Youth and Sport with a substantial budget to promote both elite excellence and mass participation. The policy was top-down. It was thought that elite athletes would make ideal citizens, act as role models for the nation's youth and stimulate participation at grass-roots. France offered a contrast with the UK where although a Minister with responsibility for Sport was appointed in 1962 it was a junior position and was continually shuffled between government departments until the 1990s. The Gaullist tradition regarding sport was not only maintained but expanded upon by subsequent administrations and between 1973 and 1992 there was an even stronger emphasis on promoting excellence through institutional means rather than relying on patriotic rhetoric. At first France had shied away from the Eastern Bloc policy of providing athletes with state subsidies because of enduring anxieties over breaching the amateur ethic. However, this changed during the following decade. In 1975 there was a separation of elite sport from physical education and its mass participation ethos. That year the Mazeuad law (named after the Minister of Youth and Sport) gave official support to the preparation of elite athletes, including the provision of financial assistance and, for the first time, set a full national sports policy. The law created the National Institute of Sport and Physical Education (*Institut National d'Éducation Physique et du Sport*, (INSEP)). It was designed to train elite, young athletes to serve the state with the assistance of professional coaches, sports scientists and sports medics.[132]

The British government also took a greater interest in sport. However, the British response, like the French, reflected its own political culture. Initially, the voluntary-based administration of British sport changed little and continued to be heavily influenced by the traditional values of amateurism.[133] Yet during the 1950s Britain shared similar anxieties with the French: loss of empire and diplomatic influence; a relative sporting decline; concerns over the health of the population and a bourgeoning youth culture. As a response to these concerns the CCPR set up the Wolfenden Committee in 1957. Not only was it concerned with elite sport but another of its aims was 'promoting the general welfare of the community through sport, games and outdoor activities'. Its report was published in 1960.[134]

In some respects 'Wolfenden' was modern and forward thinking but in other ways there was continuity with the past in terms of how people saw sport's status. Wolfenden rejected the prospect of a Ministry of Sport on the grounds that it was at odds with the traditional volunteerism of British sport.[135] But in 1965 a Sports Council was set up, receiving its royal charter in 1972. As a Quango (Quasi Autonomous Non-Governmental Organization) rather than an arm of the state, it operated on an arms-length basis from the government.[136] In France there was not only more direct state involvement but also much greater financial investment, especially in elite sport.[137]

The Sports Council had two main responsibilities: to improve the fitness of the British people and to improve the performance of elite athletes.[138] A 'Sport for All' campaign was launched to increase participation levels as well as a building programme for local sports facilities.[139] Sport for All can be seen as part of a wider drift towards what Virginia Berridge has termed a 'militant healthism' within public health.[140] The 1970s was a period of sharp growth in leisure services and the leisure industry generally, which was accompanied by the emergence of a professional class of leisure managers. Sport and leisure centres became familiar sights in many British towns. In 1972 there had been 27 but by 1981 this figure had increased to 770.[141] By the 1990s there was a shift in emphasis in the relationship between the state and sport, illustrated by two important government reports. *Raising the Game* (1995) was commissioned by the sport-loving John Major while in 2002 *Game Plan* reflected New Labour thinking on using sport in public-private partnerships to tackle health issues. In the bigger picture the sport and leisure industry now had important commercial significance. In 1997 it was the eleventh largest in the country, accounting for about £10 billion of annual consumer expenditure, employing 750,000 people and contributing £3.5 billion in tax revenues.[142]

There was a greater emphasis also placed on elite sport. When the Sports Council was set up it aimed to build up the broadest possible base of sporting participation, which it believed was related to athletic success. However, this approach proved to be hopelessly simplistic compared to the sophisticated scientific systems of the Soviet Union and its satellites (see Chapter 3). Later, based on the Australian Institute of Sport, *Raising the Game* had intended to set up a British Academy of Sport to cater for elite athletes.[143] In 1995 the Sports Council was split into two: national Sports Councils like Sport England looked after the grass-roots while UK Sport was responsible for elite athletes. Extra funding came from the National Lottery, which had started the previous year, and these initiatives had come to fruition by the 2000 Olympics.

Conclusion

Ideas linking sport and physical exercise with health and wellbeing have been promoted throughout history. However, these ideas have also been shaped through changing notions of the human body and a wider political context. The whole notion of health has been mutable; contingent not only on its contemporary context but also changing expectations of what it means. Early ideas were linked to Galenic medicine in which the attainment of health was dependent on the body maintaining its equilibrium. However, more scientific theories emerged that regarded the body as a machine and could be studied at a cellular level. In the nineteenth century these rational understandings prompted a greater intervention by Western states in improving the health of the population, usually in preparation for war. Physical culture came to be seen as an important part of wider public health policies. It was given further impetus through the emergence of eugenics, which gave a scientific justification for discourses concerning national efficiency and race degeneration due to the poor health of the lower orders. To improve the fitness of the race, therefore, greater attention was paid to the use of sport and exercise. These concerns were also commercially exploited as the rhetoric of the healthy body was turned into a profitable industry. By the inter-war period the link between exercise and health was made by most Western states but followed most avidly by totalitarian regimes. Not only was exercise regarded as part of public health but international sport was also now seen in terms of national prestige. Post-war welfare states continued to pursue the link between physical exercise and health but there was also a shift towards more consumerist attitudes to health. A fitness boom individualized health and reflected an increasing emphasis on lifestyle choice.

What did this mean for the relationship between sport and medicine? Much of the advice dispensed regarding exercise and its benefits for health was predicated on the notion of moderation. It was thought that excessive physical activity would lead to ill-health. Competitive elite sport, however, was based on the idea of excess. As a result, it meant that scientific understandings of the body gained in improving health could be applied to enhancing athletic performance.

2

This Sporting Life

Injuries and Medical Provision

Introduction

In 1897 American college football was experiencing one of the earliest of its episodic crises due to a growing death toll of players. The whole issue was sensationalized in the newspapers as part of a circulation war. On 14 November one page of the *New York Journal and Advertiser* gave graphic details, including illustrations of the injuries – a broken backbone; concussion to the brain; and a fractured skull – sustained during games by three players who had died.[1] Over one hundred years later, following a game in 2002, Alex Ferguson, manager of Manchester United, announced that David Beckham, then the world's most famous player, had broken a 'metatarsal' bone in his foot. His place in that year's World Cup was immediately put into doubt. The word 'metatarsal' was at first met with bemusement by the television broadcaster. However, the word soon entered everyday language as the media hungrily dissected the injury, its anatomical location and its consequences for the player; 'doing a metatarsal' quickly became part of the sporting lexicon. Sporting injuries have permeated other areas of popular culture. In the 1980s, on the satire show *Spitting' Image*, a headless puppet of then England captain, Bryan Robson (his head was on his lap), was asked if he was injury prone. An episode of *Quincy* was set around college football and its impact on head injuries. An opening scene in *Six Feet Under* also featured the death of a high school footballer due to a heart attack. To a certain extent the relationship between sport and medicine has been a product of modern influences and values. In this sense the media has played an important role in shaping public perceptions. The reporting of injuries sustained by athletes has not only been portrayed as a distinct feature of their working lives but through the rise of the modern media the association between sport and medicine became embedded in the popular psyche.

This chapter is concerned with the occupational life of elite athletes. This includes not only the injuries they have experienced but also the provisions sporting authorities have made for injured athletes. It also seeks to understand how the bodies of athletes have been subject to an ever-present tension between the demands and values of sport and what was deemed to be fair and safe within a sporting context, especially with regard to rules. An athlete's body is his or her only major resource. John Harding has argued that in the case of footballers – although this could apply to most if not all elite athletes – 'It is a finite resource, subject to breakdown and inevitable decline.' Footballers, Harding continues, go through a complete life-cycle before they reach early adulthood and by about thirty-five years old their bodies will no longer carry them through a season. This athletic 'death' also leads to the 'eclipse of his professional identity'.[2]

To a certain extent the emergence of modern sport in the late nineteenth century shared similarities with modern work practices. Sturdy has argued industrial work was a defining experience of the twentieth century for much of the world's population because it was located within the social categories of class, wealth and status. This social experience was bound up with the bodily experiences associated with industrial work and physical labour. Not only did this include the exercise of manual skill and dexterity but also the associated ailments of bodily fatigue, injury and illness.[3] The experiences of professional and elite athletes, therefore, not only mirrored those of industrial workers but within sport these experiences were also conditioned within a sporting environment that during the twentieth century became more competitive and the quest for sporting success put extra demands on the bodies of athletes.

'The dangers of sport'

As we have seen in Chapter 1, exercise and physical recreation were generally seen positively in terms of a healthy mind in a healthy body. However, not everyone agreed that sport was good for you, both morally and physically and criticisms of elite sport can be placed alongside debates over ideas of rational recreation. Initially, sport was seen as part of a bourgeois idealism and would play a major part in the creation of a healthy, moral and orderly work force. The failure of early rational recreation schemes accompanied greater anxieties amongst the middle classes. By the late nineteen century the extension of the franchise, the rise of 'new unionism' and militant strike action led to a more assertive working class culture.[4] Growing class tensions saw the middle classes aim to exclude the working classes from their own spheres of influence. The subsequent emergence of amateurism in sport was partly designed to assist in this process.

Professional, competitive sport, because of its association with money and the working classes – and that it was not amateur – was regularly criticized by nineteenth century cultural commentators. Geoffrey Delamayn, the main character in the Wilkie Collins' novel, *Man and Wife* (1870), was a professional pedestrian. He is represented as a 'muscular ruffian' 'who lives for the adulation of his friends, the savage enthusiasm of his fans, and above all the fascinated adoration of women'.[5] Similar criticisms of professional sport and athletes have been part of the public discourse ever since. Many socialists – but not all – because of an atheist purist tradition, did not understand sport and were ill at ease with other working class leisure practices such as drinking. Indeed, socialist ideas about leisure had a direct link to cultural commentators like Matthew Arnold and rational recreationalists. Edward Carpenter, through his utopian ethical socialism, favoured an ascetic and 'simple life'. Fabians, like George Bernard Shaw, preferred a more active lifestyle that included mixed-sex Swedish Drill while the Clarion Cycling clubs took their name from Robert Blatchford's newspaper. However, all shared a frustration in what they believed was an apathy and selfishness that ran through the working classes who preferred 'trivial' commercial pleasures.[6] Analogous socialist attitudes to sport and popular culture were evident within the Labour Party following the 1945 General Election.[7]

Physical culturalists were similarly critical of sport because its competitive nature was not compatible with the aims of bodily discipline and like amateurs they did not like the tendency towards specialization. I.P. Muller regarded 'Athletic Sports' as 'movements and exercises which are performed for pleasure or amusement in order to enable one to excel others in any special branch, or to win in competitions'. Physical culture on the other hand was about the improvement and the development of the individual. Although some sporting activities could be considered rational, Muller warned that they may prove irrational for the individual; team sports were not considered rational.[8] Sandow was an admirer of sport but he also linked its popularity to the poor physical health of the mass of spectators and argued that it would only be medically safe for people to participate 'in these strenuous contests' if they built up their bodies. He warned that those who take up football or athletics 'must first have special muscles prepared for those feats by weeks or even months of training'. If not then many could 'damage and ruin their health for life'.[9]

It was against this background that doctors made similar criticisms over the nature and competitiveness of sport. These criticisms were linked to rising anxieties over the injuries and health of athletes, especially in all codes of football and on both sides of the Atlantic. There were especial concerns over the violent nature of football played at public schools. In 1870 *The Times* published a letter from 'A Surgeon' complaining about the number of football injuries he had dealt with at Rugby School, particularly due to the practice of 'hacking'. Later that year the school's medical officer, Dr Robert Farquarhson, admitted that a boy had been killed playing football.[10]

Deaths in all footballing codes were not uncommon. In 1880 the Mayor of Southampton banned football in the town following the death of a player.[11] Between 1886 and 1895 there were 13 Yorkshire rugby players killed[12] with at least another 12 fatalities in Northern Union matches between 1895 and 1910.

John Richardson, for example, sustained his fatal injuries when he ran into one of his own players when trying to catch a high ball.[13] Fatalities and injuries in football were regularly noted in medical journals.[14] In 1894 two articles appeared in the *Lancet* titled, 'The Perils of Football'.[15] In the second it was stated that,

> Football is a dangerous game; it is also an excellent game; but if the danger can in any way be modified without spoiling the sport surely something will be gained. And if the danger is increasing, with or without a corresponding increase in the position of the game as one of skill, it behoves serious people to consider what cause the increased danger is due.

These articles had partly been a consequence of a three-year campaign against the 'dangers of football' run by the editor of the *Pall Mall Gazette*, W.T. Stead.[16]

In November 1907 the *Lancet* returned to the same subject, recording the deaths of six players in the previous few weeks. Despite stating that 'No fault can be found with football *per se*' and that 'it is pre-eminently a manly, healthy game', the journal argued that, 'none the less its perils are excessive, and those who make the laws of the game and maintain discipline among the players should see to this'.[17] The following year, after noting some reports of footballing injuries, the journal argued that football was dangerous 'due to the spirit of the game which encourages competition'.[18] Although physicians recognized the medical values of exercise, some worried about the medical implications of competition. It reflected the idea that exercise should be done in moderation. Some doctors adopted the aphorism, 'Athletics for health is safe. Athletics for prowess and superiority may be dangerous'.[19] At the 1903 annual meeting of Schools Medical Officers, R.H. Anglin Whitelocke, a Fellow of the Royal College of Surgeons, gave a paper on 'Football Injuries'.[20] In 1910 the British Medical Association's Council recommended that schoolboys participating in rowing, boxing, cross-country running and swimming should undergo medical examinations.[21] Despite these protestations and calls to ban football there was little chance of such advice being heeded. In Britain the popularity of soccer and rugby crossed the class divide. Tony Collins has argued that, despite a growing trend of rough play among northern working-class rugby players, 'violence was [also] an integral part of the "manly" philosophy of the middle-class administrators of the sport. "Rough" sports were seen as healthy and character-building.' Moreover, the threat of danger was an accepted part of working class life due to the large number of men who worked in primary industries such as mining.[22]

Sport in American educational establishments shared similar attitudes to its danger with the UK. Initially, sport replaced gymnastics as part of the American enthusiasm for maintaining health and became the preferred activities of the middle-class American male.[23] College football matches between the 'Big Three' – Harvard, Yale, Princeton – fostered intense rivalries that popularized the game.[24]

Although the sport claimed to be amateur, it rapidly developed along commercial and professional lines. This model was copied throughout the entire US university system.[25] Like its transatlantic cousins American football suffered its own periodic 'crises', something that brought similar criticisms from US medical journals. In 1903 the American Medical Association had reported that in that year there had been 35 deaths as a result of playing football as well as 11 cases of paralysis due to spinal injuries and over 500 severe accidents. Nevertheless, the game continued to be regarded as a 'passage to manhood' and its supporters claimed that 'contest victory' was paramount even if personal sacrifice was necessary. As the game's popularity increased in American colleges and high schools, fatalities and injuries mounted, and there was particular concern that these included the nation's male elite from Ivy League universities. In 1905, following meeting between football and college officials and another with President Roosevelt, rule changes were made, including the forward pass, in an attempt to make the game safer.[26]

The expansion of athletics in American universities in the inter-war years led to further criticism of college football in the shape of the Carnegie Foundation's Bulletin Number 23 (1929). While commissioned by the National College Athletic Association (NCAA) and written from the perspective of educationalists rather than doctors, the report was concerned with the health and welfare of students who played the game. The report was largely damning of football, particularly its recruitment system, which was described as 'demoralizing and corrupt' and that in all but name it was a professional game.[27] The Carnegie report found that football was the most hazardous sport within the university system, especially inter-collegiate football, with concussion injuries causing most concern.[28] This excessive incidence of injuries was put down to a number of factors. First, because of a coach's desire to win, it was suggested that his methods ignored the dangers to life and limb. This could include his tactics as well as the use of chemical substances. It was also argued that players played when not fit while there were inadequate medical examinations and supervision of athletes. Lastly, the playing schedule was found to be too rigorous.[29] These concerns – in all sports – would be echoed throughout the century. Criticism of the game extended to popular culture more widely. During the inter-war years there were a number of critical articles in women's magazines. One article in *Good Housekeeping* in 1936 warned parents that crippling injury and death constantly stalked the football field.[30] However, there was an ambivalent response to the Carnegie report. The tension between universities and their football team was deeply embedded with college pride put before the welfare of its students. Michael Oriard has argued that the corrupting 'professionalism' of college football in the 1920s formed the basis of the sport in 2000.[31]

Occupational hazards

A sporting life has offered marked distinctions with most other occupations, and living and dealing with injuries has been and continues to be one key aspect of this existence. One study has estimated that the overall level of injury to professional soccer players is 1,000 times higher than that found in other industrial occupations traditionally regarded as high risk.[32] Another has estimated that two per cent of English professional soccer players retire each year as a consequence of an acute injury, a high figure when compared with most other jobs.[33] However, Roderick has argued that what constitutes both an injury and playing or competing with pain has been shaped by a wider socio-cultural context.[34] Ideas of masculinity, for example, have been important not only in shaping athletes' attitudes towards injuries but also their own identities. As a result, it is felt that 'real men' should conceal pain as well as ignore the pain and injuries of others.

Masculinity though – and, therefore, attitudes towards injuries – has had different meanings for different social groups. Whereas middle-class sports in the nineteenth century – in theory – represented, fair play and sportsmanship and were expressions of manliness, a soccer team came to symbolize the virtues of the men who supported it, mostly from the working classes, while rugby league shared a bond with coal mining the most masculine of occupations.[35] Attributes such as hardness, stamina, courage and loyalty came to be regarded as more important than skill.[36] This perceived need to play through pain has seen the lionization of some English footballers, including Terry Butcher (versus Sweden 1990) and Paul Ince (versus Italy 1997). After bravely scoring against Austria in 1952 and then sustaining an injury, Nat Lofthouse was given the sobriquet the 'Lion of Vienna'. In the 1965 FA Cup Final, before substitutes were allowed, Liverpool's Gerry Byrne played nearly all the game plus extra time with a broken collarbone.[37] This was a common occurrence in FA Cup finals but in most cases injured players would continue to play on the wing. Byrne though continued to play on as a defender.

Ian Adams, the doctor for Leeds United in the 1970s, and who also worked in other sports, has claimed that, in his experience, there was a different psychology between footballers and rugby league players. Footballers, he felt, tended to be more introspective and were 'always looking for little aches and pains, hamstring tweaks etc'. In comparison, there was a more macho culture associated with rugby league whose players he (improbably) claimed 'probably don't feel pain anyway to be honest'. Adams cited the example of an Australian player at Leeds who during one match had his cheekbone broken. He was told to take a week off but refused as he said if he did not play he would not get paid. The following week he suffered another cheekbone fracture on his other side. Despite being a prop forward who had to scrum down, with all the pressure on his cheekbones that brought, he never missed a match when he should have been laid up for six to eight weeks.[38]

The idea of playing or competing while injured has become an accepted part of the life of the modern sporting professional. Sociologists have argued that injuries have become normalized and from an early age athletes experience 'a process of defining even serious injuries in sport as routine and uneventful'.[39] A small survey of former professional footballers concerning the injuries and medical treatment they received elicited a mixed response to the question of playing with injuries. It could be argued that this was relative to their perceptions about injuries; something conditioned by the medical advice they received (for the treatment of injuries see Chapter 6). One player, for example, who played 700 league games between 1956 and 1976 claimed that he carried an injury into three-quarters of them while another (1940–59) claimed he never did. Other respondents differentiated between serious injuries and minor ones i.e., 'niggles', with most commenting that they played with niggles. One player (1968–83) stated, 'I tended to play on through minor injuries or niggles. For most of the games I was 100% fit or 95% of the time.' However, there were various reasons for playing with a niggle. First, it was partly a process of negotiation between the player and the medical staff. Because there were only fives games of the season to go, one player (1966–76) who had pulled a muscle in his right leg had 'a jab' before each game. He said that he 'got through the games. The idea being that I had all close season to get over it.' On occasions some players would conceal injury from the club. Some did so because they thought they might lose their place in the team – and a potential win bonus.[40] Moreover, on some occasions pressure was placed on players to play from the manager and medical staff (see Chapter 6).

The main point here is that injuries within sport were institutionalized. Athletes not only sustained injuries they were aware of their consequences in terms of recovery and 'managing' them. It highlighted that sport, especially for the elite but also at recreational levels, carried different values compared to other types of physical culture. Whereas Sandow and Muller advocated total bodily health for the individual, elite sport generated notions of competition and placed an emphasis on character and courage: whereas physical culturalists and doctors generally promoted exercise in moderation, sport promoted an excessive bodily culture. This difference in attitude was illuminated by former British and Irish Lions' hooker, Brian Moore. In previewing the second rugby union test between South Africa and the Lions in 2009, he declared that for the Lions players to win, it would involve a 'fearless, even reckless disregard for their physical wellbeing'.[41]

While injuries have become an occupational hazard for elite athletes, there has been a long history of injuries associated with sport. In 1883, for example, a reader of the *Field* wrote in concerning his treatment for 'tennis elbow'.[42]

In 1887 William Renshaw had been unable to defend his Wimbledon title due to tennis elbow.[43] In 1889 *The Times* reported that hard ground due to frost had caused two 'Football Accidents'. One player, Preston North End's Jack Graham, suffered a broken collarbone.[44] These 'sporting accidents' reflected a greater awareness of accidental injuries that emerged in the final quarter of the nineteenth century. Injuries sustained on streets and in the industrial workplace, such as the mines and the railways, became sensationalized in newspapers and were read by an increasingly literate working class.[45] Moreover, just as industrialization brought particular diseases, such as phossy jaw and grinder's lung, which were contracted by workers in the match and cutlery industries, athletes now suffered recognizable sport-specific injuries.[46] However, there was a 'culture of risk' in sport not evident in other areas of industry.[47]

A greater knowledge of sports injuries had developed from the late nineteenth century. As well as 'tennis elbow' some players also suffered from 'tennis leg', which was a calf injury. 'Riders Strain' was due to a pulled thigh muscle. 'Scrum Pox', or 'Football Impetigo', was a contagious skin condition that rugby forwards contracted. Rugby scrum forwards also suffered from 'football ear' where blood collected and formed into a cyst. Meanwhile, rowers suffered from boils (probably on their backside) while boxers had 'cauliflower ears'. Following the *fin de siècle* fashion for cycling, there were initial worries that its prolonged use could result in 'bicycle face', 'bicycle hand', 'bicycle foot" or 'bicycle hump', which was an apparently painful condition caused by low handlebars. A combination of these afflictions was said to bring about the unlikely (and unknown) formation of 'cyclo-anthropos'.[48] For two years, 1907–09, the *Athletic News*, which was then considered *The Times* of football, ran a weekly doctor's column. Written by Chelsea's doctor, J. Ker Lindsay, he gave advice on subjects like treatment of injuries, the anatomy, exercise and diets. He also answered any queries from readers. In October 1907, for example, he wrote on displaced cartilages, while eleven months later the topics included bone setting and a 'study of the body'. In December 1909 he gave advice on bandaging and how to stop the bleeding.

Some sports were more dangerous than others. Boxers not only suffered black eyes, broken noses and the occasional broken jaw some also died in the ring. In 1900 Mike Riley died of an inter-cranial haemorrhage, for example, while Billy Smith died of laceration of the brain the following year.[49] As we have seen, the level of danger in American football could be judged on the levels of fatalities in the sport. In 1990 it was reported that, for the first time since 1931 'there was not a direct fatality' at any level of the game. Winter sporting accidents had their own dangers. In 1959 it was estimated that 3.5 million went skiing in the United States with injuries occurring at the rate of 5 per 1000 skiers per day. Winter sports injuries were also different in nature with some the result of striking ice or rock with head injuries common.[50]

While association football did not carry this amount of risk it was not without its dangers for professionals. During the 1913–14 season it was estimated that by New Year's Eve only 169 of the 1,701 players who had played in the first eleven of teams in the Football League, the Southern League as well as the Scottish League, had not suffered any injury. The figure dropped to 61 by mid-April.[51] Types of injuries could also be determined by how the game was played. Early football was played in rushes with an emphasis on individual play. There was also much heavy charging that could result in broken arms, legs and collarbones. As the rules of the game changed so did the nature of the injuries. In 1925 the offside law was modified and ushered in a more free-flowing game that placed a greater emphasis on athleticism. It led to more injuries as collisions between players became more violent.[52] The invention of the sliding tackle and the tackle from behind were also blamed for contributing to an increase in injuries during this period. It was claimed that these types of tackles had led to a growth in cartilage operations.[53]

The culture of football in Britain though, where the emphasis has been on the physical rather than the technical, has tended to be different compared to the rest of the world. In South America, for example, there was a dislike of the British style and the shoulder charge was particularly resented partly because of the harder grounds on which the game was played.[54] Goalkeepers were also treated differently. In Britain they could receive rough treatment and be charged (although this had radically changed by 2000). In the 1957 FA Cup Final the jaw of Manchester United's keeper Ray Wood was broken after he had been charged – fairly according to the referee – by Aston Villa's Peter McParland. By contrast, any contact with goalkeepers both in Europe and South America is deemed a foul. By the late twentieth century English football's dangers were still apparent. In 1997 it was found that over an eight-year period an average of 51 players and trainees per season (there were about 2,400 professional footballers at 92 league clubs) finished their careers prematurely as a result of injuries, accidents or sickness.[55] Footballers' injuries were also frequent. Between 1997 and 1999 it was found that approximately 75 per cent of players sustained at least one injury while 22 per cent of injuries were classified as severe and preventing the player from training or playing for at least four weeks.[56]

Injuries were not confined to contact sports. Equestrian sports, for example, were inherently dangerous. For army officers 'sport provided an arena for the demonstration of tough masculinity'. In India polo and pig-sticking were dangerous activities but at the same time were deemed an important part of a British cavalry officer's career. Not only was sport a form of thrill seeking but officers also believed that it helped to cultivate certain qualities like pluck, courage, esprit du corps, as well as leadership. Officers proudly flaunted their injuries from pig-sticking although polo was a more dangerous sport; between 1880 and 1914 thirty-six officers died from polo accidents.[57] In equestrian events serious sporting injuries could also cut across the gender divide. One of the most dangerous has been Three-Day Eventing where men and women compete on equal terms. In 1976 Virginia Holgate broke her arm in twenty-three places after a fall. The original diagnosis had been to amputate from just above the elbow but the arm was saved.[58] A show jumper, Nick Skelton, broke his neck in 2000 after falling off a horse and landing on his head. He was forced into retirement but made a comeback and was still riding in 2012.[59]

Sporting injuries have not been restricted to those that can end careers. 'Burn-out', for example, has been one sporting condition associated with young athletes. The phrase 'burn-out' itself has been in use since at least the 1920s. In America, it was observed that some high school athletes were often 'burned-out' before entering college athletic competition.[60] In Britain the 'Victor Ludorum' athletics award for public schoolboys, where boys had to run at all distances consecutively, was described as 'pernicious'. It was noted that many a promising runner's standards had dipped due to over exertion at an early age.[61] 'Burn-out' has been particularly linked with female tennis players. Martina Hingis, for example, started playing tennis at two, won Wimbledon at 16 and was forced to retire at 21. Others who followed a similar pattern included Andrea Jaeger and Tracey Austin, a US Open champion, who gave up through injury before she was 20.[62] Jennifer Capriati turned professional aged 14 but shoulder injuries eventually forced her into retirement aged 31. She speculated that these problems had been brought on by training too hard and too long, competing in too many events and 'listening to tournament organizers, sponsors and Tour officials instead of to her body'.[63]

In more recent years there has been a greater awareness that athlete's injuries are not just physical. Cricketers, because of the time they spend away from home and family, have been particularly susceptible to bouts of depression. It is also claimed (although there is little hard evidence) that the suicide rate is higher amongst former cricketers than for any other sport. In 2006 Marcus Trescothick, because of depression and homesickness, was forced to return home to England from tours of first, India and then Australia. Soon after he retired from international cricket but continued to play for his county team Somerset.[64] In addition, athletes are faced with a 'psychological barrier' after returning from injury. This could include making and experiencing a tackle in football (of all codes) or runners having to run at full stretch again following a lay-off. Moreover, in the background there is always the constant and on-going fear of an injury that may either force the athlete to miss an important event such as the Olympics or one that brings their career to a premature end. Yet a growing knowledge and acceptance about the importance of mental health in sport has contrasted with traditional notions of masculinity and of what being a professional – especially male – athlete means. These ideas have usually stressed the importance of 'character', the ability not to show any sign of weakness and when it comes to criticism from the crowd, team-mates and coaches alike to be able to 'take it'. The footballer Stan Collymore, for example, believed that he was persecuted by his manager at Aston Villa, John Gregory, for suffering from depression because it was felt that it was not 'normal' for a top footballer to be depressed.[65]

In addition to injuries, professional athletes have also had to cope with the daily grind of competing and training and the general wear and tear it inflicts on the body. There is perhaps no event that is more demanding than the Tour de France, which Christopher Thompson has shown, was 'the celebration of a distinctive Tour heroism based on suffering and survival' as much as the rider's skill.[66] In the 1920s the Tour's length exceeded 5,000 kilometres with the longest stages covering 480 kms. By 2002, however, it was 3,282 kms and the longest stage was 226 kms. While the distances had decreased, in essence, the cyclists were still riding for six hours a day virtually every day for three weeks (see also Chapter 5).

In horse-racing, in addition to the risk of falls, flat race jockeys have subjected themselves to severe regimes of wasting to make the weight, which shares characteristics similar to anorexia nervosa. Tolich and Bell have argued that while a jockey's professional skill is his/her ability to ride a horse, it is the ability to waste to make the required weight that is the fundamental skill. Wasting, therefore, is a 'work discipline and disciplinary social practice through which jockeys train and restrain their ability, their competitiveness and their psychological control'.[67] In 1850 the minimum weight for jockeys had been 4 stones and 5st 7lbs in 1875: today it is 7st 10lbs. Constant wasting weakened the constitutions of jockeys. This entailed having little to eat, long walks in heavy clothes, Turkish baths and doses of purgatives. Wasting contributed to the early deaths of Victorian jockeys, Tom French, John Charlton, Tom Chalenor and John Wells. This spartan regime was also attributed to the suicide of the most famous jockey of the nineteenth century, Fred Archer (1857–86). To lose twelve pounds in less than a week, he used 'Archer's Mixture', a very strong laxative made for him by a Newmarket physician, Dr J.R. Wright. One day he returned home ill and shot himself in a fit of delirium.[68] Bulimia has been a condition amongst top jockeys that continued into the late twentieth century. Lester Piggott's frame was relatively big for a jockey and so to keep his weight down he lived off a diet that included cigars and champagne.[69] It remains unclear though why the weights for jockeys have to be so small. In the early nineteenth century, prior to minimum weight legislation, racehorse owners sometimes resorted to child riders. This practice continued after the Second World War. Lester Piggott, for example, rode his first winner aged 12 in 1948. It was only in the 1960s that a minimum age of 15 was set (it is 16 today).[70]

While cricket would not at first seem to be an overly physical and taxing sport, the season in England is long and can be demanding. To enable them to play day-in day-out, there has been widespread use amongst modern cricketers of non-steroidal anti-inflammatory drugs to alleviate strains and bruises to get them through the game. However, this medication produces unpleasant side-effects on the stomach and the liver as well as causing dizzy spells. Ian Botham claimed that for the last ten years of his career he was taking these drugs like sweets. To counter the stomach irritation they produced, he used Gaviscon in larger and larger doses just to enable him to take the pills.[71]

The rise of sporting welfarism

Injuries and the risk of injury would nudge the sporting authorities into make greater provision for the welfare of athletes. To what extent employer welfare and its motivations were related to the productivity of workers as much as their health and safety has been a fruitful area for historians.[72] Taylor has shown how between 1900 and 1939 welfarist initiatives in British football mirrored a bureaucratization of the labour market more generally.[73] Following the 1906 Workmen's Compensation Act professional sportsmen such as footballers, cricketers and jockeys came under its remit.[74] Football clubs also resembled paternalistic employers, especially in manufacturing consent in the workplace.[75] Occupational health and safety measures, however, were uneven across the British economy until the 1974 Health and Safety Act.[76] Services were better developed in state-owned industries as private companies generally made their own *ad hoc* welfare arrangements (which in many cases included the provision of sports facilities).[77]

Almost from the outset, football clubs insured themselves against possible claims, including injured players who would lose time off work. In 1883, even before professionalism had been legalized, Aston Villa had taken out a policy against injuries with the Cyclists' Accident Assurance Corporation Ltd.[78] Insurance schemes were also common in rugby, especially in the north, where working class players predominated. In 1883 Salford rugby club set up their own insurance scheme for players, contributing 15 per cent of the gate takings from each home game to the insurance fund. In 1886 the Rugby Football Union sanctioned insurance payments at no more than 10 shillings a day.[79] The Gaelic Athletic Association, which governed strictly amateur sports, such as hurling and Gaelic football, initiated its first injury scheme in 1929.[80]

Professional football clubs were becoming more aware of the consequences of players' injuries both from the perspective of their impact on performances on the pitch and the financial implications off it. As a result, it meant that doctors were required to act as medical officers in order to fulfil contractual requirements.[81] In 1898 Middlesbrough's insurance policies stated that a player 'shall at once retire from the field and have the injuries immediately attended to and he shall not resume play without the permission of a duly qualified surgeon or medical man etc'.[82] A doctor's certificate became a condition of any compensation to footballers while Middlesbrough's players were awarded 20 shillings for injuries that rendered them unable to work for three months.[83]

Before the First World War, however, football clubs did not actually have any legal medical obligations for their employees. At an inquest following the death of the Manchester City player, Di Jones, in 1902, the club resisted claims of liability. Instead, it sought to blame Jones's insistence on walking from the field to the ambulance as having 'caused more trouble than anything else'. The jury had 'wanted to impress upon football clubs that they should not allow a man to walk off the field in a case like that'. However, the Coroner disagreed. He stated, 'Are football clubs to supply a medical staff on their field? I don't think there is any obligation on them to do that'. There was no obligation on their part for many years after.[84]

Contracts between clubs and players, however, became more complex with rule-books stipulating procedures regarding injuries and medical treatment. In 1914 any Wolves player unfit to play had to obtain a doctor's certificate from the club's own medical officer.[85] At Hull City and Wolves, players were later forbidden from riding motor-cycles; if they did and got injured they would forfeit any claims for wages. Moreover, at both clubs players had to first obtain permission from the trainer or manager before visiting the club doctor. It was also made clear that injured players now came under the control of the club. They were club assets and had to obey instructions from the club trainer.[86] As rugby league became more competitive, clubs also issued more intricate rules for their players. At Leeds this included one that stated that injuries had to be reported to the club within 48 hours otherwise the player would not receive insurance payments.[87]

In horse-racing, reflecting the patrician nature of the sport, jockeys relied more on charity. It was not until the mid-twentieth century that an insurance scheme was established for professional jockeys. In the nineteenth century both the Bentinck Benevolent and Rous Memorial Funds had been set up. In 1923 the Jockey Club inaugurated the Jockeys' Accident Fund, although jockeys did not have the right to draw upon it. National Hunt jockeys relied on charity until the Rendlesham Benevolent Fund was established in 1902. It made some provision for jockeys killed or injured but payment was still discretionary. After the First World War a National Hunt Accident Fund was set up out of jockeys' licence fees and a levy from betting. By 1955 National Hunt riders were insured for a sum of £3,000 against permanent total disablement and in the event of temporary disablement they received £8 8s a week for one year. Their dependents received £2,000 if death occurred.[88] In 1971 the Injured National Hunt Jockeys' Fund (established in 1964) was renamed the Injured Jockeys' Fund to incorporate those from the flat.[89]

The intervention of the law was a relatively rare event in sport and contributed to what Ken Foster has termed the 'myth of autonomy' regarding sport's relationship with the law; sport was seen as a voluntary activity, a pursuit for pleasure not for profit and it also had its own organizational codes and constitutional arrangements i.e., sports governing associations were considered quasi-legal bodies. From the 1980s, however, there was a decline in this autonomy and a 'juridification of sport',[90] highlighted by a growing number of court cases brought by footballers against fellow professionals for alleged foul play that had caused their retirement (for legal actions against medical practitioners see Chapter 6). Legal precedent had been set by Jim Brown of Dunfermline in 1982 when he sued St. Johnstone's John Pelosi after suffering a compound fracture of the leg. The case though was settled out of court for £20,000. In 2004 Charlton's Matt Holmes was awarded £250,000 for what was claimed to be an illegal challenge that ended his career. For the first time a player successfully sued an opponent – in this case, Wolves' Kevin Muscat – following a claim of a deliberate foul, what was deemed an 'over the top' challenge. It was also contended that Muscat was a dirty player. In court his disciplinary record was produced as evidence and other players injured by Muscat gave evidence against him. As a consequence, the case potentially had repercussions for players who were ordered to deliberately foul opponents by managers.[91]

Sport's duty of care

Because of its voluntary roots, sport in Britain was self-regulating for much of the twentieth century. But within the context of a bourgeoning welfarist ethos, there was a growing awareness amongst the sporting authorities that they held some responsibility for the health of athletes in their charge. The subsequent formation of dedicated committees and organization also placed the relationship between sport and medicine on a more formal basis. The safety procedures put in place though had a dual purpose: they were not only there to protect the health of athletes but also to protect the image of the sport. This development was linked to wider social trends such as the change in the nature of childhood. In the post-war period family life was centred more on children and accompanied by greater parental anxieties for their safety.[92] To at least be seen to be making sports safer was also necessary if these sports were to survive by continuing to attract participants and athletes in the face of competition from an expanding leisure market. Moreover, there was a now greater and ever-present threat of legal action. At first many sporting competitions had no medical attendance. However, this gap was gradually filled by voluntary organizations such as the Red Cross and St. John Ambulance Brigade, which offered basic first aid. From the late nineteenth century greater interest had been taken in the supply and organization of accident provision. By 1879 the term 'first aid' had come into regular use due to the proliferation of first aid manuals, and especially after 1887 with the formation of the St John

Ambulance Brigade.[93] They have remained a familiar sight at sporting events, especially football matches, ever since.

The concerns of sporting bodies for the welfare of athletes have manifested itself in three main areas: the establishment of bodies or committees with responsibility for athlete's welfare; changes in the rules of the sport to make it safer; and the introduction of protective equipment. One of the first sports to establish a safety code was perhaps unsurprisingly American football, in light of criticism of the sport's growing injury count. In 1922 the American Football Coaches Association (AFCA) was founded with the task of promoting safety in the sport. In 1931 the AFCA initiated the 'Annual Survey of Football Fatalities' for research into the reduction of injuries and from 1980 it was continued as the Annual Survey of Football Injury Research.[94] In the post-war period British sports became aware of the need to monitor the health of athletes (for boxing see Chapter 8). In 1950 the Amateur Athletic Association (AAA) established an independent medical advisory body 'in view of the increasing number of medical questions affecting policy which have arisen in recent years'. Its recommendations included the establishment of a medical panel of doctors to advise on athletes' injuries; the availability of medical officers and medical equipment at all major athletic meetings.[95] The death of an athlete has usually signalled a point for the sporting authorities to re-assess their regulations. In cycling, for example, there had been no restrictions on the Tour de France's overall length, the number of stages or the length of stages until after Tom Simpson died on Mount Ventoux in 1967. Following his death the Union Cycliste Internationale (UCI) progressively introduced rules about maximum lengths, rest days and the number of long races in the calendar.[96]

The medical provisions laid on at successive Olympics for the marathon have illustrated how major sporting events have not only become more aware of the health and safety of athletes but were also concerned about the image of their event. At early Olympics there was minimal medical provision. However, it was recognized by the organizers that the marathon required medical support due to the severity of the race and the hot weather it usually took place in, something that increased as the Games became more popular. For the 1896 marathon, medical men followed behind the runners in carts acting as ambulances.[97] At the Paris games of 1900, ambulances and first-aid stations staffed with physicians and nurses were set out along the marathon route. In 1904, due to the intense heat and high humidity, only 14 out of the 27 starters finished the race. The winner, an American, Tom Hicks suffered from severe heat exhaustion and required the services of four physicians.[98] The 1904 marathon was a turning point regarding the organization of medical provision for Olympic athletes. Before the 1908 marathon, runners had to send 'a medical certificate of fitness' with their entry form and prior to the start they had to undergo a medical examination by a medical officer of the British Olympic Council (BOC). With reference to the distressed state of the runners in 1904, competitors had to retire if ordered to do so by a member of the BOC appointed medical staff. Runners were also allowed two attendants to assist him throughout the race.[99]

At the 1912 Games, medical arrangements were more sophisticated. Not only did the marathon runners require examinations of the heart but so did cyclists for their road race. Doctors on the Swedish rowing team also carried out tests. As in London four years previously, runners had to send in a medical certificate of fitness and nor could they take any 'so-called' drugs (see Chapter 5).[100] For the marathon course, including members of the Stockholm Volunteer Aid Corps and the Red Cross, there were 11 doctors, 7 medical assistants, 30 sick-attendants and 2 sick-nurses on duty. Around the course, medical stations were arranged, which included ambulances and sick rooms, each manned by a physician. Refreshments were also laid on. Despite the arrangements, a runner, Francesco Lazaro from Portugal died from heat stroke.[101]

'Marathon medicine' became more sophisticated during the latter part of the twentieth century as a result of the jogging boom. At the first London marathon in 1981 there was a medical team comprising four doctors, two physiotherapists and podiatrists plus St. John Ambulance volunteers. By 2006 this team had increased to over 100, headed by Dr Dan Tunstall-Pedoe, the race's medical director since its inception. His appointment was due to criticism from some medical authorities about the dangers for 'fun runners' in this 'risky event'. As part of the service, each runner is sent medical, training and dietary advice. In addition, there is now a specialist team in cardiac resuscitation in attendance. From its beginning to 2006, 8 runners had died due to heart failure, although 35,000 people take part each year.[102]

Some of the more dangerous sports, like horse racing,[103] began to make more provision for safety measures. In motor racing, danger – and thrill seeking – rather than safety had been inherent in the sport. There was also an attitude amongst traditionalists that the better drivers coped with this danger element better than the lesser drivers. Moreover, the cars themselves were built for speed with little concern for the welfare of the driver. Between 1963 and 2000, 17 Formula One drivers were killed with another 16 fatalities made up of officials and spectators. In addition, there were many deaths in other forms of motor racing such as the Le Mans 24-hour race. A number of the circuits, especially Spa Francorchamps in Belgium and Germany's Nürburgring, were notoriously dangerous. A move towards safety in Formula One had been instigated in the 1960s by the Grand Prix Drivers Association (formed in 1961). However, it was really pushed along by Jackie Stewart who in 1969 led a drivers' strike at Spa on the grounds that it was unsafe. In 1966 Stewart had crashed at Spa and due to the poor response of the authorities to the accident, Louis Stanley, the chairman of Stewart's team, British Racing Motors, established a mobile hospital that went to all the European Grand Prix circuits. However, many circuits boycotted its use. There had been some improvements to the safety of Grand Prix racing from 1963. At the Nürburgring, for example, where once there were hedges all the way round the 28 kilometres circuit, under the initiative of Stewart these were replaced with guardrails. In 1978 medical responsibility for Formula 1 was placed in the hands of Sidney Watkins who was a professor of neurosurgery at the London Hospital. Three years afterwards the Fédération Internationale du Sport Automobile (FISA), the governing body for world motor racing, had formed its own Medical Commission.[104]

Ironically, professional football in England did not establish a medical committee until 1980, which was indicative of the FA's attitude towards sports medicine; no audit of injuries within the English game was commissioned until 1997. Rugby Union's first injury and training audit was commissioned in 2001 and the results published in 2005. Some contact sports in other countries were more pro-active. An Australian Football League Medical Officers' Association had been established in 1972 and in 1983 it instituted an injury survey for that sport. In 1992 an annual sporting injury surveillance programme was initiated.[105]

As we have seen, from the late Victorian period to the 1980s the law generally did not concern itself with the governance of sport, although the state had taken a regular interest in the regulation of leisure more generally on matters such as the licensing of music halls and public houses.[106] Despite the self-regulating modus operandi of sport and the myth of its autonomy from society,[107] there was an ever-present tension and balancing act between safety and the desire to retain aspects of certain particular sports that were deemed part of its essence and hence its attraction.

To a large extent, the regulation of violent play in association and rugby football had been ensured by amateurism. Although team games were about the giving and taking of hard knocks both the FA and the RFU deemed serious injuries from deliberate violent play unacceptable.[108] The FA had banned hacking in 1863 and in 1871 although regarded as the true mark of the 'manly' game, the practice was banned by the RFU. Hacking, basically shin-kicking, had come to be seen as unfair mainly because young men who played the game found that bruised shins acquired on a Saturday afternoon was not ideal preparation for a day's work in the office on Monday morning. Nevertheless, the mentality remained one of 'roughness within the rules', although there was still plenty of it outside them.[109]

In the 1930s there were a number of high-profile deaths in football, in particular Glasgow Celtic's John Thomson and James Thorpe of Sunderland, both of whom were goalkeepers. Perhaps more interesting than what was said at both inquests was what was not said as little comment was passed on football's wider responsibilities during these cases. It did though highlight the creeping influence of the law on sport, which had been mainly absent partly due to sport's voluntary tradition.[110] Following the death of Thorpe, the FA responded by setting up a commission. This was partly due to concerns over the question of liability as well as its position as the sole governing body of the game and law-maker. Importantly, the FA, as befitting a quasi-legal body, was keen that it should be the sole arbiter in making any changes to it laws.[111] The commission, however, conscious of the FA's wider role,[112] recommended that Law 8 be changed. It now stated that, although a player could still charge the keeper when the latter was holding the ball, the player could not now attempt to kick the ball out of the goalkeeper's hands. This was now deemed as violent conduct.[113]

Rules could also be changed if it was felt that they would reduce injuries to athletes. In 2004 the Australian Football League changed its rule relating to ruck contests due to a proliferation of cruciate ligament injuries amongst players; 16 between 1997 and 2003. There had previously been a modification to the rules, which was aimed to make the game more attractive. This rule allowed for ruckmen to gain considerable momentum when challenging for a 'centre bounce', and thus, increasing the chances of injury. The Australian Football League Medical Officers Association (AFLMOA) identified the main cause of the injury when the knee of one player made forcible contact with an opponent's shin and recommended a reduced run-up. This it was argued would still retain 'this attractive part of the game'.[114]

Innovations in equipment and their regulation have had an important impact on the safety of some sports, although this was not universally welcomed. In 1898 it was noted that with the introduction of 'safety', cycling lost much of its danger, excitement and its manliness.[115] In some sports the drive towards health and safety has changed its nature. The high jump was revolutionized due to Dick Fosbury's victory at the 1968 Olympics with his 'flop' but it had only been possible due to the invention of 'crash mats'. Another American, Clinton Larson, had attempted to use a flop-like technique in the 1920s but because of the lack of a cushion to the fall it was thought too dangerous. Instead, jumpers continued to use the straddle and western roll techniques because they landed safely in a sandpit.[116]

Safety has been the main factor behind most innovations. In 1923 the wearing of crash helmets for National Hunt jockeys was made compulsory following the death of Captain Bennett at Wolverhampton. However, this was only for racing and was not enforced for training gallops until the 1970s.[117] Their opposite numbers on the flat continued to scorn helmets until 1939. The football authorities in England became concerned over the safety of players' boots and allowed referees to inspect boots before games for any protruding metal objections on boots or shin pads.[118] Improvements in winter sports equipment also reduced the incident of certain injuries. Better designed ski boots provided more stability to the ankles but the incidences of fractures of the tibia and fibula increased while that of ankle fractures decreased.[119]

Protective equipment has been particularly important in cricket. While gloves and pads had been used in the nineteenth century, it could be argued that moves to protect a cricketer's most vulnerable parts were relatively slow in coming. It was claimed that Johnny Tyldesley, in around 1900, had invented the first abdominal protector, i.e., a 'box', when he had been out injured for six weeks after been struck in the groin. Before then batsmen stuffed towels inside their flannels.[120] However, wearing a box was not compulsory. Fred Trueman's cricket career nearly came to a premature end when as a schoolboy in the 1940s he was struck in the groin by a ball when he wasn't wearing a protector. He was rushed to hospital, underwent emergency surgery and was unable to play for two years.[121] The 1970s saw the introduction of the helmet. Batsmen now sought greater protection from fast bowlers, particularly from the West Indies and Australia, who adopted intimidatory tactics and bowled more bouncers at the head. At first wearing a helmet was voluntary. Some early prototypes only protected the temples and the batsman looked as though he was wearing a sanitary towel on his head. When helmets became standardized, for reasons of insurance it has been compulsory for international players to wear one.

Similar to changing the laws of sports, the introduction of protective equipment and its use has created tensions between doctors, rule-makers and especially coaches regarding debates over safety and maintaining sporting traditions. One illuminating example of these tensions has been the helmet in American football, both in the professional game and at college and school levels. Helmets had been worn since at least the early 1900s but it wasn't until 1939 that the modern prototype – the hard-shell helmet – was first used. To begin with it gave players more courage but coaches soon discovered it made an effective weapon. The helmet, which by the 1970s weighed three pounds, became the game's principal instrument of intimidation due to techniques such as 'butt-blocking' and 'butt-tackling'. These techniques have had long-term concerns for players. In 1968 alone there had been 36 deaths and 30 cases of permanent paralysis.[122] It was found that these cases had been as a direct result of coaches instructing players to use a tackling and blocking technique that required the use of the head. Since 1960 80 per cent of direct fatalities have been caused by head and neck injuries.[123] One doctor, Donald Cooper, then team physician at Oklahoma State, blamed the coaches for resisting safety measures, such as a padded helmet, who in turn accused doctors of meddling. Cooper claimed that coaches resisted change to helmet design because they wanted to hear noise i.e., the big whack of a hit, which was a part of the game they had been brought up with. One consequence of the increase in injuries was a growth in litigation in the 1970s with some cases brought against coaches, especially by the parents of schoolboys, because, it was alleged, they had not taught the players the dangers of tackling. Helmet manufacturers were also sued with a number forced out of business. In 1977 there had been fourteen manufacturers but after facing $150 million in negligence suits a year later there were eight. Commercial imperatives also meant that there was a lack of standardization regarding helmet design.[124]

Like American football, ice hockey has had a reputation for violent play. Drawn up in 1917, the original rules of the National Hockey League (NHL) allowed fist fights and clubs hired 'enforcers' (or 'goons') for this purpose[125] (an aspect of ice-hockey that was parodied in the film, *Slap Shot* (1977). As a fast sport the risk of injury has also been regarded as an integral part of the game. To combat this threat the sport has constantly developed and invented protective equipment since the 1920s when concerns over injuries increased. Not unlike American football, protective equipment did not necessarily lead to a safer sport; instead it made the game more dangerous. Padding in ice hockey was initially minimal with some players wearing soccer shin pads. In 1929 the first facemask for a goaltender was used in North America while shoulder and elbow pads were first worn in the 1930s. The need for further protection increased when the game moved indoors after the Second World War as play was faster, more constricted and led to greater contact. The innovation of the slap shot in the 1950s also changed the nature of the game with high-flying pucks and sticks resulting in a higher risk of injuries to the eyes, face and head. Hockey helmets were first used in Sweden in the 1950s, becoming mandatory in 1963. In 1975 the wearing of a helmet with a full facemask was made compulsory in the National Hockey League. However, this had unforeseen consequences as it encouraged a more aggressive playing style because it was believed that the head, face and throat were less at risk. The greater padding also generated a feeling of invincibility amongst players and the elbow pad, now a hard shell, became a weapon in itself. In addition, there was also an increasing incidence of minor traumatic brain injuries.[126]

In Formula One helmets were only made compulsory in 1951 when up to then many drivers had favoured a linen cap. The death of Lorenzo Bandini due to burns at Monaco in 1967 led to changes in the design of drivers' suits. Now through scientific developments a Dupont nylon material 'Nomex' was worn over a similar layer of long sleeved pants and vests and Nomex socks and gloves. The material was designed not to burn or support combustion and it was estimated that it would give the driver twenty seconds before his body was burned. Drivers also now wore a Nomex face-mask and an all-in-one crash helmet to prevent flames reaching the face.[127]

Case study: rugby union

In recent years the changing relationship between sport and medicine has perhaps been most evident in rugby union. After turning professional in 1995, the sport's rapid commercialization has had a significant impact not only on how the game itself has changed but also injuries to players. The aim here is to use rugby union to illuminate some of the issues that have been covered above in terms of injuries sustained and the attitudes of the sport's authorities to these developments.

Of course, rugby (both union and league) has always had a reputation as a rough game. Early in its amateur days, rugby footballers could be 'collared', and it was regarded by some as 'part of the game' for them to be stamped on during rucks and mauls. As Collins has pointed out, masculinity through physicality was the essence of the sport. It was exemplified by the violence in the match between England and New Zealand in 1925 but the giving and taking of it was common at all levels and this continued deep into the twentieth century.[128] Unsurprisingly, at recreational level the injuries sustained in rugby have usually been more serious and their incidence has generally been higher than in other British sports.[129] In 1970–71, in a survey of recreational sport, it had been found that the accident rate in soccer (36.5 per 10,000 man hours of play) was actually higher than that of rugby (30.5). However, rugby players' injuries were more serious with fractures and dislocations twice as common.[130] By 1991 a Sports Council survey had found that rugby (both union and league) was more dangerous: 59.3 per cent of rugby players experienced an injury every 4 playing weeks while for soccer players it was 39.3 per cent. For martial arts, hockey and cricket the figures were 36.3 per cent, 24.8 per cent and 20.2 per cent respectively. In New Zealand it was calculated that rugby injuries contributed to 49–58 per cent of all sport-related hospital visits.[131] By 2005 it was claimed that rugby union was the most 'risk-laden team sport' with professional players on average spending almost a fifth of each season on the sidelines.[132]

What changes to rugby union have taken place since 1995? First, there has been a change in the shape of players' bodies. Professionalism not only brought better paid players; they were also bigger, fitter, more skilful and more powerful. In 1991 England international forwards weighed on average 100 kilograms while backs were 83 kg; in 2003 these figures were 109 kg and 90 kg respectively. A greater proportion of this weight was also leaner body mass, allowing more force to be generated in collisions.[133] In this sense, as in American football, a player's body could act as a weapon. In addition, rule alterations altered the nature of the game as the rugby authorities attempted to make the sport more free-flowing and more attractive to television, sponsors and spectators alike. New rules were designed to reduce the proportion of static formations such as the scrum, the lineout and ruck and maul, and with more open play there has been a greater chance of high impact collisions. There was a 30 per cent increase in the ball-in-play time between 1995 and 2003, significantly increasing potential contact time and hence potential injuries per match. The introduction of tactical substitutions also allowed for fresher 'impact' players – selected for their ability to 'break' the tackles of tiring opponents – to come on late in the game; it has been these tiring players who have become more susceptible to injury.[134] In addition, it was found that there was a higher risk of injury the better the standard of rugby.[135] This greater intensity in play has been complemented with an expanding fixture list since

1995, which, due to less time for rest and recuperation, has increased the strain on players' bodies.

One outcome of these changes has been the gradual acceptance of the wearing of protective equipment for players who wished to prevent injuries. In 1996 the RFU sanctioned the use of approved head protection and in 1998 upper body equipment, i.e., shoulder pads made of soft and thin material, was incorporated into an undergarment; at first padding had only been allowed to protect an injury.[136] While scrum caps and mouth guards had been used for many years, these post-1995 developments were in contrast to rugby's traditional ethos that took pride in resisting the introduction of American football style body armour.

Attitudes towards violence also began to change, partly due to a greater media awareness of sporting injuries. One such injury was sustained by the Welsh full-back, J.P.R. Williams. Playing for his club Bridgend against New Zealand in 1978, he had his face severely raked by the studs of the All Blacks prop forward, John Ashworth whilst at the bottom of a ruck. It was claimed that Williams was lucky not to have been blinded and the subsequent damning television footage of Ashworth's foul play turned the incident into a media cause celebre. The Director of Public Prosecutions contacted Williams and asked him if he wished to press charges. Although seething over the manner of how he sustained the injury, Williams, declined because he felt as an amateur player this would not be appropriate.[137]

Despite Williams' stance, from the 1970s the medical profession was drawn to the study of rugby injuries, especially those to the spinal cord that resulted in tetraplegia.[138] These types of injuries had originally been described as 'acts of God' (it was actually the tackle that caused more paralysing injuries than the scrum). These findings as well as the growing threat of legal action from parents and also the potential damage to the image of the game had resulted in changes in the laws of the game from 1985. To protect the head and neck, scrums were to be prevented from collapsing and rucks and mauls were to be stopped from carrying on for too long, although it was not certain how effective these changes had been.[139] In 2005, following a severe neck injury to Leicester Tigers' prop forward, Matt Hampson, which had paralysed him from the waist down, there was further concern amongst the game's administrators over the safety of the scrum. The following year, James Bourke, a consultant general surgeon at the Queen's Medical Centre in Nottingham and former doctor for Nottingham RFC questioned whether the scrum was actually legal under the Health and Safety at Work Act.[140]

As a consequence of these concerns and injuries, the International Rugby Board (IRB), at the behest of its medical committee – highlighting the importance of medicine within the sport – decided to make further changes to the scrummaging laws. Law 20 had previously stated that 'Before the two front rows come together, they must be standing no more than an arm's length apart' to prevent the front rows charging at each other in forming a scrum. Instead, a scrum would now begin with the two front rows standing close enough so that the props could touch one another's shoulder before impact. It was designed to ensure that neither side had any forward momentum before the ball was put in to the scrum.[141]

Scrums had become increasingly uncontested at the lower levels of the game. Thus, there was another motive for the change. Fears over scrummaging had led to a decline in the numbers playing in that position; making it safer would encourage more to play as a prop as well as defuse the concerns of parents. Perhaps of more concern, however, was a fear that any proliferation of these types of injuries and the cost of insuring against them as well as providing care for injured players could bankrupt the game. It was estimated that the potential costs of catastrophic injuries plus lifetime care for a paralysed player was £6–8 million. Hampson had been awarded £1.125 million in compensation under the RFU's insurance policy but he also required the attention of 10 carers at an annual cost to his local health authority of £250,000 a year.[142]

Reservations were expressed, however, over these rule changes. Jason Leonard, the former England prop forward commenting on the possibility of uncontested scrums, said that 'there's a danger that we'll end up with a world-wide game of tag rugby'.[143] This comment was understandable in light of the culture of rugby union. The scrum is basically a way to restart the game. However, it carries great symbolism for rugby union aficionados. The scrum is a test of strength and as such is part of the manly essence of rugby union and at the heart of the game's identity which places an emphasis on the struggle for possession. Thus, it is what makes union distinctive and, in particular, different from rugby league. There was a fear if the scrum was taken out of union it would look like league. In addition, teams also abused the new laws. For a brief period scrums in international games were uncontested if there were not enough specialist prop forwards available on both teams. As a consequence, some teams used this law change to their advantage, especially if they were being out pushed in the scrum. Overall, however, these debates, reflected on-going tensions between how sport, particularly those like rugby union, had a culture of risk and growing safety concerns based on medical evidence.

Conclusion

The ever-present threat of injury and danger has not only been something that most elite athletes have had to deal with but it has also come to occupy the minds of the sporting authorities. As a consequence, these concerns have brought together the relationship between sport and medicine on a more formal level due to the growing regulations that governing bodies have put in place. However, these regulations have also been a product of cultural and social mores. At the outset many sports were about excess and thrill-seeking and this created the ever-present danger. Attitudes to injuries, therefore, were built on notions of masculinity and manliness and any moves to regulate sport were met with resistance and the saying cum cliché that 'it's a man's game'. However, the increasing media attention given to sport throughout the twentieth century also highlighted the injuries sustained by athletes. A greater sense of duty of care was a combination of a wider welfare ethos that began to permeate sport and practical concerns, in particular, protecting the image of sport.

While the demands of competition and the changing commercial nature of sport have been the most significant elements in shaping the bodies of athletes, the framing of sporting regulations has also been important. Of course, this has not always meant that the safety of the sport has been improved. To a certain extent, the danger in some sports has shifted in emphasis. Whereas in the football codes, there was a culture of general 'roughness' there has now been a gradual erasing of the violence that takes place. Instead, violence has become more concentrated at particular times and potentially more dangerous. In rugby union, for example, more focus is given to the technique of scrummaging rather than what the commentator Bill McLaren might have said, any 'jiggery-pokery' in the scrum. Moreover, as rugby union players have got bigger the game at the professional level has become more dangerous due to the nature and force of the collisions in tackles. In American football the adoption of 'two platoon' football in 1950 reflected the nation's more scientific and rational outlook as it created defensive and offensive specialists. In a game that was inherently violent, it meant that some players were now honing skills that were specific to one function, thus increasing the risk of danger.

3

Sports Medicine

Pioneers and Specialization

Introduction

Sport mattered to doctors more than just in a medical sense. When he was Dean of St. Mary's medical school, Lord Moran (Charles Wilson) was well known for recruiting sportsmen. It was claimed that in the middle of interviews with prospective medical students Moran would bend down below his desk and retrieve a rugby ball, which he then threw at the interviewee. If the interviewee caught the ball he was admitted; if he threw it back he earned a scholarship. For Moran, who had been decorated as a medical officer in World War One and served as Churchill's doctor, sport taught character and made for good doctors.[1] This, probably apocryphal, story gives an insight into the nature of the strong sporting tradition amongst doctors from the late nineteenth century. As we have seen in Chapter 1, Victorians were preoccupied by matters of the body and doctors were inclined to promote the benefits of exercise for physical and mental health. In the nineteenth century the cult of athleticism, with its mantra of *mens sana in corpore sano*, was an important part of a public school education which many of those entering the medical profession had enjoyed.[2] It is perhaps unsurprising that many doctors wished to continue their association with sport in some form. Although the most famous sporting doctor was W.G. Grace, the sport of choice for many doctors was rugby union. Between 1871 and 1995, when the game was amateur, doctors provided 68 England internationals; the fourth largest occupational group. Rugby union was also imbued with notions of amateurism that complemented not only attitudes towards sport but also the idea of gentlemanly medicine. The London teaching hospitals had begun playing the game in the 1860s and in 1874 the United Hospitals' Cup began. The tournament rapidly became infamous for the intensity of play and the antics of its spectators, especially at the final. The clubs and cup were both an opportunity to demonstrate athletic prowess and riotous behaviour and a vehicle for the expression of corporate pride and social – i.e., middle-class – solidarity.[3]

Sports medicine has combined the professional with the personal for many doctors. The main purpose of this chapter is to show how this personal interest evolved, which in Britain culminated with the bestowal of specialist status on sport and exercise medicine in 2005. In the quest to attain specialty status, however, sports medicine (and sports medicine practitioners) were subject to a perpetual tension and debate over its scope and definition, namely the extent to which it served the needs of both elite sport or the fitness of national populations or both. Using the British experience as the main case study, this chapter looks at how doctors got involved in sport in two ways. First, how the relationship between sport and medicine was placed on a more formal relationship through the establishment of sports medicine organizations.[4] Second, the role of the football club doctor highlights how for much of the twentieth century the practice of sports medicine was mainly undertaken by practitioners who had no association with 'official' sports medicine. Instead, the position of the football club doctor owed much to the wider social and medical context in which the role of the general practitioner developed.

The story of sports medicine not only provides an insight into its development as a medical sub-discipline but it also highlights a wider process of professionalization. Harold Perkin has emphasized that a professional society is not just one dominated by professionals. Instead, professionalism permeates society from top to bottom. First, professional hierarchies extend to most occupations as they become subject to specialized training and also claim expertise beyond the common sense of the layman. Second, a professional, social ideal, based on merit, embeds itself in society. Finally, professionalization is not a neutral process contingent solely on the acquisition of knowledge because professionals also compete for economic power, political influence and social status.[5]

Moreover, medical specialisms have tended not to have had fixed definitions. Instead they have evolved, making any definition problematic. Orthopaedics, for example, at first focussed on spinal deformities on children, hence 'paedics'. Later, the rehabilitation of injured industrial workers came under its remit. During World War One there was a major expansion of orthopaedics as a specialism as it was widely used in the rehabilitation of injured soldiers who now found themselves in specialist 'fracture clinics'.[6] In the early nineteenth century specialism had actually been associated with quackery and was viewed with suspicion.[7] The transformation of a specialism into a specialty has tended to combine scientific, political, institutional and therapeutic factors. Orthopaedics elevation to specialty status in the inter-war period, for example, owed much to medical politics.[8] It also gained academic respectability as medical schools developed orthopaedic departments and specialized surgical programmes. For orthopaedics, the establishment of the Nuffield chair of orthopaedics at the University of Oxford in 1937 was particularly important from an academic perspective.[9]

Of particular importance in defining sports medicine has been its nature as a medical practice. Unlike other specialisms, sports medicine does not lay claim to particular body parts (e.g. dentistry), diseases (e.g. cancer), life events (e.g. obstetrics), age groups (geriatrics) or functions (e.g. accident and emergency). This is because, as Vanessa Heggie has argued, sports medicine is a holistic practice.[10] Rather than a specialty in which diseases are understood in terms of processes that occur at the cellular level, sports medicine has virtually no unique diseases, treatments or technologies. Instead, sports medicine covers a wide range of interests from the treatment of injuries, to 'Sport for All' – the promotion of sport and exercise for the wellbeing of the population – to the use of and testing for drugs. Definitional difficulties, therefore, stem from the fact that it is a holism, and this has been the central issue in its struggle for recognition as a medical specialty. Any definition has been further complicated because of a 'considerable overlapping of research interests and clinical practice among the different fields'. As a result, sports medics have not been restricted to qualified doctors but have also included amongst others, coaches, trainers, exercise physiologists and psychologists.[11] In addition, there has been – and probably still is – a hazy area in knowing where sports medicine ends and where sports science begins, and vice versa. For example, two pioneers in the field, Ernst Jokl and A.V. Hill, have been in receipt of different titles. Jokl, from a physical education and physiology background, has been variously called, 'a pioneer in sports medicine'[12] and the 'father of sports medicine'.[13] Hill was a Nobel-prize winning physiologist and through his research – mainly using athletes as guinea pigs – he has gained the title of a 'giant in the field of exercise physiology',[14] although his work provided the bedrock for sports science.

The rise of the medical profession

First, it would be beneficial to place the emergence of sports medicine in the history of the professionalization of medicine. Each country has a different tradition, largely framed by its prevailing political culture. While European governments allowed self-regulation of the medical profession this took two main routes. First, those countries, such as France, that exerted tight control over all aspects of social and commercial life were more likely to regulate the medical profession through a bureaucratic regulation system in which the state identifies qualified individuals. Second, where licensed practitioners have no legal monopoly a 'modified free field' exists, usually because *laissez-faire* governments take a more relaxed attitude and are likely to grant the medical profession the right to self-regulation.[15] The second route is more applicable to the UK. In America a professional monopoly arose out of a competitive individualism in which the majority of physicians remained self-employed in the private sector. Moreover, specific legislation governed the operation of physicians in each state rather than on a national basis.[16]

In Britain, from the late nineteenth century up to 1914, the medical profession moved from 'the margin to the mainstream of social life' through a growing professionalization.[17] Roy Porter has shown how 'medicine used to be atomized, a jumble of patient-doctor transactions. Practitioners were mainly self-employed … Medicine was traditionally small-scale, disaggregated, restricted and piecemeal in its operations'.[18] The seeds of professionalization were sown first through the 1815 Apothecaries Act and then, more significantly, by the 1858 Medical Registration Act. The 1858 act provided the opportunity to develop the characteristics of a modern profession, although as it has been pointed out, this was an uneven process with some doctors, especially surgeons and physicians, having more power than others i.e., general practitioners.[19] Neither, as Saks has argued, was this process of professionalization 'objectively derived from the "scientific" or "non-scientific" status of the knowledge involved'. Rather than Western science being based on objective truth, all knowledge is provisional.[20] Instead, the process of professionalization is political. Since the 1858 Medical Act the British medical profession has attempted to extend its power and control over medicine more widely through the marginalization and exclusion of what it has deemed are unorthodox and alternative practices, such as osteopathy and homeopathy.[21] The establishment of specific medical organizations and associations, therefore, has represented attempts by doctors, in particular, to ring-fence their own specialties through the imposition of entry qualifications. Once established, these specialties have the opportunity to gain state recognition and funding. Within sports medicine, however, this particular process has been complicated due to the prominent role of non-medics such as physical educators, trainers, coaches and sports scientists and the difficulty in pinning down a definition.

Gelfand has argued that one recurrent theme throughout the history of the medical profession has been the challenge in defining who is a member and who is not on the basis of three criteria: knowledge, ethics and institutional organization.[22] It has been argued 'that sports medicine is both structurally and culturally distinct from the broader medical profession', thus highlighting that any process of professionalization is not fixed and has been subject to its own peculiarities.[23] The development of sports medicine in individual countries, therefore, has been dependent on three main factors. First, the prevailing political culture and the extent of state intervention; second, the sporting tradition of each country and the extent of its commercialization; and third, the tradition of sports medicine and to what extent it has been one based on the performance of elite athletes or mass recreation for the entire population.

The institutionalization of sports medicine

Early sports medicine organizations

Definitions of and attitudes to sports medicine have differed from nation to nation and have been dependent on the prevailing political culture. In addition, for early sports medicine doctors and organizations there was a greater focus on elite athletes rather than populations. Germany played the most prominent role in the initial development of sports medicine as a medical specialism. This was a reflection of the lead Germany had taken during the nineteenth century in medical science that led to thousands of American physicians pursuing postgraduate study in the German-speaking world.[24] In 1910 Seigfried Weissbein edited *Hygiene des Sports*, based on a collection of papers presented at a conference of the same title. It included subjects such as the effects of sports activities on organ systems and first aid for common sports injuries. Four years later one of the first comprehensive works on sports injuries, *Die Sportverletzungen*, was published.[25] In 1912 the first association of sports physicians had been founded following a Congress of the Scientific Investigation of Sports held at Oberhof. Fifty doctors attended who decided to form a permanent committee for 'the scientific investigation of sports and bodily exercise'. A 'sports laboratory' was also founded at Charlottenburg near Berlin.[26]

Other continental European countries also began to put down some sports medicine roots. In 1922, for example, the French Society of Sports Medicine published the first sports medicine journal. Sports medicine societies were also founded in the Netherlands (1922), Switzerland (1923), Poland (1937) and Finland (1939). In 1920, at the University of Giessen in Germany, the Institute for the Scientific Research on Physical Exercise was inaugurated under the stewardship of Otto Huntemüller, a professor of hygiene. He was supported by Carl Diem, then the secretary-general of the Committee on Physical Exercise of Germany and a key figure behind Berlin's bid to host the 1936 Olympic Games. One of the university's aims was to create a curriculum for German gym teachers. In 1924 the German Federation of Physicians for the Support of Physical Exercise was co-founded by Huntemüller. By 1932 a sports medicine clinic had been established at Berlin's Charity Hospital under another German leader in this field, Hermann Herxheimer.[27]

State funding was an important factor – probably the most – in shaping sports medicine traditions. In this sense, like other European countries, sports medicine in Italy – in a professionalized sense – was more developed than in Britain by the 1930s. This was partly a product of how the fascist regime had embraced sport for political ends and contrasted sharply with the voluntary attitudes to sport and sports medicine in Britain. In 1929 the Medical Association of Physical Culture was founded. A year later an Italian Federation of Sports Physicians was established, under the auspices of the Italian Olympic Association (CONI) and comprised Italy's most influential sports doctors. During the 1930s the Italian Federation became very active in sport. They organized scientific and practical courses in sports medicine for general physicians as well as courses for coaches and masseurs. In addition, the holding of national conferences disseminated scientific knowledge. Two of the most influential Italian sports physicians of this era were Giancinto Viola and

Nicola Pende who developed a biometrical evaluation schedule for athletes. The first Italian institute of sports medicine had been founded in 1929 in Bologna. Between 1929 and 1931 – as a forerunner to what later happened in Eastern Europe – its sports doctors had evaluated 2,400 boys and girls as well as 342 competitive athletes to help them choose the sport most appropriate for them. In 1930 CONI established a special hospital for traumatology in Rome to provide treatment for injured sportsmen free of charge. Also in 1930, CONI approved a scheme of the doctors' federation to co-ordinate and control all medical aspects of sport in Italy. Italian sports physicians were fully integrated into the fascist state and few opposed the measure. By 1935 2,000 members had been placed in charge of medical matters within state organizations.[28] This investment became evident in the performances of Italian athletes at the 1932 Olympics, where they finished second, and at Berlin in 1936 when they finished third.

The Soviet Union experience and appropriation of sports medicine was also shaped by its political culture. Its state-run system eventually adopted a two-tier system of sports medicine. It was the first country to provide a national public health system and sports medicine through *Fizkul'tura* (see Chapter 1) became part of this health service. However, there had been no sports science heritage in Russia and it was only in 1977 that the government first used the term 'sports medicine' (*sportivnaya meditsina*).[29] Instead, as Katzer has argued, sports medicine emerged out of 'Soviet Big Science'. Under Stalin this led to the 'scientification' of all aspects of life with the human body a subject for interdisciplinary study, which combined hygiene, eugenics, biology, medicine and physiology with the planned end product 'the perfect "body Soviet"'. As an independent discipline sports medicine had its roots in this scientific context. By the time the Soviet Union entered the Olympics in 1952 it already had an integrated and highly centralized network of sports medical centres, which drew on the Ministry of Health, the Academy of Medical Science and the State Committee for Bodily Culture and Sport. Sports medicine experts were able to advise athletes and coaches across disciplines due to their scientific knowledge and were also involved in talent spotting.[30]

International sports medicine organizations

With the growth of international sport from the early twentieth century, sports medicine was also placed on a more international footing. International medical conferences had orginally focused on matters of sanitation while the formation in 1863 of the Red Cross was an early example of an international medical body. Moreover, the aftermath of the First World War created a greater desire for international co-operation. The formation of the League of Nations combined a promotion of peace with health initiatives through its subdivision, the Health Organization.[31] Unsurprisingly, the first international sports medicine organization was formed at an international gathering of athletes. The establishment of the Association Medico-Sportive Internationale (AIMS) in 1928 took place at the St. Moritz Winter Olympics, providing a forum for collaborative research within sports medicine.

At that year's Summer Games in Amsterdam, the first international AIMS Congress was held and attracted 280 physicians from 20 countries. During the 1928 Olympics, under the direction of Professor Buytendijk, a large team of international physicians and scientists undertook some 'sport-physiological research'.[32] A laboratory was provided for testing on participating athletes, leading to the collection of anthropometric, cardiovascular, X-ray and metabolic data.[33] In his report Buytendijk outlined the research's aims:

> The purpose of these investigations was to gain a better idea of the state of training of the Olympic competitors, and to trace any disadvantages which might accrue from the exercise of the more strenuous sports. It is needless to say that such investigations were not only of scientific importance, but must also be considered of the greatest significance for the sports world and the medical advisers.

AIMS was renamed the Fédération Internationale de Médecine Sportive (FIMS) five years later.[34] The organization grew rapidly and at the 1936 congress, 1,500 physicians from 40 nations attended.[35]

Following the Second World War FIMS was recognized by the International Olympic Committee in 1952. Sports medicine gained greater credibility in 1960 with recognition from both the World Health Organisation and the International Council of Sport and Physical Education of UNESCO. In 1961 an Olympic Medical Archive was set up to collect clinical and scientific information from elite athletes around the world and used for the purposes of research on health and longevity on populations as a whole. Rather than act as a qualifying body, one of FIMS's main aims has been to stimulate both research findings and the exchange of information among sports medicine practitioners and also to foster co-operation. In addition, sports medicine courses have been set up.[36] While FIMS had benefited from post-war internationalization, its influence has diminished in more recent years due to the influence of the IOC Medical Commission and the World Anti-Doping Agency (see Chapter 5) and its main function has been to organize training courses for prospective sports medicine doctors.

American sports medicine and the American College of Sports Medicine

Sports medicine in America evolved out of a different tradition compared to most European countries. Initially, both the lack of a national health system and the country's federal structure constrained a coordinated sports medicine network. The American College of Sports Medicine (ACSM) was founded in 1954.[37] Its reliance first on voluntary contributions and then commercial investments reflected the self-help culture of American civil society. In terms of medicine the ACSM owed its roots to long-standing interests from three different areas: physical education; cardiology and exercise physiology. In Europe it was doctors who led the way and largely excluded other professions from the field. But like other sports medicine practitioners, American interest in the subject was based around the idea of studying the healthy rather than the ill. Research on elite athletes, therefore, had an ulterior motive: it was used to better understand the differences in the capabilities of performance with an eye on the challenge of keeping healthy people healthy and improving the condition of the sick and injured. Because a majority of ACSM founders were members, the American Association for Health, Physical Education and Recreation (AAHPER) played an important role in shaping the future direction of American sports medicine. In America there was less emphasis on physiology and its application to work and the environment. Instead, a common focus for research was on the relationship between physical activity and its health benefits, something which had been reflected in the growing number of departments of physical education in universities. Another area of common research, which provided further impetus for sports medicine in America, concerned the fitness of soldiers. A campaign for teaching physical fitness had been prompted by the rejection of soldiers drafted for the army in the First World War, while wounded soldiers received remedial physical therapy to accelerate their recovery. During the Second World War future ACSM members played significant roles in running programmes for the rehabilitation of convalescing soldiers. Following the war the issue of fitness switched to American children who – in a Cold War climate – were less fit than their European counterparts (see Chapter 1).[38]

Before the ACSM's formation there were other organizations that had an interest in sports medicine. The National Athletic Trainer's Association (NATA) was formed in 1939.[39] The NATA was partly a product of the boom in intercollegiate athletics and a desire for coaches for greater professional representation. Due to the link with universities there was a considerable input from the physical education profession, especially regarding the treatment of injuries through physical therapy. The NATA later developed closer relations with exercise physiologists.[40]

Because of its multi-disciplinism, the ACSM had a federal structure with its three divisions – clinical, scientific and physical education – each having a degree of autonomy. Each elected their own vice-President, with the ACSM's President alternating between each group.[41] In 1962 it adopted the journal, *Sports Medicine and Physical Fitness* as its official organ while seven years later it established a new professional journal, *Medicine and Science in Sports*. In 1963 its membership was 639; by 1976 this had increased to 3,460.[42] By then physicians composed about half of its membership with the remainder made up of physical educators and sports scientists.[43] In 1960 the Secretary-General of FIMS, Guiseppe La Cava, had commented that European medics were surprised that sports medicine was relatively unknown in the USA when it was widely practiced in countries like Italy and France.[44] By 2008 it was claimed that the ACSM was the largest sports medicine and exercise science organization in the world with more than 20,000 members.[45] After attending the 2001 ACSM conference Peter McCrory, then editor of the *BJSM*, not only described it as an eye opener because of its 25 parallel sessions but he also emphasized the gap between America and the rest of the world in terms of clinical sports medicine.[46] Nevertheless, divisions still existed within sports medicine in the US as it was run by six separate and competing disciplines. In addition, it was only in 1992 that the American Board of Medical Specialties recognized a subspecialty of sports medicine in four different disciplines – family practice, paediatrics, internal medicine and emergency medicine – while it was in 2003 that a sports medicine subspecialty in orthopaedics was recognized.[47]

Sports medicine pioneers

R. Tait McKenzie

An important figure in the history of American sports medicine was actually a Canadian who served in the British Army during the First World War. Robert Tait McKenzie's (c.1870–1938) influence, however, not only linked early thinking on physical training but also provided a line through to mid-twentieth century physical educationalists. One consequence of this lineage was the prominence of the physical education tradition within early American sports medicine. McKenzie was a professor of PE at the University of Pennsylvania in Philadelphia. His approach to exercise had been shaped by the writings of Archibald Maclaren, the Swedish Ling Gymnastics system as well as the use of anthropometry and the pulley-weight machines devised by Dudley Sargent, the PE director at Harvard. McKenzie was also a sculptor who based his pieces – 'The Sprinter' (1902) and 'The Athlete' (1903) – on a perception of the 'ideal physical form', which owed much to the classical Greek tradition. Importantly, the influence of McKenzie revealed the tension in sports medicine between elite sport and physical education.[48] While he enjoyed sport – at McGill University he had played football and athletics and in 1889 he won the Wicksteed medal for best all-round gymnast – during his medical career he felt that the priority was on improving the health of the general population.

In addition to his work on PE, McKenzie made an important contribution to the rehabilitation of injured soldiers during the 1914–18 conflict while serving as a major in the Royal Army Medical Corps. McKenzie promoted a physical form of rehabilitation, which Wrynn and Mason have argued was his most lasting impact on the medical field. Physical therapies were incorporated into the overall idea of 'active exercise' such as massage and remedial baths. Group exercises included gymnastics while individual soldiers used exercise machines. Physical therapy techniques for the rehabilitation of soldiers provided an impetus for post-war physical education and physical training programmes in America. As a consequence, argues Wrynn, 'it set the stage for the emergence of a more scientific oriented training of athletes during the 1920s and 1930s'.[49]

Ernst Jokl

One of the most prominent international sports medicine (and sports science) figures was Ernst Jokl (1907–97). Jokl was not only of the eleven founders of the ACSM but he also founded UNESCO's International Council of Sport and Physical Education in 1960 (renamed the International Council of Sport Science and Physical Education in 1982). As John Bale has alluded, Jokl's career is difficult to pin down.[50] However, through his wide-range of medical interests, publications, conferences and networking, it was marked with a great energy. It also reflected the broad nature of sports medicine itself; how it was difficult to define; how the field was open to a wide-range of specialisms and the difficulties in it becoming a medical specialty. His medical interests veered from exercise physiology to neurology to physical education to aviation medicine and anthropology.

Jokl himself was born in Germany in 1907. He was a good enough athlete to be reserve for Germany in the 400 metres hurdles at the 1928 Olympics. In 1931 he was made director of the Institute of Sports Medicine – probably the first in the world – at the University of Breslau (his hometown). But after the Nazis came to power he was dismissed two years later because he was a Jew and left for South Africa. There he was responsible for starting physical education departments at both the University of Stellenbosch and Witwatersrand Technical College, and was also appointed chief research officer of the National Advisory Council of Physical Education as well as being a PE consultant for the South African Defence Force. It was during his time in South Africa (1933–52) that he came to international attention through his call for boxing to be banned (see Chapter 8).[51] In 1947 F.M. Alexander successfully sued Jokl for defamation of character. Alexander had been credited for the invention of the 'Alexander technique'; a therapy for improving posture. Jokl accused Alexander's supporters of being irrational, neurotic and mentally unstable.[52] It was the story of the struggle between orthodox and alternative medicine during the twentieth century writ large. In 1952 he moved to the University of Kentucky in Lexington as professor of neurology and sports medicine and spent the rest of his life in America. He later produced a substantial study on that year's Helsinki Olympics, which, rather than a work of science, was a geographical study of world sporting performance. Jokl also became team physician for the United States Olympic Committee.[53]

British sports medicine and the British Association of Sport and Medicine

In her highly perceptive and critically focused history, Vanessa Heggie has argued that, in terms of specialty formation, sports medicine in Britain has been 'roughly representative of that in most other countries'.[54] When sport and exercise medicine was recognized as a specialty in 2005 the UK was one of a few countries to formally do so. However, sports medicine in Britain emerged out of a different tradition compared to other nations. A number of European nations had established sports medicine organizations earlier than Britain, which was probably a product of the European tradition of bodily instruction that stemmed from the legacy of gymnastics. In Britain the games ethic predominated. While sport was seen as healthy in a general sense it also placed an emphasis on the values of character and *esprit du corps*. Moreover, physical education lagged behind other European countries. In 1933 it was noted how PE in England had relied on schools and voluntary organizations, whereas in Germany, Italy, Czechoslovakia and Russia, the state had invested heavily in the physical education of their adolescents. 'The tension between Britain's amateur tradition and the desire to emulate the continental dictatorships was one of the most important themes in PE in the 1930s', Welshman has argued.[55] Although British pioneers played an important role in its development at an international level, sports medicine at home was carried out on a largely voluntary basis. Of course, this does not mean – as Heggie points out[56] – that doctors were no less professional in their role but it does highlight how a different political culture can shape the development of a specialty. While some of its European neighbours – despite dubious motivations – benefitted from state funding, sports medicine in Britain, like sport in general, remained largely separate from the state for most of the twentieth century.

Sports medicine's specialization in Britain can be traced to the formation of the British Association of Sport and Medicine (BASM) in June 1952. An early forerunner to BASM had been the Research Board for the Correlation of Medical Science and Physical Education, which was set up in 1946. This board participated in the Congress on Physical Education during the London Olympics two years later and the actual medical committee for the Games would include future founder members of BASM, Adolphe Abrahams and Arthur Porritt (see below).[57] Both were also part of the AAA advisory medical panel established in 1950. The post-war period had also seen the formation of more specific sports injuries clinics and 'athletic advisory' services both within the NHS and privately. Coinciding with the formation of the NHS, a sports injury clinic was formed at the Middlesex Hospital in 1948.

BASM's future direction, and sports medicine as a specialty, was determined by a variety of factors. At its outset BASM's aims were ambitious: to become the authoritative body on every medical aspect of athletics and exercise; to advise on all the general principles of athletic training and sports-related medical injuries; and to conduct research into sports injuries.[58] However, compared to the input of physical education in America, in Britain the main focus was on the clinical needs of elite athletes. This outlook was mirrored in its early membership. In BASM, doctors predominated particularly those from a physical medicine and orthopaedic background. Its first executive committee could be described as patrician and paternalistic in its social make-up. While the early executive had an interest in sport, it also represented a form of 'gentlemanly medicine' through its association with elite London hospitals, which dominated the medical profession.

BASM was akin to a pressure group, part of the British voluntary tradition, which sought a voice and influence in political circles. Its original aims also highlighted how BASM aspired to act as both an umbrella and the representative organization for medicine's relationship with sport. This was illustrated in the title of BASM. Rather than 'sports medicine' it was the British Association of Sport *and* Medicine. Promoting 'sports medicine' as a specialty was probably not considered necessary, if it was considered at all. Instead, if the relationship between sport and medicine could be furthered it was to be through the professional cachet and social connections of those early members. Yet acting as an umbrella exposed a weakness that was difficult to rectify, namely that BASM has been a largely representative body rather than a regulatory one: while it could set professional standards it was unable to enforce them within the world of sport. Moreover, because the definition of sports medicine was not fixed it would eventually allow other sports medicine practitioners, particularly physiotherapists and sports scientists, to form their own associations and act in their own professional interests. Writing in 2007, John Lloyd Parry (President of BASEM, 2003–05) could still state that 'Debates about membership of sports medicine organizations continue to plague the discipline'.[59]

During the 1950s BASM operated a restrictive membership policy. It was only open to medical representatives nominated by national sporting bodies and qualified doctors with an interest in sport; scientists with a similar interest were eligible for honorary membership.[60] There were over 100 members at the time of the first AGM but this had only risen to 130 by 1959. By 1968 an increased and more egalitarian membership of 441 reflected the multi-disciplinarity and complexities of sports medicine. About 45 per cent of its members were either doctors or fellows of the royal colleges. Other groups included those from a physical education background (20 per cent) and physiotherapy (8 per cent). Women made up approximately 10 per cent of the membership. Another group – about 30 per cent – consisted of members with no definable medical background. It also contained important figures from the sporting world including the athletics coaches Geoff Dyson, Ron Pickering, Frank Dick and Wilf Paish. The England team doctors, Neil Phillips and Alan Bass, as well as the FA chairman, Andrew Stephen, who was also a GP, represented football. Former England manager Walter Winterbottom represented the Central Council of Physical Recreation (CCPR).[61]

British sports medicine pioneers

The two most high profile figures in those early days were Adolphe Abrahams (1883–1967) and Arthur Porritt (1904–94). Both would have an important influence not only on British sports medicine but also on its development worldwide. Abrahams, the son of a Lithuanian Jewish immigrant, was the brother of Harold who won the 100 metres final at the 1924 Olympics. A consulting physician, he also served in the Royal Army Medical Corps (RAMC). Adolphe was a useful runner and rower himself at university and his initial foray into sports medicine was as the first honorary doctor for a UK athletics team at the 1912 Olympics; he later acted as the medical officer (MO) at a number of Olympics. Abrahams was a prolific writer on medicine and sport, and in particular was influential in shaping attitudes towards women's sport (see Chapter 7).[62] As part of the British amateur establishment, he was as much concerned with the moral dangers of sport as its physical ones. Young men, he felt, should keep sport in perspective or they may attain 'a disproportionate sense of value' from it. Instead, except for the professionals, athletics should be 'only an incident in life'.[63]

Arthur Porritt was born in 1900, the son of a New Zealand GP. In 1923 he went to Oxford as a Rhodes Scholar to study medicine. (He returned to New Zealand as its Governor-General, 1967–72). An all-round sportsman, he competed in the 1924 Olympics where he won a bronze medal in the aforementioned 100 metres.[64] He was later a member of the IOC. Porritt enjoyed a stellar medical career. He was surgeon to the Royal Family and, uniquely, was elected President of the Royal College of Surgeons (1960–63) and the British Medical Association (1960–61) at the same time. Some of his other interests seem to fit the image of someone who was part of the upper echelons of British civil society. Not only was he the Red Cross commissioner for New Zealand in Britain but he was also a prominent freemason who was appointed Grand Master of the Grand Lodge of New Zealand. Porritt, like Abrahams, had also been part of the amateur elite that ran British sport. He was a member of the Achilles Club and was a vigorous defender of amateurism. He served on the Wolfenden Committee on Sport and despite opposition from other committee members he stated that he would refuse to sign the final report if the abolition of amateurism was recommended.[65] The amateur ethic was also reflected in his writing on training for athletics and general health, which placed an emphasis on moderation and style. In the 1920s, in combination with Douglas Lowe – another member of the amateur elite – Porritt had argued that 'athletics was a power for the good of mankind' and that 'it must be used to develop the right kind of body governed by the right kind of mind, and embodying the right kind of ideals'.[66]

The changing direction of sports medicine

During the 1970s there was a change in the direction of sports medicine for which the newly formed Sports Council acted as a catalyst. This new direction was a product of first, a leisure boom and second, wider changes in public health (see Chapter 1): the rise of a 'militant healthism'.[67] The role of exercise and a greater emphasis on individual lifestyles were given higher government priority and was exemplified by the launch of the Sport Council's 'Sport for All' campaign in 1972. There was also a change in the nature of the post-war medical profession. The idea of amateurism came under attack and medicine was less gentlemanly in that sense.[68] Not only was the profession more meritocratic due to the expansion of the National Health Service but a greater emphasis was also placed on epidemiological research and social survey that promoted a new form of public health.[69] The formation of the quasi-autonomous Sports Council in 1965[70] – a recommendation of the 1960 Wolfenden Committee Report[71] – had brought the prospect of state funding for sports medicine organizations in the UK, if only on a limited basis when compared to other European countries. The initial focus of the Sports Council's Research and Statistics Committee was elite sport. One of the first projects to receive a grant was the joint Medical Research Council/BOA project to study the effect of altitude on athletes in preparation for the 1968 Mexico City Olympics.[72] But in the following decade, in light of the new public health, greater attention was paid to the recreational athlete.

The distribution of Sports Council funding, however, in the preceding years would be caught up in a web of politics that changed the direction of sports medicine specialization, marginalizing BASM, which made it reappraise its overall purpose.[73] The role of the Institute of Sports Medicine (ISM) proved particularly problematic.[74] Formed in 1965, it had been initially intended to act as BASM's academic arm but in 1974 BASM cut its links.[75] It was claimed that because of this split the ISM was used as an excuse by the Sports Council, stretching into the late 1980s, for not recognizing BASM as 'the' representative sports medicine organization in Britain.[76]

The Sports Council's switch in emphasis materialized in the form of a network of Sports Injuries Clinics. 'Sport for All' now translated into the treatment of 'Sports Injuries for All' rather than for elite athletes. The scheme was short-lived, mainly because of the number of already existing informal clinics, but it did signal a gradual re-definition of the specialty from sports medicine to sport and exercise medicine. This had important consequences for BASM. It was intended for the clinics to be staffed by surgeons rather than sports medicine 'experts'. Of course, at this stage sports medicine was not a specialty due to its very generalized definition and, therefore, sports medicine practitioners, especially those who ran sports injury clinics, and BASM could not claim an expertise. Now, as BASM argued for sports medicine to become a formal specialty, it promoted a model of new, specialized clinics, staffed by sports medicine specialists, rather than surgeons.[77] These developments accelerated a shift towards greater recognition of not only sports medicine as a specialty but also redefined the practice. As Heggie has argued, 'Sports medicine was closing ranks; its expertise could no longer be policed and maintained by a gentleman's agreement, an understanding about expertise and experience, it now needed to be proved to outside bodies, and protected from them, with paper certificates and even licenses'.[78]

The fragmentation of sports medicine

As a consequence of this changing political context, attempts to convert sports medicine into a medical specialty became caught up in the micro-politics of BASM during the 1970s and 1980s. During the 1970s the status of sports medicine had actually been given a boost due to government legislation, which had been aimed at raising the status of the general practitioner. Although GPs made up the vast bulk of doctors, in medicine's traditionally strict tripartite structure their status was regarded as inferior to physicians and surgeons. The 1968 Todd Report and the Health Services and Public Health Act from the same year promoted the GP's role and professional status through providing and making compulsory their attendance at postgraduate courses. As many doctors had an interest in sport they chose sports medicine and in 1975 BASM organized its first residential sports medicine course at Loughborough, which was sponsored by FIMS.[79]

Despite the potential for expansion, by the late 1970s BASM experienced a serious fracture over its future direction that revolved around a dispute between two of its most important officials: John G.P. Williams and Peter Sperryn.[80] Williams felt that academic respectability for sports medicine could only come about with a strongly doctor-led organization, and he was keen for BASM to have different categories of membership.[81] Sperryn, on the other hand, sympathized with the daily grind of sports medicine practitioners, including physiotherapists.[82] He wanted BASM to retain both its multi-disciplinary identity and role as an umbrella organization.[83] By contrast, Williams was intent on establishing and maintaining high academic standards and was frustrated with practitioners who only dabbled in sports medicine and felt that they thought of BASM as principally a club for ex-sporting doctors who saw no need for a greater recognition of sports medicine.[84] Sports medicine also began to attract sponsorship, especially from pharmaceutical companies, which increased the commercial possibilities within the discipline. As a result, different medical philosophies within BASM began to emerge with some who believed that only the overuse injuries of Olympic athletes were sports injuries whereas those who treated injuries sustained in contact sport felt that these should be given a higher priority.[85]

These developments provided the background to the formation of the British Association of Trauma in Sport (BATS) in 1980. It was a splinter group within BASM that reflected the growing frustrations of doctors who wanted to push harder for the recognition of sports medicine as a specialty. Like BATS, other splinter groups and disciplines had begun to form their own representative bodies outside the BASM umbrella.[86] The formation of the Association of Chartered Physiotherapists in Sports Medicine (ACPSM) – affiliated to the Chartered Society of Physiotherapists – in 1972 had signaled the first real split in BASM's attempts to remain as the umbrella organization for sports medicine. Although many would be both members of BASM and the new organization, this society was concerned with the professional credentials of physiotherapists who had only been accepted on the NHS in 1960.

In addition to pressures from the doctors, sports science was gaining an increasing influence within sports politics and further weakened BASM's central role in sports medicine. Sports science articles had made up a considerable proportion of those published in the *British Journal of Sports Medicine* (BJSM). In 1977 and 1984 there were unsuccessful attempts to change BASM's name to the 'British Association of Sports Science and Medicine' to reflect 'the changing nature of sports medicine towards a wider base than clinical medicine' to make it 'representative of wider interests than purely clinical ones'.[87] In 1984 the sports scientists went their own way and formed the British Association of Sports Sciences.[88] Later, in 1987 the British Olympic Medical Centre, the first sports science and sports medicine facility in the UK, was opened near Harrow. It catered for elite athletes and was founded by Mark Harries and Craig Sharp who had been a member and on the committee of BASM but described himself as a founder of UK sports science.[89] While there was much collaboration between medics and scientists within sport, this charitable trust of the British Olympic Association marked another significant moment in the development of sports science as a specialty in itself, and further diminished BASM's position.[90] Moreover, while the original idea of BASM had been to supply a pool of specialists for elite sport under its aegis, the reality was that elite athletes tended to look for their own solutions and treatments with some using alternative medicine (see Chapter 6). Partly because of this stagnation, BASM's membership fell. In 1984 BASM's membership had numbered 1,375 with doctors making up 47 per cent (644)[91] but dropped to around 800 by 1987.[92]

From sports medicine to sport and exercise medicine

In 1998, following a series of educational initiatives, an Intercollegiate Academic Board of Sport and Exercise Medicine (IABSEM) was established. This set in chain the process of specialty formation, which led to the approval of specialty status for sport and exercise medicine (SEM) by the Department of Health in 2005. In addition, not only was SEM to treat injuries of those who undertook physical activity but stress was also placed on injury prevention and encouraging the wellbeing of the general populace through exercise and physical activity.[93] In anticipation of the change in sports medicine's direction, BASM changed its name to the British Association of Sport and Exercise Medicine (BASEM) in 1999.[94] Despite the struggles within BASM, there had been a growing demand amongst doctors for sports medicine qualifications. This need also complemented the boom in the leisure and fitness industry and the growing sales in sports medicine products such as sprays and bandages.

Moreover, the Government was paying ever-closer attention to wider trends in public health, especially obesity, and the virtues of physical activity. As Zweiniger-Bargielowska has shown, these anxieties were not new and had existed since the 1890s when the sedentary lifestyles of the middle classes was cited as a cause for expanding waistlines.[95] Over one hundred years later, a report, *Forecasting Obesity to 2010*, predicted an obesity epidemic.[96] In 2006 the Parliamentary Health Select Committee estimated that the full cost of obesity and overweight people to the NHS was £7 billion per year.[97] Set against this increasing awareness of obesity, there has been a trend against participation in sport.[98]

An early qualification in sports medicine had been the London Hospital diploma established in 1981. Many of the GPs who took this diploma then went on to undertake other courses. These included the Society of Apothecaries' diploma in sports medicine, which was established in 1989. Another diploma was offered by the Scottish Royal Colleges Board for Sports Medicine. This board had been set up in 1986 mainly through the efforts of Donald McLeod (President of BASM/BASEM, 1995–2002) and gave the discipline greater credibility.[99] At first these courses only catered for a relatively small number of sports medicine specialists. Higher degrees in sports medicine later became available at Nottingham and Glasgow. In 1994 the Royal Society of Medicine's sports medicine section was established with Roger Bannister as the first president. By 2005 there were eight Master degrees being offered in sport and exercise medicine. Educational developments led to the emergence of two distinct groups: first, those practitioners working in the NHS and who had an interest in sports medicine; and second, those, especially doctors, who worked privately in sports medicine, had their own clinics and whose sole source of income was the discipline. Accompanying BASM's name change to incorporate exercise medicine, there were also changes in membership regulations. Now only doctors could have full membership rights while, unless they were already full members, those from the allied professions were offered only associate membership whereas previously they had enjoyed equal rights with doctors.[100]

Despite the membership changes in favour of doctors there continued to be tensions amongst this group. In 2001 there were 760 members of BASEM with 517 doctors (approximately 65 per cent of the membership), physiotherapists numbered 123 (16 per cent) with the rest comprising sports scientists, chiropodists, educators, osteopaths (who had been banned 30 years previously), dental and veterinary surgeons and students.[101] For those sports medicine doctors working in the private sector, the lack of specialist recognition caused problems over insurance. Because of government legislation, to qualify as a consultant a new specialist qualification – Certificates of Completion of Specialist Training (CCSTs) – had been introduced as a mandatory requirement from 1997. Insurance companies, like BUPA and PPP, now required that doctors work six years full-time to gain this recognition (or ten years part-time). Norwich Union would not accept anyone working in sports medicine or in musculoskeletal medicine, which threatened the financial future of those working in this area.[102]

The medical care of elite athletes was now firmly the responsibility of the governing bodies of sport and backed up by UK Sport. In this sense, BASEM had little input bar its representation on various committees. With a growing emphasis on promoting exercise for the population, the change to 'sport and exercise medicine' seemed inevitable. The scientific scope of sports medicine was also changing and now extended to other specialties such as cardiology, respiratory medicine, gynaecology, rheumatology and neurology. Moreover, there were growing calls for the use of evidence-based medicine in research to further improve the status of sports medicine within the medical profession as well as with sporting bodies.[103] Nevertheless, the shift towards sport and exercise medicine had marked how sports medicine had evolved from a largely voluntary activity pursued by doctors who had an interest in sport to a specialty that was now under state control with a clear career path for highly trained professionals.

Sports medicine practitioner: the football club doctor

Some of the first sports medicine practitioners were football club doctors.[104] Doctors and others such as coaches, trainers and physiotherapists (see Chapter 6) were practicing sports medicine long before attempts were made to specialize the practice. Most of these practitioners did not contribute directly to this process. Instead, the role of the club doctor in British football highlights how much of sports medicine has developed outside of any institutional framework.

The role of the football club doctor emerged from a culture of voluntarism that was a feature of Victorian society. Most football doctors were general practitioners (GPs). After the 1858 Medical Act they found that their role had been diminished within orthodox medicine's tripartite division of physicians, surgeons and GPs.[105] It reflected more generally how the middle classes were not a monolithic entity but subject to fragmentation. During the first half of the nineteenth century GPs (aka apothecaries) had been denigrated for their association with the drug trade and their low social origins.[106] Moreover, it seems that the economic struggle associated with general practice meant that many GPs were themselves in poor health during the nineteenth century.[107] Doctors though shared a growing middle-class propensity for joining associations, and becoming a football club medical officer was part of this urban civic process.

The process leading to the appointment of football club doctors has traditionally been informal and held little financial reward. For some doctors sport raised medical questions and interest. Following a head injury playing rugby, Neil Phillips questioned why his neurosurgeon forbade him from ever playing the game again when some years afterwards he started to play once more.[108] Ian Adams developed an interest in soft tissue injuries during his national service in the Paratroops because of the similar type of injuries sustained in both sport and parachute jumping.[109] Many clubs enjoyed long-term associations with their doctors as well as a particular practice. For some doctors the job held the potential for social climbing. Andrew Stephen, a Scot, became a club doctor at his local club, Sheffield Wednesday, just after the war when the senior partner in his practice, and the club's previous MO, had been made a club director. In 1949 Stephen himself became a club director and in 1955 its chairman. He claimed that he had 'drifted into football rather by accident than by intention' but subsequently became chairman of the FA (1967–73).[110]

From the 1960s there was a gradual change in the role of the football club doctor due to attempts to improve medical care within football. In 1961–62 the Football Association held a series of regional conferences of Football League club doctors. It culminated in a brief report that included some recommendations for future practice. Furthermore, in 1963 Alan Bass was appointed the first team doctor for the England national team, and medical appointments were made at under-23 and youth team level. Meetings of club doctors also took place but little seems to have come from them. In 1976 it was commented that the FA had 'little control of the medical credentials of those who move to the aid of most players injured on football pitches',[111] and, as we have seen in the previous chapter, it was not until 1980 that the FA had established a medical committee. While doctors were professionals with a general background in medicine, there was little or no systematic training for this position. Both Stuart Carne of Queen's Park Rangers and Barrie Smith of Aston Villa commented that 'by and large one learns on the job'.[112]

The demands of the job differed from club to club. Most of the early club doctor's work took place during the week. West Bromwich Albion's Issac Pitt, for example, would usually hold a weekly clinic with injured players, report their state of fitness to the board and sometimes accompany them on visits to specialists.[113] One doctor currently working part-time for a medium-sized Midlands' club is present at the training ground for two hours 3–4 times per week, plus 'as and when needed'.[114] He would also cover all home games for the first team and the reserves. Moreover, as very few medical officers traveled to away games the home team doctor would deal with the medical problems of both teams.[115] During the 1970s Leeds United's doctor, Ian Adams, would go in five days a week for about 45 minutes. In addition to covering all first and second team games, he traveled with the team for European games. He was only able to do this, he said, because he had very understanding practice partners.[116] During the period they shared the job at Aston Villa, David Targett and Barrie Smith had busy full-time jobs in general and hospital practice respectively. It was not possible for both to attend the training ground on a regular basis and so they split the responsibility.[117] It has been a complaint by some doctors who have an honorary position that clubs have still demanded 24-hour attention. The few club doctors employed on a full-time basis are on call around the clock; they travel everywhere with the team and attend all the matches.[118]

For much of the time the job, even on match days, was relatively routine. Stuart Carne has described how he and other medical practitioners would sometimes discuss local medical politics during dull games.[119] At times, however, it could be uncomfortable. John Rowlands, a GP from Formby, said that on one of the few occasions he deputized as a club doctor – it was a legal requirement post-Hillsborough for a doctor to be in attendance two hours before kick-off otherwise the match could not proceed – he 'just didn't feel on top of the situation'. For one match at Macclesfield (where Chester City then played) there was a spate of major injuries; a broken ankle, a broken cheekbone and a player split his head open requiring stitches. At his next match there he was faced with the potential of a major crush in the crowd, and 'felt that the whole thing was not right, and not organized, and a disaster waiting to happen'. Rowlands had made a round trip of 160 miles, used up his half-day off, the club had denied him a free ticket for a friend, and then offered him a paltry £5 for expenses.[120]

In 1989 the FA established a Medical Education Centre, located at Lilleshall in Shropshire.[121] According to its head, Alan Hodson, there remained resistance to the development of sports medicine in British football when compared to foreign competitors.[122] Nevertheless, from 1990 the FA began to run sports medicine conferences. One was organized with the Royal College of Surgeons in Edinburgh, comprising surgeons, doctors and physiotherapists. Another two annual meetings were directed at those specifically in football.[123] After the Hillsborough Disaster in 1989 the FA also ran courses for crowd doctors. A number of club doctors, such as Mike Stone at Manchester United and Arsenal's John Crane, gained the sports medicine diploma through the Scottish colleges, highlighting the growing specialization of the role.

It is likely that more football clubs will appoint doctors on a full-time basis. Moreover, the threat of litigation will perhaps force football club doctors to obtain a sports medicine qualification in future as medical defence unions may have issues about supporting them if they do not.[124] Nevertheless, the professional soccer market for sports medicine qualified doctors remains a very narrow one. A few doctors have combined work as a club MO with running sports injury clinics available to the general public.[125] However, it is unlikely that most GPs would give up their lucrative practices to specialize.[126]

Conclusion

The development of sports medicine, as a specialism, over the twentieth century can also point to wider trends within medicine, health and the role of the state. First, the demand for sports medical services has been largely commensurate with both the intensification and internationalization of sporting competition. Whether for commercial reward or national prestige, sports medicine was regarded as a vital component to achieving these goals. Second, sports medicine's growth was also a product of the spread of welfarist ideas concerning public health. Physical education gained a greater importance and exercise was seen as a cheap form of preventive medicine. Third, partly because of this growing demand, the function of sports medicine was constantly redefined. Not unlike how other specialisms have developed, particularly in Britain, sports medicine was subject to medical politics that altered its original purpose. While sports science took care of the performance of elite athletes, recreational athletes became the responsibility for sports medicine in the shape of sport and exercise medicine. This scenario, where the elite-recreational athlete split was devolved, to a certain extent, was played out in most countries albeit subject to a different political culture. Because of its constantly changing nature, it further underlines Heggie's argument that sports medicine is a holistic practice. Finally, the growth of sports medicine also reflected the growth in the consumerism of medicine, especially in America where 'fitness' has become a cult and a business.[127] This in itself has highlighted prevailing discourse, and its construction, around the whole question of health. As Roy Porter argued, immense pressures had been created by a combination of interested parties – the medical profession, medi-business, the media and the advertising of pharmaceutical companies – and as a consequence, doctors and patients become locked into a scenario where everyone has something wrong with them.[128]

4

Science and the Making of
the Athletic Body

Introduction

At the 1960 Rome Olympics Britain's Don Thompson won gold in the
50 kilometres walk. Nicknamed *Il Topolino* (The Little Mouse) by the
Italian press, Thompson's victory was proclaimed heroic and 'plucky' in a
quintessentially British way. His preparation had been unconventional to say
the least. Thompson, who was an insurance clerk, had collapsed in the heat at
the Melbourne Games in 1956 and in order to prepare himself for the humidity
of Rome he created a steam-room effect in his bathroom using kettles and
heaters, and walking up and down continuously on the bathmat.[1] His feat
though was set against the growing rivalry in international sport between
America and the USSR where greater resources in terms of coaching and
sports science were being dedicated to the preparation of their athletes for the
Olympic arena. By contrast, Thompson's preparation reflected British sport's
amateur tradition.

This chapter charts the evolution of athletes' training methods since the
early nineteenth century. At the root of this process has been an on-going
tension in the relationship between coaching and science. The relationship
between sport and science rather than a story of unhindered scientific
progress has been a process shaped by its prevailing social and cultural
contexts. Roy Porter has pointed out, because of a two-way cultural traffic
in knowledge, much of modern scientific medicine owes its foundations
to traditions that have been described as folk, popular or rural in origin.[2]
Tensions between coaching and science, therefore, need to be placed in
the context of not only scientific developments but also changes in the
sporting world. In addition, the development of training methods reflects
the recurring issue over the definition of sports medicine itself; in other
words, where does medicine stop and science begin? Track and field athletics
is used as the main case study because it has been this sport more than
others where the relationship between sport and medical science has been
not only the closest but also has had the most dramatic effect on athletic
performance.

Early trainers and coaches

Ideas on what constituted the athletic (or sporting) body had begun to take shape in the late eighteenth century. The gambling on sports such as prize-fighting and pedestrianism generated not only a competitive impulse but also a greater demand to improve the performance of athletes through more systematic training regimes. To begin with, instead of scientists, it was the coaches and trainers[3] of prize-fighters, pedestrians and rowers from the late eighteenth and early nineteenth century who were first practitioners of bodily instruction. Coaching itself is a process of 'knowledge transfer' but one subject to its own cultural and social context. Coaches and trainers have acted as 'gatekeepers' by exercising a large influence over their sports both socially and in sporting terms. Through their attitudes to coaching, which have been moulded by their own experiences, coaches have transmitted values as well as knowledge to athletes, and shaped the way that sports have been played. Although many early coaches/trainers were poorly educated they were also autodidacts and to a certain extent scientists in their own right. Their training theories were empirically-based deriving from observation, experience and an oral tradition where they learnt by 'stealing with the eyes'. Coaches formed their own communities of practice where information was only passed on within tight social networks and was not chronicled for fear of rival coaches gaining an advantage.[4]

Two of the earliest books on athletics training included John Sinclair's *Results of the Enquiries Regarding Athletic Exercises* (1807) and Walter Thom's *Pedestrianism*, published in 1813. From his investigations Sinclair concluded that there was little difference in the training of horses, fighting cocks, pugilists, greyhounds and runners.[5] Galenic humoural theory (see Chapter 1) formed the basis for the training regimes of early modern athletes. Medical treatment, therefore, was through either changing the lifestyle of the patient or by restoring the humoural balance.[6] Trainers had two main aims. The first was to achieve this balance in the body by removing impediments through a programme of diet and exercise. Thus, at the start of training athletes first would have their body cleansed of gross humours through the standard means of purging, vomiting and bleeding.[7] This cleansing could involve the taking of three purgatives, such as Glauber's salt, over a four-day period as well as any other emetics thought appropriate.[8] The second main aim was to improve the wind, i.e., stamina, of athletes through exercise, which mainly consisted of walking or running. Any additional sweating, purging or even bleeding was undertaken when deemed necessary.[9]

The most famous pedestrian of the early 19th century was Captain Robert Barclay who, for a substantial bet, walked 1000 miles in 1000 hours on Newmarket Heath in the summer of 1809. A Yorkshire farmer, Jackey Smith, who it was claimed was 'very knowing in all sporting science', supervised his daily regime, which lasted for three to four weeks.[10] Smith controlled Barclay's sleep patterns and woke him up at 4am to move him from his bed to a hammock as it was felt that this would loosen his muscles ready for training. His day began with the taking of emetics to purge the body of toxins. Running started at 6am with Barclay wearing layers of clothes including two pairs of breeches, which were designed to make him sweat. A massage followed and then a rest in a heated bed. His sweat would be replaced by a tankard of strong malt liquor followed by an hour of relaxed walking in warm dry clothing. In the afternoon there was more running, including sprinting uphill. He ate a high-protein diet that consisted of undercooked beef, mutton and raw eggs. During the challenge itself Barclay was assisted by a medical attendant, William Cross, who was responsible for treating injuries and perhaps more importantly ensured he didn't fall asleep before or during the walk.[11] Barclay himself turned trainer and used similar methods in preparing the pugilist Tom Cribb for his fight against the former American slave, Tom Molineaux, in 1811. Tom McNab has argued that Barclay's methods lingered on well into the twentieth century in many sports.[12]

Early 'scientific' training 1870–1914

During the final quarter of the nineteenth century there was a growing reaction against the training methods of Barclay. From around 1870 onwards the term 'scientific training' was gradually used to refer to the training of athletes. However, this was a reference to regular and systematic preparation rather than biomedical science. Instead 'most training methods continued to rely heavily upon the accumulated experience of successful athletes and trainers'.[13] These changing attitudes to the training of athletes had been buttressed by the emergence of scientific (or Western) medicine during the nineteenth century.[14]

Since the Renaissance period rational theories of the body began to challenge and replace Galenic-based ideas. With the discovery by William Harvey (1578–1657) of the circulation of blood, hydraulic models of the body emerged. In the seventeenth century Rene Descartes (1596–1650) argued that the human body was a machine operating according to mechanical laws and principles while the soul operated autonomously. Previously, Galenic ideas of the body had viewed the attainment of health holistically. Now Cartesian dualism saw the body as being no longer determined by 'virtues' of mysterious *vires* but instead by technical concepts such as motion, size and temperature. The professionalization of science during the nineteenth century created an institutional framework for the spread of scientific ideas. Western medicine established a reductionist approach in which the examination of bodies and their diseases were localized and analysed into ever-smaller parts. This reductionist approach led to the employment of machine models of the body that integrated anatomy, mechanics, physiology and psychology into the study of human sporting performance.[15] The invention of medical instruments, such as the microscope, enabled physiological researchers to analyse changes in the pressure and flow of body fluids, to measure changes in body temperature, isolate and stimulate tissues and glands. This allowed investigation of bodily functions and to explore the chemical and nervous pathways by which the body's functions co-ordinated.[16] Through further developments in physiology, such as the work of Claude Bernard on metabolism, the body was seen as a self-regulating mechanism that needed to be kept in good running order by exercise and diet.[17] From a scientific point of view it became more acceptable for athletes to work their bodies harder and to push themselves to the limit. Sport and especially track and field athletics provided ideal material for scientists interested in bodily functions and movements.[18] However, as with most theories, there was a lag before new ideas were put into practice.

Scientists were originally more interested in studying athletes for the purposes of physiology generally rather than consciously attempting to boost their performance. As Cronin points out, up to 1914 the worlds of sport and medicine saw little value in engaging with the other. A few scientists were interested in athletes but only as subjects for medical research.[19] Phillipe Tissié, for example, was interested in the physiological impact on the body of a French cyclist in his (failed) attempt to break the record for the 24-hour distance event in 1893.[20] In 1906 a Dutchman, Van den Berg, also examined the effect of cycling on the heart.[21] Other pioneers included Etienne-Jules Marey (1830–1904) who through contemporary photographic technology developed an interest in the biomechanics of sport.[22]

Scientific experiments were generally of an *ad hoc* nature. There was no critical mass of scientific knowledge and medical debates continued over the amount of stress that physical activity could place on the body. Tissié, for example, reflecting contemporary attitudes, actually opposed competitive sports due to their apparent 'medical dangers'. Of particular concern among scientists was the condition commonly referred to as 'Athlete's Heart'. Because of its vital function, debate continued over the consequences of competitive sport on the heart throughout the twentieth century.[23] 'Athlete's Heart' first became associated with sport following the 1867 university boat race between Oxford and Cambridge. Writing in *The Times*, the physician, F.C. Skey, denounced the competitive nature of such contests and their consequences for the body.[24] By the 1980s, however, the Athlete's Heart had become 'normalized'. While the enlarged Victorian Athlete's Heart was regarded as pathological and unhealthy, it was now seen as fit and physiologically adaptable.[25]

Of perhaps more long-term importance to the relationship between athletics and science was the development of anthropometry. During the Victorian era there was an increasing obsession with measuring body parts and body types, and in particular to identify the 'normal body'. This 'normalcy' through the application of anthropometric techniques aimed to determine the 'athletic body' through physiognomic schemes.[26] These ideas had their roots in early nineteenth-century theories about heredity and breeding, which were used in horse racing and cock fighting. However, with the emergence of eugenics and racial theories they were now given a greater scientific platform. A leading proponent in America was Dudley Sargent, Harvard University's director of PE. He had instituted a programme of exercises, known as the 'Sargent System', based on a dynamometer and lung capacity tests.[27]

The growing literature on physical culture produced by the likes of Sandow and Müller provided ideas for bodily instruction through weight-training and exercise programmes plus advice on diet and lifestyle as well as providing visual representations of ideal body types.[28] In 1901 another prominent physical culturalist, Eustace Miles, in conjunction with F.A. Schmidt, wrote *The Training of the Body*, which was more of a coaching manual. It analysed mechanical movements of athletes in activities as diverse as bowling and climbing. Miles was also a champion rackets player and had added information derived from his own experiences.[29] The muscular ideal mainly promoted by Sandow still remained central to physical culture but others as well as doctors advocated a less muscular physique, and this advice spilled over into sport. The male body was now of neo-classical proportions, which balanced height, weight, muscle development and mobility. The ideal athlete, therefore, was neither too tall nor too small, too thin nor too fat.[30] At the same time, and seemingly running in contradiction to the growing scientific evidence, there was a growing emphasis on moderation regarding training and competition. But this reflected 'an evolving amateur attitude amongst doctors which saw "staleness" as the physical manifestation' of an unhealthy obsession with sport and placing too great an importance on winning.[31] These doctors adopted the aphorism, 'Athletics for health is safe. Athletics for prowess and superiority may be dangerous.'[32] Staleness amongst athletes, its causes and the quest to cure it, would continued to be a topic of debate deep into the twentieth century.

In light of the emergence of scientific medicine and new ideas regarding the body, unsurprisingly, there was much criticism of old-style trainers. In particular their use of purgatives and other home-made concoctions, which were originally thought to prevent the 'staleness' of athletes through over-training.[33] Archibald Maclaren's *Training in Theory and Practice* (1866) made this particular point. As well as physical education, Maclaren also had a background in medicine.[34] For him, rather than excessive exercise, and ultimately injury, it was purging, vomiting, the denial of liquids and eating semi-raw meat that led to athletes 'training off'. Maclaren further argued against the use of heavy clothing to reduce weight through perspiration. Basing his argument on physiological knowledge, he argued that this would not affect fatty tissue as changes in the tissues were dependent upon changes in respiration and circulation.[35] Maclaren was also interested in different body shapes, reflecting the Victorian fascination with the ideal of the symmetrically appropriate body.[36]

The Lupton brothers made a strong case for athletics to develop links with the medical profession and also criticized the traditional methods of trainers.

> These antiquated ideas are not fossilized yet: men exist who prescribe raw meat as food and withhold drink from parched lips; who reduce the body 'to get off substance' far below its natural weight. By these means weakness not strength is induced; the man so trained cannot win.[37]

While acknowledging the skills of professional coaches and trainers, the Lupton brothers also bemoaned the lack of orthodox medical input. They admitted that the surgeon lacked the practical knowledge of training that professional coaches possessed but it was hoped that 'if the science of the one could be blended with the practical experience of the other in one individual, we should then be able to give the world assurance of a trainer'. In addition, 'Medical students might with advantage educate themselves to this end, and in a very short time the athletic world would possess men capable of giving practical and scientific advice and training quarters'.[38] However, there was little cross-over between professional coaches and trainers who continued to rely on traditional methods and the growing number of doctors who had played sport at public school and university and were imbued with different sporting values. Professional coaches and trainers continued to rely on their own 'eye' and tacit judgement. Their knowledge base was wide and included an eclectic range of sources such as medical science, physical educators, animal trainers, circus performers, newspapers, sporting journals and magazines. Because they heavily favoured empiricism to experimental science, coaches felt that, rather than anthropometric techniques, each individual had their own complex psychological make-up and that this was just as important in assessing the potential of athletes.[39]

Some athletes also had their own individual training programmes with little input from coaches. Walter George, who set a world record for the mile in 1886 that lasted for nearly 30 years, was famous for his 'hundred up exercise' where he would chalk a line on the floor in the pharmacy where he worked and prance on the spot, lifting his knees high.[40] Later, George's training was based on running every morning and afternoon where he mixed up his regime. He alternated slow runs of one to two miles with faster stretches of 400 to 1,200 yards with a series of short sprints.[41] While George had turned professional to race, Arnold Strode-Jackson, winner of the 1,500 metres at the 1912 Olympics, embodied the British amateur ethos. Educated at a public school and then Oxford, his approach to training was casual, consisting mainly of massage, golf and walking. However, he had an abundance of natural talent.[42]

Successful British coaches by the early twentieth century included Sam Mussabini and Harry Andrews whose methods were largely based on their own observations. Andrews was renowned for training professional runners like Alf Shrubb who at one time held every world record from 2 to 10 miles. Like many trainers he promoted the virtues of walking. For training for the longer distances, he advocated that runners wore plenty of clothing to lose fat.[43] Mussabini coached Olympic champions like Reggie Walker (South Africa), Harold Abrahams, both in the 100 metres, and Albert Hill, who won the 800 metres and 1,500 metres in 1920. Another Mussabini athlete, Willie Applegarth, won a gold in the 4 × 100 metres relay in 1912. In addition to the preparation of athletes, Mussabini was very interested in the biomechanics of running and used slow motion film and photographic sequences to study athletes in action. He was also interested in the stride length of sprinters especially their arm swing and various phases of the sprint race, and he recognized through trial and error that sprinters decelerated during the race.[44] Both also believed that athletes needed a good constitution with a strong stomach and sound digestive organs. For constipation, for example, Mussabini recommended one of his home-made laxatives called 'Black Jack'.[45] Both Andrews and Mussabini were also strong advocates of the use of massage for runners as well as an adherence to hygiene.[46] However, they were also alive to modern developments. Andrews, for example, was not averse to administering drugs like strychnine to his athletes, albeit in exceptional circumstances.[47]

International sport and the rise of coaching

Although Britain had been the pioneer, from the late nineteenth century modern sport began to take on an international dimension. Football was being exported to Europe and South America while cricket and rugby were played in the British Empire. America, through professional baseball and inter-collegiate sporting competition, was establishing its own particular sporting culture as was Australia. In addition, there was growing competition between Britain and America in sports such as athletics, swimming, rowing and cycling. Moreover, the inauguration of the Modern Olympics in 1896 provided a platform for national pride and from 1908 they were increasingly fuelled by nationalism. As a consequence, national sporting performance became an important indicator of a nation's health. With this growth in competition, there was a greater demand for athletes to have the best possible preparation for the Games.

International sport began to unravel British amateur attitudes towards coaching. Fears over the perceived consequences of any sporting decline can be traced back to at least the 1906 Intercalated games in Athens where blame was pointed at the lack of organization for British athletes. This had contrasted sharply with the more systematic approach of the Americans and Scandinavian countries.[48] After the 1908 Olympics, where the American team had won thirteen out of the twenty-three track and field events, it was commented that the British were amateurs and had to be more 'business-like' like the Americans who were regarded as professionals.[49]

Following a disappointing performance in Stockholm in 1912, further questions were raised about Britain's lack of coaching expertise and preparation in comparison to other nations. The hosts, for example, had appointed Ernie Hjertberg as its chief athletics trainer. A Swede by birth, he had lived in America for forty years coaching in universities and private athletic clubs. For the Stockholm games he had organized the training and selection procedure for Swedish athletes in 1911.[50] The British response was to put a national scheme of coaching in place, highlighting a shift away from 'pure' amateurism towards a greater emphasis on the pursuit of excellence. In addition, a Canadian, William Knox was appointed as national athletics coach. He was well known on the (professional) Highland Games circuit and specialized in field events. The preparations for the 1916 Berlin Olympics were linked to anxieties over Britain's sporting prestige, racial hygiene, social Darwinism and Britain's place in the world order.[51] Germany itself had been given an incentive to improve its sporting performance when Berlin was awarded the Games. In addition, up to 1914, Germany had been the leader in experimental physiology, partly because of the amount of testing taking place on its soldiers. In Britain there was a fear that their scientific discoveries would be applied to German athletes.[52]

It was in America though where the greatest developments in coaching were being made. Here coaching had flourished under the collegiate system through the likes of Walter Camp, Clyde Littlefield and Brutus Hamilton.[53] Inter-varsity competition provided a structured and highly competitive sporting environment that fostered a large pool of athletic talent and created a demand for coaches. Importantly, these educational institutions became sites for experiments and the advancement of coaching knowledge and practices. American coaches adopted a more specialized and systematic approach to coaching that reflected more generally the growing influence in America of F.W. Taylor's ideas on 'scientific management'.

Walter Camp, recognized as the 'father of American football', also explained American football in terms of rational efficiency. Influential in writing (and re-writing) the laws of the game between 1878 and 1925, he was also the (unofficial) coach of Yale for twenty-five years and the 'leading foot-ball expert in the country'. For Camp, American football was a game of tactics and leadership and this notion was passed on to other sports like baseball and basketball. As a result, in American sports the emphasis on the coach orchestrating games from the sidelines has offered a striking comparison to sport in other countries.[54] The importance placed on the coach in American sport was in direct contrast to attitudes to coaching in Britain.

On Roger Bannister's lack of a coach, J. Kenneth Doherty commented that (half tongue-in-cheek):

> To an American this is heresy. No coach to make decisions, to seek aid for financial problems ... No coach ... to influence the faculty in shifting exam schedules, to suggest that the girl friend might well stay until after the big race is over ... No coach to scare away the heebie-jeebies of doubt and fear by quoting medical authorities that "physical activity", no matter how strenuous, cannot harm a healthy heart or other vital organs of the body.[55]

By contrast, the strong strain of anti-coaching in Britain was summed up by Ronald Kittermaster, headmaster of King's School in Worcester. He believed that:

> The training of athletic champions for national or international sport is entirely foreign to the British educational-athletic tradition ... The view that the object of all sport should be competition ... is an un-British and anti-educational view, a denial of all that is best in sport.[56]

While there is more than a little amateur myth-making to this statement, it does give an indication about the different attitudes towards coaching in different countries, and hence the relationship between sport and science.

Before 1914 the pre-eminent American athletics coach was Michael Murphy who was credited with the invention of the crouch start for sprinters. Selected to coach the American Olympic teams in 1908 and 1912, he had previously worked at a number of clubs and was also coach at the University of Pennsylvania. Although Murphy had undergone some medical training and was a friend of R. Tait McKenzie, his methods were based on his own observations rather than any experimental studies. His attitudes to physical conditioning, for example, placed an emphasis on cleanliness, deep-breathing, at least eight hours sleep, bathing, massage and simple calisthenics. In addition, he stressed that athletes should not over-train.[57] Dean Cromwell (1879–1962) was another eminent American coach. He coached ten Olympic champions, including Charley Paddock in the 100 metres in 1920. Although he was dismissive about the myth over the athlete's heart, his training motto was about 'moderation' as he did not want his charges to overextend themselves in training.[58]

Science and sport in the inter-war period

During the inter-war period a greater rational-scientific approach to sport emerged. A 'paradigm shift' took place in the scientific understanding of the training of athletes and a scientific body of knowledge was built concerning human physiology through recorded observations related to exercise, human anatomy and physiology.[59] Cronin has identified the period from the 1920s as one when medicine begins to use sportsmen as guinea pigs to determine what a healthy body was and to develop theories of athletes as distinct and special.[60] Nevertheless, there was still a considerable lag between the discovery of this new science and its application in elite sport. While the twenties and thirties were important decades in the development of sports medicine through a greater physiological understanding of athletes' bodies, practice was and continues to be ahead of theory. Arnd Kruger has argued that even as late as 1979 'the practice of training was still ahead of theory'.[61]

The two leading nations regarding this relationship between science and the training of athletes were America and Germany who established the foundations for the discipline of exercise physiology.[62] Following the 1924 Olympics, scientific studies were published by a number of American scientists that used athletes as subjects. These included the successful eights crew at the 1920 and 1924 Olympics where Yale University physiologists set out to measure 'the maximum that the human engine can attain in any form of exertion'. Tests included measurements of rowers' mechanical efficiency whilst on the water and oxygen consumption through the 'Douglas Bag' while the crew rowed on an indoor rowing machine. From their results they claimed that a man could use fat as the exclusive fuel for intense exertion.[63] As we have seen in Chapter 3, the 1928 Olympics provided the first opportunity for doctors and physiologists to undertake anthropometrical and cardiological tests on competitors – mainly runners and sprinters.

A significant event in the history of sports science was the establishment of Harvard University's Fatigue Laboratory in 1927. Research on fatigue had at first been directed towards the fitness of workers through the use of ergogenic aids but was given further impetus following a demand for greater knowledge on soldiers and battle fatigue after the First World War; its impact on athletic performance was incidental.[64] Founded on the principles of F.W. Taylor's scientific management and Frank Gilbreth's time and motion studies, the laboratory became one of the main sites for research into human performance based on physiological responses to activities involving endurance, strength, altitude, heat and cold.

One of the most influential scientists on human performance was the British physiologist Archibald Vivian Hill. With the German biochemist, Otto Meyerhof, Hill had been awarded the 1922 Nobel Prize for Physiology and Medicine for discovering the distinction between aerobic and anaerobic metabolism.[65] In 1925 Hill's scientific achievements had been given world-wide recognition with his Presidential address to the section on physiology of the British Association for the Advancement of Science, 'The Physiological Basis of Athletic Records'. In 1927 he published both *Muscular Movement in Man* and *Living Machinery*. Hill had been a keen runner in his earlier years and this had given him an interest in the study of the physiology of athletes for the benefit of the wider population.[66] In 1923 he explained that:

> Athletics, physical training, flying, working, submarines or coal-mines, all require a knowledge of the physiology of man, as does also the study of conditions in factories. The observation of sick men in hospital is not the best training for the

study of normal man at work. It is necessary to build up a sound body of trained scientific opinion versed in the study of normal man, for such trained opinion is likely to prove of the greatest service, not merely to medicine, but in our ordinary social and industrial life.[67]

Hill believed that athletes were easy subjects to experiment on as they could repeat exactly their performances. At Cornell University in 1927 he measured the acceleration of sprinters – who were wearing a magnetic band – through the use of a galvanometer. Large coils had been set up at 1 to 10-yard intervals alongside a track and each time a runner passed by a coil a deflection was recorded with the velocity computed by dividing the distance between each coil by the elapsed time. But another motivation for him was that the study of athletes was 'amusing'. It again highlighted the novelty of the relationship between sport and medicine, and his digression into applied exercise physiology was said to be puzzling to his peers.[68]

Between 1922 and 1924 Hill's research had focussed on the relationship between muscular exercise, lactic acid and the supply and utilization of O_2 – oxygen deficit and debt – when athletes had been running. In stressing the importance of 'maximal O_2 uptake' ($VO_{2\,max}$) Hill was able to show how it determined athletic performance; the longer athletes were able to sustain their $VO_{2\,max}$ for extended periods, the better their performance. In order to obtain high levels of $VO_{2\,max}$ and at the same time prevent the build up of lactic acid within their muscles, athletes required a systematic training regime, or as it was termed, 'the steady state of exercise'.[69] Hill's research not only formed the basis for sports science and exercise physiology but his work also provided a medical basis for coaching texts that were able to take into account the physiological limits and potential of athletes' bodies.

The core of Hill's theory – that the athletic body's capacity for stress was greater than it was first believed – was put to the test by athletes and coaches in Northern Europe. Finland's Paavo Nurmi was amongst the first to recognize that athletes could increase their training workload. He was famed for his even-paced front-running that was built on a three-times a day training regime.[70] Uniquely, Nurmi won the 1500m and 5000m at the 1924 Olympics on the same afternoon. His training was built on the principle of running different distances including repeated sprints. The pioneer in this area of training was the Finnish coach, Lauri Pikhala. What he called 'Terrace Training' stressed a balance between work and rest.[71] Yet Nurmi only trained in the spring and summer as winter training was not considered necessary.

Nurmi's principle of alternating work with recovery periods was built upon by the German, Dr Woldemar Gerschler. He was the head of the Freiburg Institute of Physical Education and also the coach of Rudolf Harbig. Using Harbig as a guinea pig, Gerschler was an early promoter of interval training – resistance through repeated speed. This training system basically aimed to alternate hard, measured runs with recovery runs over a set time. It could then be tweaked through manipulating distances, repetitions and the recovery interval. Using this regime Harbig set world records for both the 400 metres and 800 metres in 1939.[72] Gerschler worked in a three-man team. The other two were a cardiologist, Herbert Reindell who provided Gerschler with scientific research on the effectiveness of interval training, and a psychologist called Schildge.[73] One part of Harbig's training included a workout of ten repetitions of 400m. Through measurements of his heart rate after a run, they were able to calculate the optimum rest period before Harbig should run again. As Nicholas Bourne has argued, the close monitoring of heart rate and division of time within time to form intervals represented 'a significant increase in the level of sophistication and objectivity of the training process'. The use of 'measured work intervals' now allowed athletes to increase their training intensity above race pace. This translated into better performances on the track. In 1930 the Swedish coach, Gosta Holmer, invented an early form of interval training, the fartlek system. It was a form of endurance training that systematically alternated different running speeds – sprinting, striding and easy running – over varied terrain. Its most famous exponent was the Swedish middle-distance runner, Gunder Hagg. During the Second World War he broke fifteen track records. His world record for the mile, 4:01.4, lasted from 1945 until 1954. Interval training still forms the bedrock of training programmes for many athletes.[74]

Coaching and the British amateur hegemony

During this period British athletics was dominated by an amateur elite, in particular, the Achilles Club. It was formed in 1920 and comprised a network of Oxbridge old boys. Successful members of this club at Olympic level included Douglas Lowe and Lord Burghley. However, while amateurism remained the dominant sporting ideology, there was a growing awareness of Britain slipping further down the international sporting pecking order. One member, Harold Abrahams, famously employed Sam Mussabini as his coach in preparation for the 1924 Olympics, signalling a shift from the ethic of pure amateurism. In addition, there was an evolution in athletics training literature, which was dominated through the publications of Achilles members.[75] Some were based on the latest scientific research, such as that of A.V. Hill, and criticized past methods, reflecting wider debates between orthodox and unorthodox medicine. In *Training for Athletes* (1928) Adolphe and Harold Abrahams stated that, 'Quacks and charlatans … know that the best appeal is the introduction of something mysterious cloaked in pseudo-scientific phraseology'.[76] By contrast, they advocated a study of an athlete's tissues to understand muscular activity.[77] Although it tried to debunk some myths, *Training for Athletes* was not a complete break from past practices and ideas on the preparation of athletes.

While it advised against the use of alcohol as a tonic for athletes, alcohol was also seen as a medicine and as a way of averting occasional bouts of staleness.[78]

New developments also blended with a traditional British aversion to professionalism and specialization. Sport was still regarded as a force for good in terms of participation, which was preferable to the pursuit of winning. In 1929 Douglas Lowe and Arthur Porritt declared that:

> We want our athletic "giants" just as we want our great "brains" but we want them as incentives and as examples, not simply as perfected mechanisms through which to advertise. We feel sure that those who have the cause of athletics most deeply at heart will endorse the opinion that if athletics are to retain their very definite ideals they must be thrown open more and more to the average man – to all men! And surely enough in the process, the great athletes will still be found, without the selfish hot-house production by today's specialisation methods.[79]

Lawrence and Mayer have identified the inter-war years as a period when scientists and medical doctors were in a contest with their rivals and peers in the arts and other professions, and perceived part of 'their moral duty to publicize their social and moral insights'.[80] Porritt saw athletics as a power for good for mankind, and advocated a 'sensible' training programme and to 'Mix' with your fellow athletes, remembering that if there is a greater gift than health it is friendship.[81]

In addition, despite the appreciation of the new science and in contrast to the training regimes of athletes such as Nurmi, moderation was still a key theme in British literature.[82] To develop stamina, for example, Douglas Lowe, winner of the 800 metres at the 1928 Olympics, stressed 'never do too much in training'.[83] In *Athletics* Lowe and Porritt state that, 'The essence of ... training should be embodied in the word moderation'.[84] Much emphasis was also placed on the importance of style over training for endurance and stamina.[85] On the matter of training school boys Webster and Heys advised against an arduous schedule and believed that a coach who sets a boy 'to run a fast mile on five days out of seven is nothing less than a criminal lunatic'.[86] Instead, the advice was 'Little and often'.[87] The Cambridge-educated Irishman Robert Tisdall advised that 'Style comes first'.[88]

The leading British thinker on coaching in the inter-war years was F.A.M. (Frederick Annesley Michael) Webster. Almost uniquely among British coaches, he brought a rational and scientific approach to the field events, which because of the British harrier tradition had been the bridesmaid to those on the track. He also was familiar with A.V. Hill's work on oxygen debt as well as drawing on the work of Pavlov to theorize about the effects of anxiety on the efficiency of an athlete's circulation and digestion. In 1934 he was appointed the first director of the AAA summer school at Loughborough. However, Webster was a relatively lone voice and there was a lack of a coaching culture in Britain. Following the success of German athletes at the Berlin Olympics and the fear of an impending war, the British government did place a greater emphasis on coaching through the formation of the National Fitness Council. The AAA saw this as an opportunity to revive the idea of a national coaching scheme and a head coach. Interestingly, the candidate the AAA chose was an Austrian, Franz Stampfl, indicating the lack of suitable British candidates.[89]

The athletic mind

Similar to attitudes towards training the body for competition, coaches were also aware of the importance of the preparation of an athlete's mind. While the methods of modern sports psychologists may reflect a more scientific approach, those employed by traditional coaches shared a desire for a similar outcome for their athletes. The notion of the 'will', therefore, has been a recurrent theme in sporting discourse and is reflected in its current use through words such as determination and commitment. In the nineteenth century the 'will' was largely expressed in terms of 'character', 'courage' and 'pluck'. In Britain these qualities were to take on a distinctly British edge. Playing sport itself, for example, had been thought to be character building, especially within public schools. In his book on boxing A.J. Newton claimed that 'Courage, British bulldog hanging-on pluck wins many a fight against superior odds'. Importantly, 'there must be no element of funk'.[90] There was also an awareness of funk (panic or cowardice) in athletics and how nerves played a part before a big race. Harry Andrews suggested that a coach should talk to the athlete about anything but the race itself to keep his mind occupied.[91]

For those belonging to the amateur elite the motivation of athletes remained a personal matter. Lowe and Porritt were generally dismissive of the views of trainers and instead it was advised that athletes should develop their own powers of rational judgement and weed out what was useful and what was not. As a consequence, the mental side of training involved 'the cultivation of self-discipline and will power', i.e., 'pluck'.[92]

Sports psychology as a medical sub-discipline was pioneered in America by Norman Triplett. In 1898 Triplett, a cycling enthusiast, observed that social influence, through a pacing machine and competition, seemed to motivate cyclists to better performance.[93] Coleman R. Griffith became the first person to conduct systematic sport psychology research and practice. Between 1925 and 1932 he was the director of the Athletic Research Laboratory at the University of Illinois as well as working in professional sport. On one occasion he interviewed Red Grange following a Michigan-Illinois college football match who told Griffiths he could not remember a single detail of his performance; highlighting how some top athletes play on instinct alone. Griffiths also corresponded with Knute Rockne on the psychology of coaching and motivation. In 1938 the Chicago Cubs hired him as a team sports psychologist.[94] Sports psychology in Germany was also being developed, first by August Bier and then Robert Schulte. Initially, it reflected a form of constitutional psychology, which was largely based on racial anthropology where performances it was thought were due to an athlete's fixed temperament.[95]

While there was an awareness of the 'mental side' of sport, the psychological methods used in British sport were mainly non-scientific and could be described as cod psychology. During the 1930s a number of football clubs experimented with 'psychological methods'. Some clubs, including Arsenal, Brentford and Sheffield Wednesday, used the Reverend M. Caldwell, a chaplain to two large London 'mental' hospitals who was described as an expert in practical psychology and gave lectures on what he termed 'psychotactics'. At one time, Wolves players also attended regular sessions at a local psychologist in an attempt to build up their confidence.[96] The *ad hoc* nature of these experiments reflected not only a growing acceptance of Freud's ideas from the turn of the century but also a popularization of psychology. As a consequence of a lack of authority within psychiatry, it had allowed a host of people to practice and disseminate their own brand of psychology through classes, magazines and books.[97]

The Football Association's first coaching handbook also placed an emphasis on the need for the coach to apply a psychological approach and identified 'types' of players. One was the 'timid' type another the 'strong, eager, thrustful type', plus the player who 'gives up' easily was seen as another problem. While it was felt necessary to instil self-confidence in timid players, 'thrustful' players required 'firm but tactful handling'. Those who give up were deemed to lack 'backbone' and at times 'a really sharp word' was necessary.[98] In general, psychological techniques in football were relatively rudimentary and for many years managers based their ideas largely on traditional masculine values. It was in the 1990s, following the large injection of television money and the arrival of foreign coaches, that saw the introduction of sports psychologists into British football.

Sports science in the post war period

Following the Second World War elite international sport was transformed. Due to the onset of the Cold War there was an intensification of sporting competition. Although it never escalated into a full-scale military conflict, 'it did become a "hot war" in the context of sport, where superiority was not an abstraction, but a reality to be demonstrated repeatedly and conspicuously'.[99] It was particularly the Olympic arena where rivalries between East and West were played out. These developments further stimulated ideas about enhancing performance that were increasingly based on a physiological paradigm.

The major characteristic of the training schedules of athletes, especially middle- and long-distance runners was the increase in the volume of their workload. No-one epitomized this more than Emil Zátopek. Whereas in Britain emphasis was placed on the importance of style, Zátopek was known for his ungainly gait. After winning the 10,000 metres at the London Games, he then, uniquely, won the 5,000 metres, 10,000 metres and marathon at the 1952 Olympics. He aimed to dominate races from the front and this entailed training every day.[100] He did so without a coach or stopwatch but his schedule was so gruelling that the coach Fred Wilt described him as the 'originator of modern intensive training'.[101] It was claimed that Zátopek trained for five hours a day, seven days a week, and his daily workout consisted of twenty repetitions at 200 metres; forty runs of 400 metres before finishing with twenty repetitions at 200 metres. Each interval was followed by 200 metres of jogging and the time taken for the intervals after a 400 metres was 75–90 seconds.[102] Zátopek was the example that others such as Peter Snell and Jim Ryan followed in pushing back the barriers of human endurance and the stresses on the human body.

Of course, there was always the possibility that athletes could over-train. The British marathon runner Jim Peters was one who had increased his training workload to Zátopek-like levels. In 1951 he had stated that he trained five or six times a week, and on a Sunday he pushed his son's pram on a three hour walk. In 1949–50 his annual training mileage had been 1,400 (2,253 km) from 190 runs but by 1952–53, this had increased to over 4,000 miles (6,400 km) from 500 training runs. In 1953 Peters set a world best for the marathon of 2 hours 18 minutes 40.2 seconds. However, based on Peters' insatiable appetite for training, Harold Abrahams declared that 'Jim Peters' Plans Frighten Me'. He offered no scientific evidence for this and recognized that standards had improved but he believed that Peters was pushing himself too far.[103] Abrahams' words were prophetic. At the 1954 Empire Games Peters was leading the marathon when he entered the stadium. However, under a hot sun he was a ghostly figure who staggered towards the finish and fell over six times. He never reached the tape and eventually became unconscious. He was put on a saline drip as his life hung in the balance. Peters never ran again.[104]

One of the most acclaimed sporting achievements in the early post-war period was Roger Bannister breaking the four-minute barrier for the mile in 1954. In the process Bannister beat his main rivals, America's Wes Santee and John Landy from Australia, to the mark. In some quarters it was declared amateurism's final hurrah. The main protagonists, Bannister, Chris Chataway and Chris Brasher, were represented as sporting gentlemen and a throwback to an age of amateurism that was now under threat from a sporting nationalism stoked by the Cold War; a popular perception that still persists.[105] However, much of this rhetoric concealed the reality of a well-planned and well-executed race that had been underpinned by modern training techniques. In the first instance Chataway and Brasher were pacemakers and pacemaking was illegal at the time under AAA rules. Moreover, they had all received tuition from the Austrian coach, Franz Stampfl (although he was not their full-time coach).[106] Bannister himself was a medical student on the cusp of an outstanding career and was able to apply scientific principles to his training. Although his observations on his training were regarded as largely subjective, Arnd Kruger has concluded that his training theory was ahead of its time.[107] He was familiar with the literature in experimental physiology and ran experiments on himself to enhance his performance, which included treadmill runs with oxygen-enriched air. He also used the Swedish fartlek and interval training techniques as well as the most advanced technology available.[108]

Athletes of all disciplines also began to adopt weight-training programmes after 1945. These naturally included the throwing events but even runners like Zátopek used weights to strengthen themselves.[109] As we have seen, an early promoter of weight-training was Eugen Sandow. Thomas Delorme later developed resistance weight-training programmes for the rehabilitation of World War Two veterans. These had helped restore muscle strength and speeded up their recovery. Furthermore, Peter Karpovich helped to debunk the muscle-bound myth of weight-training and outlined how a systematic programme could increase speed, reduce injury and improve flexibility.[110]

The growing acceptance of the benefits from a more scientific perspective led to the emergence of sports medicine and sports science as academic disciplines in the post-war period. These developments were now driven by the idea of excess rather than moderation.[111] Beamish and Ritchie have argued that in the 1960s the modern principles of athletic training became 'scientifically entrenched'. This created a further paradigm shift that led to 'the application of physiological principles to understand and enhance performance in athletics'.[112] Mignon has added that 'Sports medicine of the 1960s saw the emergence of a new type of individual, "the trained athlete", different psychologically and physiologically from the man in the street'.[113]

A number of physiological studies – of how cells and organ systems of the body perform their functions – had had an important impact on coaches and their approach to training athletes. First, Thomas Cureton in his study of physical fitness that had been conducted at the University of Illinois's Physical Fitness Research Laboratory linked body build with athletic performance.[114] More significant to the understanding of training and improvements in performance was the work of Hans Selye (*The Stress of Life*, 1956) on the body's adaptation to stress. Selye's work allowed coaches and athletes to better understand the limits of an athlete's performance especially in light of the increased training workloads they now were undertaking. Selye advanced the theory of the General Adaptation Syndrome in which stress was regarded as 'the wear and tear caused by life' with life itself seen as 'a process of adaptation to the circumstances in which we live'. It was found that through internal organs such as the endocrine gland and the nervous system the body adapted to stress. At first the body would be in shock to any form of stimuli but there would then be a process of counter-shock, which enabled it to adapt and resist until it reached a stage of exhaustion.[115] Thus, for athletes it was necessary to build up their reserves of resistance.

In the early 1960s biomechanics also emerged as a sub-discipline within exercise and sport science, partly due to the technical advances in film, which allowed coaches to now view the movements of athletes in slow motion. One of the pioneers was Geoff Dyson, chief national coach of the AAA from 1947 to 1961. His *The Mechanics of Athletics*, based partly on Newton's laws of motion, was regarded as the most authoritative text on the subject.[116] While Tom McNab has described Dyson's rational, scientific approach to coaching as transforming the post-war British athletics literature, it also brought a devaluation of practical experience. As a consequence, there was a biomechanical bias to the coaching literature.[117] A conversation between Dyson and Cureton highlighted these on-going tensions between the practical and the scientific. Whereas Cureton had insisted a particular high jumper could have jumped higher if he had been fitter, Dyson argued that this was simplistic and a more intuitive approach was required that took into account age and the technical abilities and deficiencies of the jumper.[118]

Despite British sport's prevailing amateur ethic the 1968 Mexico City Olympics signified a closer relationship with science. In 1965 the British Olympic Association organized a party of doctors, scientists and athletes to investigate the effects of altitude on athletic performance in readiness for the 1968 Games, which were held at over 2000 metres above sea level. While thinner air was expected to assist sprinters and athletes in the field events, it was thought to be detrimental to those in endurance races. Interestingly, these were not only expressed in terms of the health of athletes but also that the choice of Mexico City was unfair and contrary to amateurism and the Olympic spirit. The British Olympic Association (BOA) subsequently concluded that a minimum of four weeks training at altitude was needed. The International Olympic Committee (IOC) had previously set a maximum period of four weeks in a pre-Olympic training camp but it signified that even amateur athletes now required regimented and scientific training.[119]

Coaching in Australia

Coaches in Australia were also beginning to adopt nascent sports science techniques after 1945. Largely unaffected by the war, the early post-war period was a golden period for Australian sport, particularly in tennis, swimming and athletics. Coaches though provided the cutting edge. These included Harry Hopman in tennis, June Ferguson in athletics and swimming's Forbes Carlile.[120] In particular, Australian coaches – in all sports – collectively rejected the idea that heavy training created staleness in athletes. Instead, there was a growing belief that they should be trained to the point of exhaustion.[121] While different coaches utilized science in different ways, an application of scientific principles was at the heart of these developments.

Chief among these were Australian swimming coaches, especially Forbes Carlile. Carlile was an early advocate of Selye's General Adaptation Syndrome and had also been a pupil of Professor Frank Cotton, regarded as the 'father of sports science in Australia' who had developed a connection with the Harvard Fatigue Laboratory during the 1930s. Carlile, a lecturer in physiology at the University of Sydney, provided a bridge between 'hard' science and coaching in Australian sport. Carlile had gained a master's degree on 'Studies in the physiology of muscular exercise', which included evaluations of body measurements, the effects of heavy training and changes in athletes' blood profiles. As a consequence, in his book *Forbes Carlile on Swimming*, he firmly sets out what this meant for swimmers: 'Let us get this straight from the start – preparation for top competitive swimming must be a well-planned, year-round process'.[122] While acknowledging that every athlete was different and that many coaches could tacitly recognize the signs of exhaustion and over-training, he argued that 'the challenge for the physiologist was to be able to measure the amount of general and specific adaptations to stress and to find reliable tests of how long an individual was able to resist a given stress'. He identified a number of the stresses of the swimmer in training, like muscular exercise and bacterial infections, and a list of symptoms of failing adaptation, such as chronic loss of body weight and psychological unrest.[123] While Carlile had been a professional swimming coach since 1955, ironically, he did not receive universal (and Australian) recognition for his methods until 1962 after his success with the Dutch national team at the European championships.[124]

The two most significant coaching figures in Australian athletics during this period held ideological differences in the training of athletes. Whereas Franz Stampfl advocated a rational and scientific approach, his great rival Percy Cerutty favoured one based on naturalism. As we have seen, Stampfl first coached in Britain and was associated with Roger Bannister. However, he eventually settled in Australia where he trained the likes of the multiple world record holder Ron Clarke and the 1968 Olympic champion at 800 metres, Ralph Doubell. While he did not adopt scientific principles to the same extent as Carlile, Stampfl's approach was a combination of Newtonian principles of motion and Hans Selye's theories of stress adaptation. His preferred training method though was interval training. He also argued that athletes suffered from too little training and that, staleness, the bogey of athletes and coaches could be avoided by a gradual build up in the volume and intensity of training.[125]

In addition to John Landy Percy, Cerutty also coached Herb Elliott, arguably the greatest miler in history. His philosophy of training shared similarities to the counter-culture and a rejection of Western materialism as well as with early twentieth century physical culture. He largely rejected new scientific fashions and derided Stampfl's methods as boring and regimented. Cerutty developed his training ideas from experimentation on himself and applied many of the principles derived from studying the movement patterns of race horses and big cats. He was also in debt to the physical culturalist George Hackenschmidt as a teacher of living, both physical and mental. Cerutty developed his own philosophy called 'Stotanism' – a derivative of Stoic and Spartan based on his reading of medieval writings on religious asceticism – which placed great emphasis on combining the natural environment with the training of athletes. He set up a seaside training camp in Portsea in Victoria where his athletes famously trained on its steep sand dunes as well as golf courses and forests. There were also a variety of activities that mixed running, including fartlek, on different surfaces with weight-training and swimming and were set to music from Calypso to Beethoven. At the centre of his methods was a belief that life's realization could be developed through running.[126]

Boxing and sports science

The adoption of sports science throughout the sporting world was never universal and in fact was very uneven. Its reception was dependent on the financial means and will of individual countries, which partly reflected the importance they placed on sport as well as the extent of cultural resistance within individual sports. In boxing, for example, training methods could be termed traditional, which reflected the working-class backgrounds of both trainers and fighters. Few had access to medical journals and trainers worked within their own communities of practice in which methods were passed on by word of mouth. However, even boxing's citadel was beginning to be breached by the 1980s. The film *Rocky IV* offers a contrast between traditional and modern training techniques (and also an allegory for the Cold War). In their preparation for their fight, Rocky Balboa adopts traditional and natural methods that utilizes nature, the American Great Outdoors, whereas his Soviet opponent's training is given a sinister spin as it is undertaken in laboratory-like conditions using modern sports science techniques, including illegal drugs. Of course, Rocky wins but in reality sports science was now been advocated for boxing in America.

However, scientific methods were not widespread. In 2002 it was stated that 'the use of so-called "old-school" training methods such as long distance running and the avoidance of weight-training still persist in boxing today'.[127] More boxers, however, have employed strength and conditioning experts who have begun to replace the all-round role of the trainer. Whereas previously the trainer dealt with every facet of the boxer's regimen, the roles of cornermen have become more specialized. One of the first American boxers to adopt sports science techniques was Evander Holyfield. In 1986 he teamed up with a strength and conditioning specialist, Tim Hallmark. Essentially, Hallmark transformed Holyfield's preparation. Out went the traditional miles of roadwork and hours of sparring. In its place came a comprehensive weight-training programme, sprints and plyometrics – exercises that incorporate jumps and hops to enhance speed and strength. Conditioning drills would be followed with the monitoring of Holyfield's heart rate to assess workrate and recovery as well as analysis of his blood, urine and saliva to give hormonal and metabolic feedback on his state of health and response to training.[128]

Sports science in Eastern Europe

Following the Second World War Eastern Europe, led by the Soviet Union, largely rejected its former ideological commitment to non-competitive physical, cultural activities and embraced the previously tainted 'bourgeois' sports. In particular the Olympics were seen as an arena to display the virtues of communism as a superior way of life compared to the decadent West. This use of sport as a political tool by the Eastern bloc was highly successful in terms of the results achieved. When communist countries first made their debut at the 1952 summer Olympics they won 29 per cent of the medals; in 1976, it was 57 per cent. The USSR 'won' every Olympics, summer and winter (bar 1968 and the winters of 1980 and 1984) while between 1956 and 1976, the German Democratic Republic (GDR) advanced from 15th to 2nd in the medal table.

There has been a popular (mis-)conception that this success was solely achieved through a systematic drugs programme (see Chapter 5). While drugs were certainly a factor, this view fails to take into account that the structural foundations of sports medicine were deeply embedded within the state machinery of Eastern bloc countries. Interestingly in Eastern Europe, like the West, there was disagreement over what constituted sports medicine. While the USSR (see Chapter 1) primarily saw it as part of a wider health agenda, reflecting a pre-war tradition of physical culture, in the GDR, reflecting a wider German tradition, the priority was sporting performance and hence there was a greater emphasis on sports medicine as science.[129] By the 1960s the focus of GDR sports medicine was on discovering talent, planning individual training regimes and treating sports injuries. In the Soviet Union, from a total of 3 million full-time athletes, each one was attached to one of 400 sports medical dispensaries, which employed 5,500 doctors; 14 for every dispensary.[130]

The communist sports system contrasted with attitudes in the West where coaches still regarded their practices as an art rather than a science, and continued to work alone utilising knowledge within their own 'communities of practice'. The success of athletics and sport in general amongst Eastern bloc countries was due to a greater scientific approach, and in particular, the idea of periodization. Periodization prepared athletes for competition using a highly sophisticated system involving training cycles and a variation in the volume and intensity of workouts, which was designed to bring athletes to a peak for a particular event, such as the Olympic Games. Of course, this was the aim for the vast majority of coaches. However, periodization was the product of an all-encompassing theory of sport and training, which was the work of the Soviet training theorist, Lev Pavlovich Matveyev, published in 1965. Through periodization an athlete's training programme was divided into specific cycles of time and was another by-product of Soviet planning science. Matveyev incorporated aspects of Selye's work on stress and adaptation but this was to be part of an overall coaching system that allowed athletes to peak for competition.

It was only in 1975 that periodization entered the lexicography of Western coaches through Britain's Frank Dick's critique of Matveyev's theory.[131]

In Eastern Europe a totally different approach to training also emerged as coaches worked together with scientific researchers. Instead of looking solely at physiological responses to exercise, a more holistic view was taken.[132] Nicholas Bourne has argued that in 1969 the Soviet coach V. Popov was the first to advocate the comprehensive planning of training, and that this was 'a watershed moment that demonstrates how the planning of training and theory began to be recognized as an independent discipline in its own right'.[133] His plan featured a division of labour where training was broken up into specific yearly, monthly and weekly cycles.[134]

The state-sponsored athletic body

In response to the sporting success of Eastern European nations, the governments of Western countries also began to develop a fixation for sporting success on the international stage. As a consequence, the state began to intervene in the development process for elite sports. To gain state aid, national governing bodies now had to adopt professional management structures as well as high-quality coaching and talent identification schemes.[135] It was argued that for nations to 'optimise their chances of winning medals' at Olympic Games on a consistent basis they need to 'develop, operate and provide funding for an efficient Elite Athlete Development (EAD) system'.[136] In 1976 Australia failed to win an Olympic gold medal. It produced much navel gazing and in response – which was a cultural response, highlighting the national importance that country places on sport – in 1981 the Australian Institute of Sport was founded. It marked the start of the nationalization of elite (Olympic) sport in Australia.

In Britain this process did not start until the 1990s when it was bolstered by funds from the National Lottery, which began in 1994. However, since then the increased state investment in elite sport has required that each national governing body has a talent identification and development strategy, something that was set out in the 2002 government report, *Game Plan*.[137] As a consequence of this political outcome, British elite sport, in addition to EAD systems, has become aligned to sports science through the adoption of a generic model for developing athletic potential, Long Term Athlete Development (LTAD). LTAD systems are predicated on notions that it takes 8 to 12 years of training or 10,000 hours for a talented athlete to reach elite levels.[138] The LTAD model has outlined a comprehensive and structured training programme, competition and a recovery regime to ensure optimum career development, and has been developed by Istvan Blayi, a sports development expert, on the basis of research into physiology, physical development and the analysis of training/competition outcomes. Under this system, sports are classified as either early specialization, which require early sport-specific specialization in training or late specialization sports, which require a more generalized approach to early training.[139] The LTAD is essentially a rationalized, scientific and mechanistic paradigm that now drives performance sport. There is also an insistence that coaches fully integrate sports science and sports medicine into their programmes. In particular, a great deal of emphasis is placed on physiology with successive stages of the model described as 'building the engine', 'optimising the engine', and 'maximising the engine'.[140] At the centre of the LTAD's methodology is a belief that anthropometric measurements and physiological evaluations enable the accurate assessment of an individual's suitability for an event and allow potential athletes to be counselled towards appropriate sports.[141]

However, to what extent is the LTAD a new departure or does it reflect on-going tensions over the rational scientific model and the intuitive skills of the coach? Perhaps surprisingly Steve Cram, given his status as chairman of the English Institute of Sport, but maybe less so considering his experience as an athlete, has reservations over this approach. He has argued that the emphasis on the 'hot-housing' – i.e., scientific evaluation – of athletes devalues individual motivation as the main attribute of a top-class athlete.[142] There is also a sense that the LTAD is an unwieldy, one-size fits all model, which has been used for the benefit of government because of its quantitative, easy to measure function that suits large bureaucracies. In one study on football, despite the failure to find any significant variables the authors still concluded that anthropometric measurement should remain an integral part of a performance profiling programme.[143] Instead, Dave Day has argued that research findings should remain part of the toolbox of coaches, which should be used intuitively, instead of being imposed on coaching.[144]

Conclusion

By the twenty-first century, one of Britain's most successful athletes was a woman, Paula Radcliffe. World record holder in the marathon, it has been estimated that in 2003–04, she earned over £2 million per year. But these commercial rewards have only been achieved through a mixture of natural ability allied to a strenuous regime that has reflected the greater scientific attention that athletes give to their training. Through a mixture of trial and error and advice from coaches, sport scientists and sport medics, Radcliffe trains on an eight-day cycle, which includes two long runs, a hard session every other day and a rest day. Every morning she checks her pulse and if it is over a certain mark (45 beats per minute) it signifies she has not fully recovered from the last hard session and hence she regulates her training accordingly. Her weekly distance is around 145 miles, which equates to over 6,000 miles per year, a figure exceeding that of Jim Peters in the 1950s, when Harold Abrahams declared that his plans scared him. Radcliffe has regularly trained at altitude in the Pyrenees and in the American Rockies, a route that many modern athletes have taken since 1968. Training at altitude increases red blood cells in an athlete's body, which in turn maximizes his/her oxygen carrying capacity. She also maintains this 'oxygen debt' by sleeping in a low oxygen tent. Four times a week she endures an ice bath to aid recovery and reduce any inflammations. She also has regular massages. Whereas previously athletes used goose grease as an agent, Radcliffe uses emu oil, the modern equivalent.[145]

To what extent does Radcliffe's preparation differ from that of Captain Barclay? Since the nineteenth century sport has applied scientific principles to the training and preparation of athletes. This application, however, has been contingent not only on prevailing scientific knowledge but also the wider sporting context in which the intensity of competition has shaped the demand for this knowledge and resources. In their preparation of athletes early trainers relied on their own intuition and based their judgement on personal experiences. By the Cold War era the Soviet Union especially felt that nothing could be left to chance and poured in vast state resources in the pursuit of Olympic medals. In the West sport has not only become a lucrative commercial activity but, through the intervention of the state, it has become subject to unwieldy managerial and administrative structures that order and organize the lives of those athletes in its pay.

At the same time, scientific knowledge has changed the athletic body, both physically and psychologically. Whereas the mantra of moderation brought fears of staleness from over-training, a greater awareness of the body's ability to endure fatigue and other extremities gave coaches the confidence through this knowledge to place excessive demands on athletes' bodies. While the athletic body may have become a distinct clinical entity by the 1960s, caution should also be taken in using catch-all phrase as social factors, such as gender, ethnicity and class, can also shape an athlete's identity. In particular, for much of the twentieth century the athletic body was constructed in technically and scientifically advanced nations. In large areas of the globe, athletes have not had access to these resources.

5

Testing Times

Drugs, Anti-Doping and Ethics

Introduction

'If it takes ten to kill you, I'll take nine.'

This quote, with reference to amphetamines, has been attributed to the British cyclist Tom Simpson and highlighted Simpson's obsessive search to improve his performance. In 1967, during the Tour de France, Simpson died on Mount Ventoux. Following an examination of his body, traces of amphetamine were found in his blood. Tom Simpson did not die solely because of the dose of amphetamine he took, however, his death became associated with drugs and for some this has tainted his memory ever since.[1] Over thirty years later the British magazine *Cycling Weekly* named Chris Boardman as the best British cyclist of all time in its 2001 poll. Simpson was second. A debate ensued in the magazine's pages over the choice of Boardman instead of Simpson in which the main issue revolved around Simpson's association with drugs. One contributor who supported Simpson posed the question, 'Why not Tom?' answering it rhetorically, 'We know why, don't we?' Another contributor argued that, 'Chris Boardman deserves his accolade as the top British rider, if for no other reason than he was, by general consensus, the cleanest rider in the peloton'. On his reasons for not selecting Simpson, he added that he 'was a man of a particularly black time in the history of our sport. He died as he had lived, with amphetamine coursing through his veins and a selection of pills in his racing jersey pocket'.[2]

In Chapter 4 the focus was on how the athletic body was shaped by developments within medicine and science. Here, while acknowledging how the use of drugs has also contributed to the enhancement of performance, this chapter is more concerned with the ethical reaction that drugs in sports has evoked, which has led to an anti-doping discourse and ideology.[3] The aim is not to provide a polemic on the use of drugs in sport, which has been the main focus for much of the literature on this subject. Instead, the chapter aims to show that as much as a scientific process, medicine – through drugs in sport – is also a social and cultural construction that has been shaped by wider political and economic factors such as the rise of the pharmaceutical industry and the influence of governments.

The emergence of an anti-doping discourse

No topic in modern sport has been more emotive than the use by athletes of performance-enhancing drugs nor provoked as much debate or as much literature.[4] As Paul Dimeo has shown, this debate has largely taken place within a moral and ethical framework that has tended to see drugs 'as a problem' and a form of cheating, which has led to an anti-doping discourse throughout sport.[5] As a result, there has been a tendency to evoke value-laden terms such as 'civilization' and 'dehumanization' when discussing the impact of drugs in sport on modern society. Even John Hoberman, perhaps the leading historian in this field, has tended to place the issue in these terms.[6] More emotive accounts[7] have highlighted how the debate has been a product of late-twentieth-century modernity. Invoking moral and ethical terms implies that contemporary society is, or is becoming, more civilized than in past eras. Instead, it could be argued that the notion of civilization is a very thin veneer. Moreover, this approach, when looking at the history of sport and drugs, can lend itself to teleological tendencies. In particular, the debate is judged against sporting values and standards of fair play and sportsmanship from a mythical Golden Age of sport.

Why then has drugs been such an emotive issue? First, it invokes wider cultural implications. The issue of drugs in sports, for example, has reflected human fears of the unnatural. In this case, the spectre of athletes taking on the appearance of muscle-bound mutants 'drugged up to the eyeballs'. Throughout history there have been anxieties over scientific developments, which have created myths and been reflected in literature such as the legend of Prometheus, Mary Shelly's *Frankenstein* and *Brave New World* by Aldous Huxley. More recently through innovations such as IVF, genetic engineering and cloning, familiar tropes within the media have questioned how 'natural' these discoveries are, further highlighting humans' ever-evolving definitions of life and as a result, what is 'normal'.[8] Mike McNamee, one of the most ardent academic opponents not just of the use of drugs in sport but also other biotechnologies, has admitted he finds 'the unfettered use of technology to augment human nature utterly repellent'.[9] Of course, perceptions of what are either 'natural' or 'unnatural' are conditioned by wider cultural ideas.

Importantly, the ethical and moral dimension surrounding 'drugs in sport' has mirrored historical anxieties over addiction to social drugs and alcohol since at least the nineteenth century.[10] As a result, the controversy over doping has displayed the characteristics of a moral panic, i.e., an hysterical (over) reaction from critics and the media leading to both national and international debates fuelled by politicians. At the same time the medical profession has been at the centre of debates in framing what is meant by addiction.

However, debates over athletes taking drugs and the emergence of an anti-doping ethos have also been located within a specific sporting context and as such it has been perceived as a type of 'sporting disease'. In particular, this discourse has revolved around the notion that taking drugs is a form of cheating; that it is contrary to the principles of sport and can been seen through the continuous invocation of phrases such as 'fair play', 'sportsmanship' and 'a level playing field'. As Dimeo has argued, a good-bad dichotomy emerged. Sports doctors and policy makers, working on promoting an anti-doping ethos, have been imbued with a Christian morality and self-belief that athletes who take drugs are 'evil' and that they are doing good work in protecting both the health of athletes and the integrity of sport.[11] In 1962, for example, an article in the *Olympic Bulletin* was titled 'Waging War against Doping'. It read:

> One of the plagues of modern times is the disastrous practice of doping which unfortunately has been adapted to sport. The use of drugs and artificial stimulants nowadays are the chief evils from which one must protect athletes.

Writing over thirty-years later in the *British Medical Journal* (*BMJ*), Domhnall MacAuley, a former rower and drug-sampling officer but then editor of the *British Journal of Sports Medicine* (*BJSM*), similarly proclaimed that,

> Though an athlete's motivation in taking drugs is understandable, we cannot condone it. Firstly, it can be dangerous to the athlete's health and, secondly, it is against all principles of fair play.[12]

Similarly, in 2005 Yesalis and Bahrke simply stated that their concern over the use of anabolic steroids in sport was because 'it is cheating – the use of these drugs violates the rules of virtually every sports federation'. This concern was also founded on a number of moral and ethical issues including harm to the health of the athlete, and that athletes who use drugs gives them an unfair advantage over athletes who do not.[13]

As we have seen though any notions of fairness in sport are themselves social and cultural constructs. Perceptions of cheating have been products of the values and beliefs of a largely self-selected sporting elite in which the ideology of amateurism has been central to this ethos. At one time even training and coaching, especially in rugby union, were deemed as a form of professionalism and therefore, cheating. This was partly because it was associated with the working classes but also because sport was believed to be who was the best on the day. Of course, amateurism itself is full of contradictions having mutated over the twentieth century. But if amateurism has declined as an ideology it is interesting that its legacy in the form of an anti-doping ethos has persisted. It is perhaps also unsurprising that leading amateur administrators and doctors in British sport were at the forefront of devising drug-testing policies. In addition, there was a wider political context at work. In particular, the growing sporting strength of communist countries during the Cold War caused a great deal of angst amongst Western nations that they were not 'playing the game'. However, as Dimeo has pointed out, we should be wary of being drawn into any simplistic narratives of West good, East bad, as it has been Western countries that have been at the forefront of the relationships between drugs and sport. Moreover, it was government intervention that led to the formation of the World Anti-Doping Agency in 1999 as international attitudes to drugs began to change.

Popular medicine and the quest for success

There has been a long history of athletes and coaches experimenting with various substances in their quest to find a cutting edge. The diet of early athletes, for example, was supplemented with various tonics and potions in an attempt to stave off the effects of staleness and to instill character. Professional endurance sport during the second half of the nineteenth century was characterized by the use of strychnine, caffeine, cocaine, nitro-glycerine, alcohol, ethyl ether and opium.[14] Rather than seeing the use of these substances as akin to late twentieth century systematic doping, their application needs to be seen in their contemporary context. Alcohol, for example, was a particularly common part of an athlete's diet in the nineteenth century as it was thought to give strength and stamina. On occasions it was given to pugilists to give them extra 'bottom'. However, the use of alcohol should be seen in light of a society in which many people utilized alcoholic drinks as thirst quenchers or for physical stamina. In addition, because these drinks had been filtered they were regarded as less dangerous than water, which was scarce in rural areas and contaminated in the growing urban centres.[15]

In 1900 there were no doping regulations and stimulants of all forms were openly used by coaches and their athletes, such as in the 1904 Olympic marathon won by the American, Tom Hicks. During the race he had received several injections of strychnine as well as eggs and some brandy. In the report of the Games it was noted that 'from a medical standpoint, [the marathon] demonstrated that drugs are of much benefit to athletes along the road'.[16] As we have seen, scientists and physicians were then more interested in studying athletes to further medical research than consciously attempting to boost their performance.

How then did an anti-drugs discourse in sport emerge? It was in the 1800s that the first synthesized drugs were produced, making artificial substances more potent than natural ones. In addition, their application was made easier with the invention of the hypodermic needle in the 1850s. From the late 1800s concerns over drugs in society in general had begun to grow and were linked to contemporary attitudes towards progress and the superiority of the West. In particular, the Temperance Movement gave a moral authority to the campaign against drink, which was then applied to other stimulants. As a consequence, narcotics, such as opium and cocaine along with alcohol, became associated not only with addiction and degeneracy but also crime and vice.[17]

Because of the growth in the use of opium – following the Opium Wars (1840–42 and 1857–60) with China – and other substances, restrictive legislation on over-the-counter medicines was first passed in Britain in 1860.[18] Heroin and morphine were now prescribed more and more as sedatives. After 1900, due to pressure for reform, there was a clearer demarcation between what was considered illegal and legal drugs as the 1906 Pharmacy Act restricted the sales of some drugs. In addition, the use of cocaine and opium as stimulants declined after the Dangerous Drugs Act of 1920, which made them available only on prescription in Britain.[19] In America a similar 'drugs problem' was framed around an idea developed by doctors and psychiatrists: the 'addict type'. Addiction became defined as a disease. In 1914 the Harrison Anti-Narcotic Act criminalized drug addiction and made opiates and other narcotics legally available only on prescription for treating illness. During the inter-war years addiction became associated with a psychopathic personality as an addict was considered a potential criminal and diagnosed with sociopathic tendencies.[20] Thus, there was an increased awareness not only of drug use but also that it carried a social stigma. Any association between sport and drugs presented problems for those who saw the nineteenth century cult of athleticism as having potential public health benefits at recreational level with its mantra of a healthy mind in a healthy body. Moreover, it also created anxieties over modernity and it was against this background that the roots of anti-doping ideology were planted.[21]

The first sport that introduced rules over doping controls was of the equine kind rather than the human variety.[22] In 1903 the Jockey Club banned the doping of horses. Unsurprisingly, as pre-modern coaches and athletes had based their training ideas on training racehorses, using stimulants in horse-racing had a long history. With racehorses, because of gambling, there were two forms of drugs: those that enhanced performance and those that impeded it. In 1838 it was claimed that horses were doped with opiate balls and that this would hamper their performance; other stimulants through the use of hypodermic needles worked in improving performance. For the Jockey Club, horse doping became an increasing problem in the 1890s, although its response smacked of anti-Americanism. American trainers had gone to Europe around the turn of the century. Because of their success, especially those who trained for fellow American owners, William 'Betcha Million' Gates and James Drake, they became known as the 'Yankee Alchemists' who brought with them their own more 'scientific' stimulants, such as purified cocaine and morphine. Importantly, they were more successful in their use of stimulants than English trainers who were more likely to use a bottle of port. Weary of American success, a leading English trainer, George Lambton, purchased some of the Americans' medications and announced to the press that certain horses in certain races would receive stimulants. This forced the Jockey Club to act. It was not until 1910 though that a saliva test was developed to detect the most common drugs used. Since 1930 drug testing in horse-racing has been introduced for all races organized under the auspices of the International Horse Racing Organization.[23] To a certain extent there is an irony here as it was this overtly commercial sport, rather than an amateur one, which had first established testing procedures in order to present the public with an impression of fairness. The betting industry otherwise would have collapsed if gamblers felt the sport was corrupt and not a level playing field.

By the 1908 Olympics enough concern had been raised about the use of stimulants in athletics for a rule to be included that stated no marathon runners either at the start or during the race could take any drug, otherwise this would lead to their disqualification. What drugs were referred to is unclear but it indicates that drugs were seen as a means of cheating as well as producing physical side-effects. Without any tests, in an age of amateur hegemony, organizers were perhaps appealing to the athletes' sense of fair play and sportsmanship. The race itself was won by an American, John Hayes. The Italian runner, Dorando Pietri, when leading the race, had collapsed and was helped over the line after suffering from heat exhaustion. It has since been claimed that this was partly induced from taking strychnine, although there is no evidence for this. Even amongst those in sport there was growing criticism of the use of drugs. In 1911 the trainer Harry Andrews stated that, after testing some of his athletes, 'From America, whose citizens are far ahead of us in most training, has come one most injurious practice, namely, the use of drugs as stimulants'.[24]

Sport, science and chemical assistance

As we have seen, the inter-war years were a formative period in the development of sports science. One result of the research around fatigue was the production of amphetamines.[25] Amphetamines, or pep pills as they became known, would become the drug of choice for a growing number of athletes. Scientists also experimented with other potential chemical stimulants for athletes. The German physiologist Hermann Hexheimer, for example, was conducting experiments with the effects of caffeine on the performance on track sprinters and cyclists.[26]

It was also during the 1920s that a perceived stigma between athletics and the use of drugs was more publicly asserted. The growing knowledge of athletes taking drugs drew critical reactions from British commentators. Lowe and Porritt stated that their use was 'absolutely to be deprecated'. They argued that not only was it medically unsound but there was the consideration of possible disqualification and 'not playing the game'.[27] Similarly, the Abrahams brothers rejected the use of drugs on medical grounds. They believed the practice was not widespread in Britain but had been puzzled by a recent announcement by the German authorities who warned their athletes against the 'dangers of doping'.[28] Although Germany may have been a pioneer in exercise physiology, not all German doctors approved of the use of drugs when it came to sport. In 1924 one physician commented that,

> there is nothing more reprehensible than using pharmacological substances in an attempt to improve one's performances in competition with others who bring to the sporting encounter only that fitness they have achieved through training.[29]

Of course, for some amateurs training was a form of cheating.

The use, availability and reception of drugs in sport during this period, at least in Britain, needs also to be understood in the context of drug use more generally. Recreational drug use in the *fin de siècle* was popular amongst a small literary sub-culture. The main drugs of choice were hashish and opium, although cocaine had been brought to the public's attentions through Arthur Conan Doyle's Sherlock Holmes. There was generally little comment on this as it was restricted to a small elite. During World War One, however, there was hysteria in the press over a so-called cocaine epidemic when it emerged that prostitutes were selling drugs to soldiers, although Harrods had actually included cocaine in a special kit to send to soldiers at the front.[30] It brought fears that the recreational use of cocaine was spreading in the British army. Cocaine though did become the popular substance for those in the 'drug scene' during the 1920s and show business stars such as Cole Porter used it as a means of relieving depression. In Britain, under the Dangerous Drugs Act of 1920, there were prosecutions for those found in possession of illegal drugs, especially cocaine, and this led to growing concerns over the consequences of addiction. While recreational drug use remained relatively small-scale into the 1930s, an increasing hostility to narcotic drugs was fostered by the popular press.[31]

These public anxieties were also now being mirrored in sport. In 1926 the German athlete Otto Peltzer inflicted a rare defeat on Finland's Paavo Nurmi. The following year it was alleged – seemingly incorrectly – that Nurmi had accused Peltzer of using artificial stimulants in beating him. There then followed some discussion in the European press.[32] Interestingly, the following year the International Amateur Athletics Federation (IAAF) introduced the first anti-doping regulation in sport in which suspension was threatened to anyone who used drugs, although there was no list of banned stimulants. Although Vettenniemi has argued that 'the IAAF decision can only be understood as a solemn but vacuous declaration of intent', in light of the absence of testing, the manner of the IAAF's response reflects how the matter was then perceived. The ban though soon fell into obscurity and no athletes would be suspended until the introduction of urine tests in the 1960s.[33]

'The Monkey Gland affair'

During the inter-war years some British football clubs, reflecting the growing research on fatigue, experimented with ergogenic aids like ultra-violet light rays and also pep pills.[34] One of the most high-profile cases was the use of so-called 'Monkey Glands' by the footballers of Wolverhampton Wanderers.[35] The implantation of 'Monkey Glands' had been popularized by the Russian Serge Voronoff in the 1920s. It was alleged that an injection of testicular implants would rejuvenate the patient.[36] However, based on moral grounds, there had been a great deal of opposition in Britain to the treatment. For a start, anti-vivisectionists opposed the slaughter of monkeys to allow the treatment. In 1928 MPs had protested against granting permission for experiments and it was duly denied by the Home Secretary, Joynson-Hicks. The Breeders Association also rebuffed Voronoff's plans for the gland-grafting of British racehorses. But as much as the science it was the perceived unknown consequences of this treatment that stirred public sentiment. Voronoff's ideas also carried eugenicist overtones. In 1927 he proposed that bright children should be grafted with the glands of monkeys. This, he argued, would endow them with greater physical and mental powers, which would eventually create a 'new super-race of men of genius'. It led to calls within the press for both a moratorium on such research and for scientists to demonstrate a social responsibility.[37]

The Wolves' manager, Frank Buckley, had been behind the idea to administer gland treatment. In 1937 he had been approached by Menzies Sharp (it was claimed he was a scientist but it is difficult to clarify his position). Rather than monkeys, extracts from the glands of slaughtered cattle were used. These included the pituitary, suprarenal, thyroid, mid-brain extract and embryonin. The players were given twelve injections over a six week period, which was to last them over the whole season. The main idea behind their use was to prevent staleness within players as well as improve their mental speed, stamina, physical fitness and resistance to illness. Buckley also claimed that some of players had gained weight and had grown taller as a result of taking the treatment.[38]

Because of the improved form of Wolves, other clubs experimented with the gland treatment, including Fulham, Preston, Portsmouth and Tottenham Hotspur. Within the popular press the matter became sensationalized. Interestingly, during the same period the *Daily Mirror* ran a series of articles written by Dr Friti Moderni on the use of gland treatment.[39] Ironically, the 1939 FA Cup Final was contested by both Wolves and Portsmouth and has since been known as the 'Monkey Gland Final', which Portsmouth won 4-1. The matter was raised in Parliament and the Football Association later held a conference and decreed that while the treatment was permissible, individual players had the right to refuse it. A proposed investigation by the British Medical Association (BMA) did not take place due to the war.[40]

While the whole episode caused a major stir in the football world, it also reflected contemporary anxieties over drugs. In 1938 one (anonymous) famous player was quoted as saying: 'We're not blooming guinea pigs.'[41] Harry Goslin, the captain of Bolton Wanderers, condemned the treatment, arguing that it was 'selfish'. Rather vaguely, in which he may have confused the idea of doping leading to deterioration in performance rather than enhancement, he stated, 'If you are going to dope a set of fellows, I think that is pretty bad.'[42] Some clubs though such as Arsenal refused to use gland treatment. Following some experiments, the club trainer Tom Whittaker claimed that while it may help in cases of illness there would be little effect on healthy players.[43]

The emergence of a sports drugs culture

In the post-war period developments in the pharmaceutical industry were vital in changing the relationship between sport and drugs. The Second World War had provided a period of increased experimentation and collaboration and brought about the industrialization of the pharmaceutical industry. As a result, sales of prescription drugs began to vastly outstrip those medicines that were a combination of natural preparations; the industry now also spent twice as much on marketing as it did on research. The discovery, production and marketing of the antibiotic Penicillin (developed during the War) were crucial to this change. Other important developments included anti-depressants like Valium, Beta-blockers, which treated cardiovascular diseases, and steroid drugs, such as cortisone.[44] By the 1960s, according to a survey, more than thirty types of pharmacological agents could be found in the average American household.[45]

The use of amphetamines, or 'pep pills' like Benzedrine, had become increasingly popular amongst American and British athletes as a result of being brought back into the country by returning soldiers from the Second World War.[46] These drugs and other stimulants were later on offer through various forms of 'underground' networks, which varied from local gyms, cycling teams to research laboratories (and from 2000 the internet would be an important, perhaps the most important, source).[47] Amphetamine use was becoming common if not widespread also within European sports including rowing, cycling and track and field. In Italian football it was found that in 1961 36 per cent of footballers tested had taken the medication, while in England Everton Football Club admitted to their players using mild stimulants in the early 1960s.[48] The use of amphetamines or 'little balls' as they were known was also widespread in Brazilian football in the 1950s.[49]

The use of artificial aids though also continued to arouse scepticism and criticism. One ergogenic aid for athletes that became widely used in the 1950s was 'oxygenation'. As a student in 1951, Roger Bannister had used other athletes at Oxford as guinea pigs on treadmills to test the control of breathing.[50] On the issue of oxygenation, Bannister contributed an article to the *Olympic Bulletin*. He claimed that 'all records would be beaten were we to administer oxygen to athletes in a manner similar to the one used in connection with ... the

Everest climbers'.[51] Footballers from Brazil, Argentina and Chile received inhalations of oxygen while it was reported that Mr. Scopelli, the trainer of the Spanish side, Espanol, gave his players inhalations during half-time and at the end of games. Interestingly, German footballers were forbidden to use oxygenation while some French doctors had condemned its use.[52]

Cycling and the culture of drugs

Perhaps in cycling more than any other sport there was not only a culture of drug-taking and stimulant-use but the entire sport seemed to operate on the level of the Omerta in which all the sport's secrets were kept within the cycling fraternity. It perpetuated a culture of denial that persisted (and perhaps still persists) up to the early twenty-first century. Within the context of a commercialized team sport that relies on sponsorship, it is unsurprising that no-one – teams, riders, race organizers as well as the cycling authorities – was willing to go against the system due to the risk of losing commercial revenue. Furthermore, the whole concept of long-distance cycling and the Tour de France in particular necessitated the need for some form of stimulant.

A complex – and contradictory – mythology had been constructed around the race by its organizers, the media and especially its founder, Henri Desgrange. His idea of a perfect Tour was when only one rider finished. Because of the excessive distances involved it was a race for 'supermen', 'giants' who though only normal men were able to endure unparalleled suffering and without the help of any chemical assistance. At the same time, if this image was not maintained there was a risk that it would undermine the Tour's unique appeal but if cyclists didn't take any stimulants it would have been difficult for them to finish the race. The organizers realized this and so initially ignored warnings about the hazards of drugs.[53] Cyclists have claimed that taking any form of stimulant or drug is not so much about enhancing performance but just getting by on a day-by-day basis. The Irish rider Paul Kimmage who rode in three Tours in the late 1980s described himself as 'desperately naïve' in thinking he could ride a Tour de France on two multi-vitamin tablets each morning. As a consequence of riding six hours a day for twenty-three days, it was not possible without vitamin and mineral supplements, chemicals to clean out a tired liver, and medication to take the tiredness out his legs. For greater efficiency, medication was injected. This was not doping according to Kimmage because he was just replacing what had been sweated out. However, he soon realized that when he started accepting medication the line between what was legal and what wasn't became very thin. 'Most fellows cross it without ever realizing it', he added.[54]

Cyclists had been using stimulants since the late nineteenth century. Racers experimented with substances such as caffeine, nitroglycerine, opiates, cocaine, arsenic and ether as well as alcoholic beverages. Their medicine was a mix of the modern and old wives' tales. One of the most popular was *le vin Mariani*, which combined wine with coca leaves and had been recommended by the medical establishment.[55] One persistent idea was that fluid replacement was not necessary during a race. In 1924 one of the cyclists, Henri Pesslier, showed his bag of medicines to a journalist. It contained: one bottle that he claimed had medicine that was 'cocaine for the eyes' and 'chloroform for the gums'; a cream to warm up his knees; plus some pills, called 'dynamite'.[56] At first the French public did not object to the idea of sports doping. Many substances used were unregulated and on sale at the local pharmacy and spectators often gave cyclists a swig of champagne, which was believed to be a stimulant. It can be argued that the public generally have been relatively ambivalent about doping in sport ever since.[57]

Soigneurs, a personal assistant, played a key role in the preparation of cyclists. It was they, before the employment of team doctors, who would offer advice, massage and secret home-made remedies that included stimulants. They relied on experience-based methods and their trade secrets were handed down through the generations by word-of-mouth. Their home-spun ideas continued right through until the 1980s. One soigneur gave his riders boiled cattle feed; the idea being that it would sit in the stomach as it was absorbed and prevent the stomach muscles from tensing and using energy. Riders also had their own idiosyncrasies. Tom Simpson obsessively drank carrot juice, for example, and was even prepared to try hypnotism. He also recommended 'the cold water sit'. This involved placing the buttocks and crotch in a bowl of ice-cold water followed by the use of cocaine ointment to toughen up the crotch.[58]

However, Simpson also had a strict training regime and his medication was designed to support this in anticipation of a grueling schedule. In 1967 he spent £800 – a huge chunk of his earnings – on Tonedron, an amphetamine considered a superior type of stimulant. The drugs usually came from Italy after being couriered over the border by some of the cyclists.[59] Two years earlier he had outlined the tonics and medicine, based on the advice of two doctors, he was to use to get him through a Tour. He had a special box that contained small ampoules. Their contents included vitamin B complex, liver extract and a muscle fortifier, which could have been a steroid. There was only one early hormone extract, Serodose A+B, widely available in cycling from about 1962; another Decca-dorabulin had been on the market from 1959 and available in Simpson's hometown of Ghent from the mid-1960s. At the time though neither product had been banned.[60]

The rise of anti-doping ideology and practice

Cycling would be inextricably linked with the emergence of an anti-doping ideology in the post-war period. Dimeo has argued that as an ideology anti-doping was a social and cultural construction, which reflected the social and sporting values of those who drove the thinking behind anti-doping. But up until the 1960s there were no doping controls or tests in place to identify athletes using drugs. Instead, criticism of drugs in sport would revolve around the notions of fairness and the health of athletes.

Criticisms and concerns had begun to harden from the 1950s in both America and Europe.[61] In 1957, echoing earlier criticism of the 'professionalism' of American amateur college sport, the American Medical Association had passed a resolution condemning the 'alleged widespread use of amphetamine substances by coaches, trainers and athletes to improve athletic performance'. Two years later a special edition of its journal was devoted to the use of amphetamines in sport.[62] The Italian sports medicine authorities were also showing a growing interest in doping in cycling. In 1955 the first ever anti-doping convention was held after a number of incidents in cycling had brought 'unhealthy practices' to the attention of scientists.[63] Highlighting the shifting climate on the issue, Fausto Coppi, after his retirement in 1958, was actually questioned on the subject during a television interview. He was asked, 'Did you take drugs?', to which he replied 'Only when necessary.' When asked, 'And how often was it necessary?', Coppi hesitated, smiled and said, 'Practically all the time.'[64] The IOC was also aware of doping in sport. In 1950, for example, it was alleged that the Danish team doctor, Axel Mathiesens, provided the rowing team with Androstin in a 12-day period leading up to the European Championships.[65] The issue of doping even received papal intervention when in 1956 Pope Pius XII contributed an article titled, 'Let us condemn the practice of doping.'[66]

Attitudes within the medical profession were ambivalent towards anti-doping; there was no universal medical policy on the issue during this period. In his book, *The Human Machine* (1956), Adolphe Abrahams gives a critical analysis of the use of certain stimulants, which included caffeine, strychnine and amphetamines. He was actually sceptical about their ability to 'increase athletic efficiency'. However, there was little sense of any moral opprobrium about their use, although he admitted that the sporting authorities wanted to forbid them and had wanted him to provide a definition of drugs. Abrahams admitted that this was difficult. He even admitted to having experimented with one of them on himself, sodium phosphate. He added that:

> It would be impossible to eliminate these indispensable constituents that occur in Nature. Is their additional administration in the form of tablets, capsules, mixtures, or injections to be permitted, encouraged, deprecated, or forbidden?[67]

When using drugs, Abrahams' advice was 'use your common sense'. In *Sports Medicine* (1962) J.G.P. Williams similarly argued that:

> The moral objections to "doping" are somewhat difficult to define. It is all very well to say that anybody who artificially improves his performance by taking drugs is "not playing the game" but where is the line drawn in the case of a drug which has a therapeutic as well as stimulant effect?[68]

While acknowledging the potential enhancing qualities of amphetamines, Williams pointed to the potential of addiction not in a public health sense but with reference to athletic performance. At this stage there was little scientific evidence on the effectiveness of these substances.

The ossification of anti-doping as an ideology and a practice was dependent on a number of factors. First, as we have seen in Chapter 4, the Cold War had created a sporting arms race as well as a nuclear one. Second, the death of the Danish cyclist Knud Enemark Jensen at the 1960 Olympics also brought the issue of drugs to a wider public audience. Whatever the real reasons for Jensen's death,[69] it was partly attributed to his use of drugs. As a result, however, it forced the IOC to engage with the perceived dangers posed by unregulated doping.[70] Finally, the counter culture emerged in the 1960s. With a rise in the consumption of recreational drugs, highlighted by the 'hippy revolution', a desire for a more natural existence grew.[71] The passing in Britain of the Misuse of Drugs Act in 1971, a relatively punitive piece of legislation that was a legacy of James Callaghan, Home Secretary for the previous British Labour government, was essentially a reaction to the explosion of cannabis and heroin use in late 1960s London.[72] While the use of drugs in sport were for totally different philosophical reasons compared to the consumption of drugs such as cannabis, it added to a general climate of anxiety within society about their use and created a reaction amongst establishment groups that 'something must be done'.

After hoping the issue would go away, the IOC, under the Presidency of the American Avery Brundage (1952–72), set up a doping sub-committee in 1962 headed by Arthur Porritt who had expressed anti-drug sentiments in the 1920s (see above). The first European Conference on Doping and the Biological Preparation of the Competitive Athlete was the following year and the definition of doping that it came up with formed the basis of anti-doping throughout the world. The United Nations Educational, Scientific and Cultural Organization (UNESCO) also established a sub-committee on doping. In 1965 the British scientist Professor Arnold Beckett devised the first testing procedures, which were first introduced in British cycling's Milk Race in 1966. Testing was also conducted at the 1966 football World Cup.[73] The involvement of British scientists and administrators in designing the initial anti-doping schemes reflected wider social and sporting traditions. They were men of a certain generation who felt that sport meant something more than winning. As Dimeo argues, they belonged to elite social groups who 'wanted to fashion sport in their image: the established amateur traditional culture'.[74]

Despite these initiatives, there continued to be uncertainty over what constituted a banned substance. In 1966 the IOC doping commission presented a preliminary list of substances that would be prohibited at the Mexico City Olympics. Anabolic steroids were not on it as there was no test for them. On the use of the anabolic steroid, 'Dianabol', BASM stated that, while its use should be discouraged, it was also of 'no practical value'.[75] Reflecting the IOC's paternalistic sensibilities, it was stated that the 'problem of doping can be met only by a long-term education policy stressing the physical and moral aspects of the subject'.[76] In 1967 the IOC established its own Medical Commission, headed by the Belgian aristocrat, Prince Alexandre de Merode. Hunt has argued that under Brundage the IOC had dragged its feet in setting up the Commission because there was a tendency amongst its members to see doping as 'a problem of image management rather than a medical or ethical issue'.[77] Initially, de Merode had intended for the IOC itself to act as the central anti-doping agency. Instead, Brundage gave power to the international sporting federations and at a stroke diluted the IOC's attempts to control and influence the issue and which weren't revived until the formation of the World Anti-Doping Agency (WADA) in 1999.

In France there was direct government action. Following a campaign led by Dr Pierre Dumas to raise awareness of the health risks of doping from the 1950s, legislation was passed in 1965 that targeted the use of stimulants in sport. In line with the French government's interventionist policy on sport,[78] doping was seen as a public health matter because, it was believed, athletes, especially cyclists who enjoyed great popularity, acted as role models for young people. Anti-doping laws were also passed in Belgium (1965) and Italy (1971), the two other major cycling nations. However, the French government soon turned over its responsibilities for drug tests to the sports federations, which as with the IOC's actions led to conflict of interest: sporting bodies would not want to attract negative headlines and jeopardize the future of their sport by exposing widespread doping.[79] Image management became a major priority for sport and its governing bodies when facing the problem of doping.[80]

During the Tour de France in 1966 riders resisted testing and they staged a go-slow in protest against these measures. Also that year the first five in the world championship all refused to take a drugs test, including Jaques Anquetil, five times winner of the Tour de France who in 1988 admitted to drug use.[81] However, the death of Tom Simpson in 1967 gave a greater urgency amongst sporting administrators to make testing stricter. Importantly, his demise on Mount Ventoux took place in a different media environment with his death not only making the front pages in France, Britain and America but it also featured grim images of Simpson's last moments. His collapse was also captured by French television, giving the whole issue greater amplification and heightening public fears around drugs more generally.[82] At the autopsy amphetamine was discovered in Simpson's body, which further demonized the use of performance-enhancing drugs and led to further criticism of cycling, especially the Tour and its excesses.

In addition to the health of athletes, fairness was another ideal that was promoted as part of the IOC's rhetoric concerning anti-doping. It was also used with respect to two other issues that emerged in the 1960s. First, gender testing was introduced (see Chapter 7).[83] Second, with the 1968 Olympics being held at altitude in Mexico City there were concerns about how athletes would perform. However, as we have seen in Chapter 4, the IOC continued to see the issue in terms of amateurism and restricted athletes preparation.[84] Nevertheless, fuelled by Cold War rivalry, there had been an exponential increase in the use of drugs amongst athletes both in Western nations and then in Eastern bloc countries from the 1950s. Instead of amphetamines the drug of choice now was anabolic steroids. In 1954, at the world weightlifting championships, the US team physician John Ziegler had been told by his Soviet counterpart that his athletes were taking testosterone. On his return Ziegler began to experiment with testosterone and the anabolic steroid, Dianabol. News of its success in weightlifting spread to athletics and American football.[85] At the 1972 Olympics it was claimed – by their own doctor – that every American weightlifter was using some sort of performance-enhancing drug.[86]

Whereas athletes in the West generally relied upon informal networks for their drugs, in the communist countries drug use was state sponsored. During the 1970s the German Democratic Republic emerged as a sporting superpower. There has been a popular perception that its success was built solely on its state-sponsored doping programme that was run by the Stasi, the country's secret police.[87] From 1974 a work group 'unterstutzende Mittel' (uM) was given responsibility for overseeing the planning and distribution of drugs to all sports. Recent research by Barbara Cole and Dimeo and Hunt, however, has pointed to a more nuanced interpretation of the GDR sports system and the role of doping. Instead, it was part of a comprehensive sports medicine system, which included other aspects of sports science as well as talent identification programmes. Moreover, athletes were largely positive about their experiences of the East German system, many were aware of what drugs they were taking and their motivations were mostly personal rather than politically inspired.[88]

So efficient was the overall GDR system, built on a population of 17 million, that even the Soviet Union began to see it as much of a rival as Western nations.[89] The effects of using anabolic steroids also brought about changes in the physiological make-up of some of the athletes, especially women. At the 1976 Summer Games East German swimmers made a considerable impression both in and out of the pool. Kornelia Ender won four gold medals but both her and her teammates were described as having an 'incredible physical discrepancy' compared to their American counterparts. While senior GDR female athletes were sworn to silence about taking what were termed 'performance-enhancing supplements', those under eighteen were told that their 'little blue pills' were vitamins.[90] They were not only physically bigger but also begun to develop some of the visible side-effects that would be associated with the use of anabolic steroids, especially a deep voice and the growth of body hair. It was later discovered that some of the adverse effects on female athletes were not reversible. These included menstrual abnormalities, shrinkage of the breasts and male-pattern baldness.[91]

By 1975 a test had been devised by British scientists to detect anabolic steroids, like Dianabol, and these were added to the banned list. However, those countries with sophisticated medical support found it relatively easy to find loopholes in the system. Most importantly, testing was not done outside of competition, therefore, if athletes stopped taking the anabolic steroids three weeks before the test they could not be detected. In addition, what was becoming clear was that athletes were being assisted in their attempts by the sporting authorities to get around the tests. Some national bodies, including the United States, looked upon the new testing protocol as a way to beat the system. East German scientists devised a 'testosterone loophole' in which detectable synthetic anabolic steroids were replaced with injections of testosterone-depot, in the final few weeks. As testosterone was naturally occurring these doses could not be differentiated from hormones normally found in the body.[92] Despite the new test few athletes tested positive at the 1976 Montreal Olympics. Again, it stemmed from both the lack of a universal central body solely responsible for drug testing and a nationalist impulse, which meant that to keep up with your sporting competitors the need to take performance-enhancing drugs became greater.

In their efforts to catch up with the USSR and increasingly the GDR, Hunt has argued that American sporting bodies were complicit in their attempts to make the LA Olympics in 1984 a success. The Soviet authorities had been similarly complicit in making Moscow 1980 the 'purest' Games ever due to the tampering of samples and the integrity of the testing. On being warned of changes to drug testing protocols at the 1983 Pan-American Games, the US chef de mission advised his athletes to go home if they had been taking drugs: twelve members of the US track and field team did so to avoid the new testing procedures but of those that remained several were caught. One episode in sporting relations between East and West verged on black humour. It took place at the 1986 Goodwill Games in Moscow; a competition that had been organized to repair sporting relations after the boycotts in 1980 and 1984. To cement this goodwill the Soviet authorities forewarned the travelling US athletes that they would be subject to rigorous drug testing. This allowed the Americans time to cease their anabolic steroid cycles well before competition and thus when they were tested they would be 'clean'. On their arrival the US athletes discovered that there was to be no testing at all, allowing Soviet athletes to take their medication as late as possible and giving them a competitive advantage.[93]

Drug use in British sport

In Britain, perhaps more than in other countries, given its sporting heritage, the calls for banning drugs were very vocal and were combined with a strict moral dimension. In 1987 Arthur Gold, the chairman of the Sports Council's Drugs

Advisory Group, invoking a moral form of rhetoric, referred to the issue as 'a battle for the hearts and minds of men'. He continued to vigorously argue that, 'No one will defend in public the illicit use of drugs. It is dishonest. It is cheating and unhealthy. The person taking drugs is not only a rogue, but a fool'.[94] But the whole issue continued to expose many contradictions regarding the role of science and medicine in sport. In 1986 Sebastian Coe, winner of the Olympic 1,500 metres in 1980 and 1984, somewhat puzzlingly 'urged competitors to use scientific research to improve performances rather than cheat by taking drugs.' It is of course stating the obvious that the use of drugs in sport was due to scientific research. Coe further argued that, 'Not to use the latest scientific research is a willful refusal to think. It is intellectually bereft'. Again highlighting the grey area between what constitutes the difference between legal and illegal, Coe argued that blood chemistry analysis and isokinetic assessment were examples of 'valid ways' for athletes to improve their performance. 'Let us make the doctors and scientists work for us rather than the other way around', he added.[95]

Rumours charges and accusations were later made that the British sporting authorities were corrupt and had been complicit in dampening efforts to catch those British athletes using illegal performance-enhancing substances. In 1987 the Minister for Sport, Colin Moynihan, claimed that some British governing bodies had 'made deals' to ensure that certain competitors would not be tested for drugs at important events. Moynihan along with Coe had conducted their own inquiry and found considerable evidence of malpractice regarding testing procedures. One of Moynihan's main criticisms revolved around what he believed was a national governing body's conflict of interest in being responsible for the testing system, which left it open to possible corruption due to pressure from commercial sponsors anxious to exploit television opportunities. Instead, echoing international criticism of the drug-testing system, he advocated the establishment of an independent body.[96]

Moynihan's claims were supported in two reports. First, an independent investigation by *The Times* and then the AAA sponsored Coni Report. As Waddington has argued, both found that an informal doping infrastructure existed,

> consisting of networks of relationships between athletes, coaches, doctors and ... some sports administrators who were involved in supplying, using, monitoring and concealing (or at least 'turning a blind eye' to) the use of drugs.[97]

While the Coni Report agreed with many of the newspaper's findings it was a public relations exercise, which aimed to dampen *The Times'* conclusions. It also argued that partly because of the implementation of out-of-competition testing in 1986 in British athletics and the side-effects due to prolonged use of anabolic steroids, the use of drug in sport was in decline. Instead, there was no evidence of this. Afterwards it was revealed that the British sports doctor,

Jimmy Ledington, had provided steroids to British athletes and gave advice on how to avoid testing positive.[98]

'Snooker loopy, nuts are we': Beta-blockers and Bill Werbeniuk

For the most part the controversy around drugs since the 1970s has been centred on the use of drugs in sports, such as athletics, cycling, swimming and weightlifting, which required either endurance or explosive qualities. In the 1980s though with the extension of the IOC's list of banned substances more sports were drawn into anti-doping debates and the accompanying anxieties about drugs in society more generally. One such sport was snooker. Snooker, it can be argued, is the antithesis of a healthy body; it has been said that to be good at snooker is a sign of mis-spent youth. However, mainly due to the influence of television, it was one of the boom sports in Britain during the 1980s. On the face of it, its connection with drugs may seem surprising as it was a game without any physical contact and through marketing had carefully built a reputation as a gentlemanly one with a high-level of sportsmanship.

However, this squeaky-clean image began to change in 1985 when the IOC added beta-blockers to its banned list of drugs. Unofficial tests at the Los Angeles Olympics had indicated that a majority of athletes competing in the modern pentathlon had used beta-blockers during the shooting event. Before the Games the IOC medical commission had permitted their use but only if prescribed by the athlete's doctors. Beta-blockers have been used in the treatment of hypertension and heart disease but can be effective for those athletes in so-called target sports like archery, golf, shooting and snooker. The drug reduces muscle tremors for prolonged periods and can suppress adrenalin flows, thus helping players cope with the pressure when faced with a particular putt or shot.[99] But after 1985 even medically-prescribed beta-blockers were banned by the IOC and then the UK Sports Council.

In 1985 a number of players had tested positive for beta-blockers at that year's Snooker World Championships, although the results were not made public at the time.[100] At the outset the World Professional Billiards and Snooker Association (WPBSA) resisted calls for the drug to be banned. At the same time as the story over beta-blockers broke, the sport was embroiled in a sensationalized story concerning the addiction to cocaine of another player, the Canadian, Kirk Stevens. Ironically, an opponent Silvino Francisco, who after defeating Stevens had exposed the story, was fined by the WPBSA.[101] The entire episode though brought the issue of drugs in the sport into the media glare. This spotlight had been intensified through the prevailing rhetoric of the Conservative government on drugs in society. It railed against the legacy of the permissive society from the 1960s and instead preached individual responsibility and restraint, especially the use of social drugs, which was believed to be part of a wider decline in moral values.

Prominent among the players who had failed the test in 1985 was Rex Williams, the chairman of the WPBSA itself. Williams claimed that he was prescribed beta-blockers because of depression and had been taking them over a number of years.[102] Like Williams, those who were thought to take beta-blockers were middle-aged. Two years later, however, Neal Foulds who was then aged 23 admitted to using beta-blockers on doctors' orders.[103] The WPBSA had not banned beta-blockers and it had actually reduced the number of drugs tests. Instead testing was undertaken according to the rules of the association. Of course, snooker was not an Olympic sport and did not have to take its lead from the IOC. In addition, it also reflected how international federations, rather than a centralized body, had sole authority over how they ran their sport. However, the Sports Council did have to take its lead from the IOC and it also disbursed money to individual sports for testing. The sport, therefore, had to comply with its rules, which included drug testing based on the IOC's procedures, mainly to maintain its public image.[104]

In 1988, after the Sports Council had threatened to withdraw funding for the sport's drug testing system, the WPBSA banned certain types of beta-blockers and even Williams had agreed to come off them.[105] One player though stubbornly refused – Bill Werbeniuk. Werbeniuk suffered from Familial Benign Essential Tremor.[106] It was a hereditary tremor which meant that his cueing arm shook when playing a shot. The only cure doctors prescribed was to drink copious amounts of alcohol; sometimes up to forty pints a day.[107] His alcohol intake though produced a rapid heartbeat. In an attempt to steady this he began to use the beta-blocker drug, Inderal.[108] To try and get around the problem, the World Professional Billiards and Snooker Association's (WPBSA) medical advisor recommended that he take another beta-blocker, Atenolol, but Werbeniuk claimed that his doctor would not prescribe it for him. Werbeniuk continued to play on but was eventually fined for refusing to take a test. He was subsequently suspended and played his final match in 1990.[109]

The issue of the use of performance-enhancing drugs in snooker, however, not only reflected the growing anxieties concerning drugs in sport but it also exposed many of the contradictions. When the story first broke there was a sense that 'these things did not happen in snooker'. Former world champion Terry Griffiths casually remarked about the introduction of drug testing at the 1985 World Championships that, 'I suppose it is a good thing. It clears everything up officially'. Moreover, the sport's governing body buttressed the announcement of the tests with a suitable public relations campaign that attempted to take the moral high ground and demonstrate snooker as a 'clean sport'. Importantly, it was mindful of 'preserving the good image of snooker' because it wanted to illustrate 'to the millions of *young people* (my italics) playing snooker all over the world that the illegal substances will not be tolerated in our sport'; this re-affirmation of course was also aimed at their sponsors. Predictably perhaps press muck-raking was blamed for the rumours.[110] Once the revelations of the use of beta-blockers became public though there followed the familiar unsporting, anti-drug rhetoric. Former world champion, Ray Reardon, said that he had been unaware of any players using this medication but if they had done so he felt that it was 'most unfair' even if they were on beta-blockers on medical advice as it was helping their game. He added, 'I know the pressures of snooker. Lately there have been many times when I have needed something. But I love this game too much to do so.'[111] In Parliament Colin Moynihan accused Neal Foulds of cheating.[112]

The glaring irony (or hypocrisy) throughout the entire episode was that at the time three of the game's main sponsors were tobacco manufacturers: Embassy, Rothmans and Benson and Hedges. After stepping down as the WPBSA chairman, Rex Williams suggested that smoking during tournaments should be banned because nicotine had steadying qualities.[113] Werbeniuk almost perfectly summed up the complexities and contradictions about those drugs which had been banned but had been prescribed for a medical condition: 'Inderal [the beta-blocker] is not a performance-enhancing drug, it is a performance-enabling drug for me.'[114] From the perspective that doping controls were designed to protect the health of athletes, it is not without irony that the snooker authorities had deemed that it was permissible for someone to smoke and drink forty pints per day in front of the television cameras but not to take one little pill. Instead, of course, of more concern to them was the sport's image and its appeal to television audiences and sponsors, and at this particular time drinking and smoking despite their public health issues were deemed more acceptable than what was perceived as the smear of drug-taking.

Ben Johnson, WADA and the political fall-out

Throughout the 1980s the drip-drip effect of scandals and rumours had meant that, 'Increasingly, doping scandals were perceived as damaging to international sport'.[115] The disqualification of Ben Johnson at the 1988 Seoul Olympics though, because of the publicity and scrutiny it brought, proved to be a turning point. The now instant global visibility of sport through television had also increased its political value. A new political climate emerged in which governments began to take a greater interest in anti-doping for reasons of expediency. It was within this context that a more autonomous anti-doping agency, the World Anti-Doping Agency (WADA), would (eventually) be established in 1999.

Because of this changing perception regarding sport and drugs, governments played a greater role in shaping not only anti-doping policies but also reinforcing the whole rhetoric around the subject. The establishment of the Dubin Commission by the Canadian government to investigate the Ben Johnson affair had set the precedent. The end of the Cold War had also signaled the end of the GDR sports system. In addition, by the end of the 1980s the Soviet Union began to suffer a decline in its global sporting status. Because it was unable to keep up with developments in Western pharmacology it now wanted reform of doping regulations. At the 1988 Seoul Games, in the spirit of *Perestroika* perhaps, the Soviet President Mikhail Gorbachev had ordered that all Soviet competitors had to pass a pre-competition test before they were allowed to compete.[116]

Later China brought itself into the anti-doping fold. When China first returned to the international sporting arena there were fears that it would embark on a GDR-style, state-sponsored drug system. These fears seemed to be confirmed with the success in the early 1990s of Chinese athletes and swimmers, and their subsequent disqualification. In March 1995, however, following international criticism China enacted a series of strict anti-doping regulations on its own initiative.[117] Ironically, it was now complying with the sporting values that were associated with Western liberal democracies. It again reflected the growing perception of the importance attached to sport by national governments; while during the Cold War success by any means was all that mattered, it was now important that a country's athletes – who were both representing their country and receiving money from the state – should be seen to be 'clean' as well as successful.

Importantly in America, where its sporting bodies had been as complicit as any other country,[118] there was a change in the political climate that reflected a shift towards the 'moral right'. In the 1990s Bill Clinton appointed Barry McCaffery as the White House 'drug czar' to fight a 'War on Drugs'. McCaffery identified drugs in sport as an aspect of a more general drugs problem amongst young Americans not one limited to the world of sport. For McCaffrey, doping set a bad example for American youths and he did not differentiate between doping and recreational drugs. Moreover, McCaffrey regarded top athletes as role models and they needed to be 'clean' to set an appropriate example – rhetoric that had echoes of the French government in the 1960s.[119] In 2000 a report by the Office of National Drug Control Policy stressed the value of sport to society and urged a tightening of doping policies. Three years later George W Bush's State of the Union Address referred to anti-doping and signaled the US government's increasing role in enforcing anti-doping procedures.[120]

Calls for change in the anti-doping sporting landscape were given a further boost after the much-publicized Festina crisis in the Tour de France of 1998. It not only highlighted the deeply rooted drug culture within the sport but the subsequent police investigation revealed an extensive, incestuous network of relationships between riders, coaches, doctors and officials that had contributed to a particular cycling culture. This network was uncovered a few days before the start of the 1998 Tour when Willy Voet, a soigneur for the Festina team, was arrested by French police after crossing the border from Belgium. The police found 250 batches of anabolic steroids and 400 ampoules of EPO – the new drug of choice for cyclists – in his car. The team's headquarters were searched soon after and the police found other suspect products.[121]

WADA was formed in November 1999 with Dick Pound as its first President. There had been a push for a more centralized anti-doping body since 1988. It had taken over ten years for it to be established, partly due to resistance from the IOC President, Juan Samaranch, who was more concerned about the damage that doping scandals could inflict on the Olympics carefully nurtured image and therefore its commercial potential. But with the impending departure of Samaranch in 2001, the election of Jacques Rogge signaled a much more determined anti-doping campaign. Pound believed deeply in the ideals of the Olympic movement and he approached his job with a certain evangelical zeal. He viewed drugs in sport as a 'disease' that had to be eliminated. Yet Pound was also a realist and had been critical of the previous inaction on doping. In particular, as early as 1989 he pointed out that, 'We [the IOC] still have no clearly stated definition of what doping is'.[122]

WADA's formation had also been a product of increasing distrust of the IOC within America, its biggest financial donor, and also the European Union following the 1998 Salt Lake City Scandal. In 2001 WADA made a hugely symbolic and significant statement by moving its headquarters from Lausanne, the home of the IOC, to Montreal, which also reflected a shift in power of anti-doping policy from the IOC to North America. As a consequence, American sports, such as baseball and football, which had not been part of the Olympics and had generally ignored any doping regulations, now came under the same scrutiny as the Olympic sports. At WADA Pound aimed to introduce a robust transnational doping policy. In 2003 the Copenhagen Declaration on Anti-Doping in Sport committed the world's leading athletic bodies (including the IOC) to the World Anti-Doping Code. Pressure was applied to those sporting federations, like the International Cycling Union, who had initially baulked to sign up. The code was later ratified by UNESCO as well as national governments. It reflected how responsibility of the issue was now being taken out of the hands of sporting federations and being placed with more powerful political bodies.[123]

Conclusion

In 2008 the British sprinter Dwain Chambers lost his appeal to overturn the ban imposed by the BOA to prevent him from competing at future Olympic Games. Chambers had been banned because he was a 'convicted drugs cheat' – in the words and eyes of the media and many of the public – and the BOA had a policy of not selecting anyone who had been banned for this offence. Chambers had been one of the athletes caught up in the BALCO scandal. BALCO (Bay Area Laboratory Co-operative) was a San Francisco-based company. Between 1988 and 2002 it was accused of supplying performance-enhancing drugs to elite athletes, including Major League Baseball players. A federal investigation of BALCO and its owner Victor Conte began in 2002, which tested 550 athletes; twenty were found to be taking tetrahydrogestrinone (THG), a type of synthetic steroid, and undetectable until then. Other athletes who were implicated included Olympic sprint champion, Marion Jones and Barry Bonds, holder of baseball batting records.[124] Afterwards, in response to the moral opprobrium that had accompanied his actions, Chambers was more penitent. He accepted his 'guilt' after realizing his 'mistake' because taking drugs was wrong and he later spread 'the message' amongst young people about the 'dangers' of using drugs on behalf of UK Athletics. It was a message imbued with a morality that echoed past cries about the unfairness of athletes taking drugs.

It is perhaps ironic that when the consumption and production of medicine has increased sport is the one area that is trying to eradicate its use. Or at least, it is trying to control its use in line with what it deems acceptable. This sense of 'acceptability' though has its roots in ideas that can be traced back to notions of amateurism. Despite the shifting politics in the anti-doping landscape, it is unlikely that the authorities will be ever able to eradicate drugs in sport as much because it is difficult to define what is meant by artificial enhancement. Moreover, as Thomas Hunt points out, we live in a performance-enhanced society where the use of stimulants abound in other areas of life from air force pilots to students revising for exams. It begs the question where does treatment stop and enhancement begin?[125] Like a number of commentators, Andy Miah has argued that because of a combination of the volume of new scientific research, particularly with reference to new genetic technologies, and sport's commercial demands we should give up the fight to distinguish the line between fair and unfair advantages. Instead, there should be a greater concentration on making sport safer.[126]

Where will all this end? It won't of course – at least while modern sports continue to be invested with the values of competition. As per Tom Simpson's opening quote, athletes have been willing to push their bodies to the limit since the onset of modern sport. Health risks, in what ever context, have been eschewed in the quest to gain an edge over an opponent.

6

Repairing the Athletic Body

Treatments, Practices and Ethics

During the 1988 Seoul Olympics the British middle-distance runner Peter Elliott sustained an injury to his groin. In order for him to continue competing at the Games he was given a cortisone injection before each subsequent race. Even though he could now race, it meant that the injury would be exacerbated and it would eventually keep him out of athletics for more than a year. For Elliott the knowledge of the consequences of this injury was compensated with the silver medal that he won in the 1,500 metres.[1] The case in point highlighted not only some of the dilemmas that athletes faced regarding injuries, particularly how far can they push their bodies before they sustain serious injury but also that essentially elite sport is about excess rather than the cultivation of a healthy body. The bodies of professional sportsmen and women have a limited amount of 'athletic capital' that allows them to compete for a certain number of years. Any 'athletic death' is not only conditioned by the ageing process but also by the wear and tear inflicted on them through training and competition. 'Body management', therefore, and the recovery from both minor and serious injuries has been a crucial and accepted part of an athlete's working life. These demands further highlighted the unique needs of this particular patient – the athlete – and the difficulties of the medical profession in treating them. George Sheehan, an American cardiologist and a runner who wrote a training book on the subject, believed that 'the athlete is medicine's most difficult patient'. He mused that:

> Physicians who handle emergencies with éclat, who drive fearlessly into abdomens for bleeding aneurysms, who think nothing of managing cardiac arrest and heart failure, who miraculously reassemble accident victims, are helpless when confronted with an ailing athlete. They are even less able to counsel the athlete and [answer] his never-ending questions about health.[2]

Whereas the previous two chapters concentrated on enhancement, here we are more concerned with the enabling of athletic performance; how the day-to-day practices concerning injuries and their treatment have developed. As a site for medicine, sport has operated outside the control of the medical profession, if not the influence of medical professionals. Instead, individual sports have developed their own medical sub-cultures. Not only has this been evident in the treatments and practices that athletes have experienced but also through the particular tensions that have revolved around the ethics of the practitioner-patient relationship within elite sport.

In conjunction with the sporting medical sub-culture that athletes have inhabited, we can also see the treatment of athletes' injuries in light of the shifting boundaries between orthodox and alternative medicine since the nineteenth century. In essence, since the nineteenth century, medical orthodoxy has been based on its political legitimacy while alternative medicine has been demarcated in terms of its political marginality. As Saks has argued, definitions of both are relative to their political importance and not necessarily 'objectively derived from the "scientific" or "non-scientific" status of the knowledge involved'.[3] For example, the dismissal by doctors of some treatments as 'quack remedies' reflected the on-going professionalization of medicine as the medical profession attempted to marginalize 'alternative' practitioners. Alternative medicine had not officially existed in Britain before orthodox medicine came into being with the 1858 Medical Registration Act. As a consequence, herbalists, midwife-healers, bonesetters and others competed for custom with physicians, surgeons and apothecaries in an open market. Until then there was no national unified, enforceable legal monopoly of medicine despite the existence of various organizations for physicians, surgeons and apothecaries. Even after 1858 the market did not disappear. While in some European countries the doctor was under direct state bureaucratic control, in Britain there was a 'modified free field'. By contrast, the demand for the services of alternative healers in America, especially osteopaths, has been greater, reflecting the lack of a national health service and also a more liberal medical marketplace.[4] The medical profession in Britain had been granted the right to self-regulate but the government did not award it a legal monopoly as alternative/unorthodox healers were still allowed to practice under the common law. However, it was now illegal for these practitioners to claim that they had any medical qualifications they did not possess. Instead, a *de facto* monopoly emerged that put alternative practitioners at a competitive disadvantage. In addition, specialization within medicine was not an inevitable process. Instead, it was a political one with each specialty struggling with one another in the pursuit of state recognition and funding.[5] These tensions have also been evident in sport's medical marketplace.

As with the training of athletes, early methods for the treatment of injuries were initially carried out by trainers and coaches. They usually had little formal medical training and used popular forms of medicine to treat minor ailments.[6] For corns and bunions, leeches could be applied to the feet while, following a couple of days of rest, the treatment of strains and bruises involved rubbing the injured area frequently with spirit embrocation, and then holding the leg under a cold water tap for as long and as often as could be tolerated.[7] Boxing trainers, many of whom were former fighters themselves and predominantly from working class backgrounds, similarly used traditional methods that persisted deep into the twentieth century. In preparation for fights, for example, trainers would 'pickle' the faces and fists of boxers to harden the skin against blows to prevent cuts.[8] A common remedy for black eyes was the application of raw steak while to treat a boxer's cauliflower ear one trainer would 'bind a freshly roasted white mouse tightly over it'.[9] During fights trainers used a variety of substances, some that doctors might have termed 'quack remedies', such as cow dung, spiders' webs, tannic acid and nitric acid, to stem the blood from cuts that boxers had suffered.[10]

In 1920s America the trainers of college football teams were from similar backgrounds to those in Britain. It was claimed that the trainer's role lacked definition because of the growing importance of the coach in the sport and they had been reduced to minor duties such as tending equipment as well as providing medical care under the direction of the team physician. The Carnegie report on *American College Athletics* noted that few trainers had 'any scientific training' and that 'tradition, superstition and prejudice have usurped the place that should be filled by scientific reason and knowledge'. It was said that,

> the trainer's locker has become a quack cabinet overflowing with proprietary ointments, liniments, and washes, and his quarters a museum of old and new appliances for applying heat, water, light, massage, and electricity.[11]

Sports medicine has also been shaped by national cultures and attitudes to medicine more generally. In Irish sport, for example, the tradition of alternative practices has persisted. For example, Billy Ritchie, the trainer of Glentoran FC in east Belfast, was a bonesetter and ran a successful sports injury clinic from his home.[12] Ossie Bennett, a self-taught masseur, worked with many GAA teams and athletes while Dan O'Neill was a farmer who also ran a busy bonesetting clinic. His clients included both athletes and animals.[13] Sean Boylan, a manager in Gaelic football, was also a practicing herbalist. He was manager of Meath for twenty-three years and used various herbal remedies for the alleviation of players' muscle fatigue and other ailments. In 1988, a week before the All-Ireland Final replay, one player, Liam Harnan broke a bone in his shoulder. After applying a comfrey poultice and some physiotherapy, he was able to play without any injection.[14]

The British football trainer

One of sports medicine's most emblematic images has been that of the football trainer running on the field to treat a player with his so-called magic sponge.[15] More than any other role, the football trainer has highlighted both developments in the treatment of athletes and the management of injuries. It also provides an insight into the history of the relationship between sport and medicine, especially with regard to physiotherapy, as well as on-going tensions between orthodox medicine and alternative practices. While the image of the football trainer with his bucket and magic sponge has been both mythologized and derided, it is important to put his role into context. Football clubs were professional and commercial operations and generally sought the best available medical care for their players. However, the demand for medical care was also shaped by firstly, football's production process, which in turn was largely a product of the changing nature of the game's commercialization; and secondly, a footballing sub-culture that in Britain has been built on a practical tradition, placing the virtues of experience over those of qualified expertise.[16]

A demand for football trainers had emerged after the FA had legalized professionalism in 1885. Initially, there were limited ideas on what comprised training for footballers and the first generation of football trainers was largely made up of ex-professional athletes and athletic and rowing trainers.[17] Their job was initially divided up into a number of duties: day-to-day responsibility of the players; getting players fit; and treating their injuries. The only organization that offered training that would have been any use to a football trainer was the Society of Trained Masseuses, formed in 1894.[18] Massage had been part of the British medical scene for many centuries but in the late Victorian period it had enjoyed a revival. Heggie has argued that this revival reflected wider trends in modernity and massage was part of the uptake of 'scientific' training and medical treatment.[19] However, the Society was dominated by women and given the masculine nature of football it was unlikely that clubs would employ qualified female masseuses.[20] Athletic coaches in Britain, such as Harry Andrews and Sam Mussabini, were fulsome in their praise of massage's 'health-giving' qualities. Massage for athletes was also widespread in America and Australia. In addition, highlighting the huge trade in 'quack remedies' during this period, a niche market for massage liniments, herbal potions, patent pills and tonics opened up and was directed in part at the sporting world.[21] In 1899, for example, it was claimed that every side that had won the FA Cup since 1893 had used Gratton's Embrocation.[22] Although football and athletic trainers shared similar medical techniques, the Society of Trained Masseuses showed little interest in their work or recruiting them. Instead, it had been too concerned about establishing the Society's own professional credentials.[23]

During the inter-war years the trainer began to take on a more physiotherapeutic role. In one newspaper article under the headline, 'Diplomat and Psychologist', it was said that a trainer 'must be a masseur [and] conversant with every form of modern electrical device'.[24] While massage was still part of the job, this change owed something to the legacy of physiotherapy from the First World War. Physiotherapy had enjoyed a 'good war', mainly because of the rehabilitation of disabled soldiers through physical therapy that placed an emphasis on active treatment.[25] The attitudes of the medical profession to physiotherapy began to shift and many orthodox practitioners had gradually come to accept its benefits. Physical medicine had also emerged as a specialty amongst some doctors and there had been a move towards the use of electrical treatments. However, physiotherapy itself continued to occupy a subordinate status within medicine.[26] A larger body of expertise on the treatment of injuries had emerged during the inter-war years that incorporated physiotherapy. Dr Charles Heald, an advocate of physiotherapy and also the physician in charge of the electro-therapeutic department at the Royal Free Hospital, wrote a pioneering book entitled, *Injuries and Sport: A General Guide for the Practitioner.*[27] In addition, the surgeon, William Eldon Tucker, contributed an essay on 'Athletic Injuries' to *The British Encyclopaedia of Medical Practice.*[28] In the late 1930s the Football Association published its first coaching manual, which contained a chapter on the treatment of injuries.[29]

During the inter-war period most football trainers came from the first generation of former players. Some had also gained medical experience during the war[30] and by 1938 it was claimed that the medical knowledge of a growing number of trainers was supported by diplomas in massage and physical instruction.[31] The most famous trainer during the inter-war years was Tom Whittaker of Arsenal, then the most successful and modern club in England. After retiring from the game through injury in 1925, he was sent by the club 'to take a course of lessons' under the tutelage of Sir Robert Jones, the pioneering orthopaedic surgeon, in which he studied 'anatomy, massage, medical gymnastics and electrical therapy'. Whittaker was later the regular trainer for the England team.[32]

Because they were now insured employees under the 1906 Workmen's Compensation Act (see Chapter 2), the medical care offered by clubs exhibited the characteristics of occupational health.[33] The bigger clubs, unsurprisingly, were able to afford the best medical facilities. Up to 1914 Aston Villa was the wealthiest club in the land and in that year it outlined proposals to build 'a special room for the doctor' to be fitted up with 'X-rays, radium and other modern appliances'.[34] The growing use of electro-medical apparatus, such as sunlamps, reflected how clubs were employing a more scientific approach to treating injuries.[35] Electrotherapy, hydrotherapy and exercise machines were the fashion at first, followed by the use of ultraviolet light treatment.[36] These new methods were employed in combination with what could be termed more traditional applications. One treatment for pulled muscles was for players to sit all afternoon with towels over their legs and pour boiling water over the towels. These types of practices continued after 1945. One player has described how during the 1950s he sustained a twisted ankle and had to keep dipping the ankle into a wax bath until it had a thick coating.[37]

Paradoxically perhaps, while there had been a shift to more modern methods, it was during these years that the image and mystique of the football trainer and the magic sponge became firmly established, usually via the press, in the popular consciousness. The perception that was created had begun to raise concerns among mainstream physiotherapists who were then trying to establish their own medical credibility and professional credentials. J.W. Mowles complained that the lay press were conveying to the public an image that 'trainers are great experts in dealing with all forms of injury at sport'. He particularly singled out 'the use of the magical wet sponge by trainers when dealing with injuries on the field of play; following its application, many players apparently helpless and crippled by injury are cured in a matter of seconds'.[38]

Following the Second World War a growing, if small, number of football clubs began to hire qualified physiotherapists. Gradually, 'physiotherapist' began to replace 'trainer' as the term for the practitioner who dealt with players' injuries, although 'trainer' was still in use in the 1980s. In 1953 it was claimed that 7 out of the 92 Football League clubs had a physiotherapist.[39] An FA survey in 1961–2 revealed that 12 out of 45 clubs employed full-time qualified physiotherapists – or remedial gymnasts – with another 11 employed on a part-time basis; there were none at all at the 22 other clubs.[40] Moreover, with the expansion in coaching there was a growing division of labour within football clubs as coaches had responsibility for players on the training ground while the treatment room was the trainer's domain. Different attitudes to sports medicine within the sport had been underlined with the abolition of football's maximum wage in 1961 and the modification of its retain and transfer system two years later. The subsequent rise in transfer fees and wages saw players become increasingly valuable assets. These events accelerated commercialization within the game as well as stimulating the emergence of a football technocracy in which qualifications in coaching and medicine gained in importance.[41] From the 1950s through to the 1970s FA News, an in-house journal, regularly published articles on the treatment of injuries as well as advertising products like ultrasonic therapy machines.

Moreover, there was an influx of trainers now with a background in remedial gymnastics. The establishment of the School of Remedial Gymnastics at Pinderfields Hospital in Wakefield acted as a de facto training school for future football club physiotherapists.[42] The college's first two principals, John Colson and William Armour, wrote a sports medicine text, Sports Injuries and Their Treatment,[43] while Armour ran the FA's treatment of injury course. The initial in-take at Pinderfields of 115 men formed the nucleus of the Society of Remedial Gymnasts.[44] They brought new approaches to handling footballers' injuries, which highlighted developments within physiotherapy more generally. Remedial gymnastics had largely been a product of the war and placed an emphasis on exercise-based methods for rehabilitation, especially for injured servicemen, amputees and paraplegics.[45] Remedial gymnasts brought a more active form of treatment for footballers' injuries. Similar developments were taking placing in America as a number of athletic trainers became involved in 'corrective therapy' during the 1940s.[46] It signalled a shift away from the previous machine-oriented approach of those physiotherapists who were members of the Chartered Society of Physiotherapists. Importantly, because of the physical nature of this technique, it was better suited to men than women.[47] Moreover, since William Armour was running the FA course, football trainers gained some knowledge of remedial gymnastics. Norman Pilgrim, Coventry City's physiotherapist from 1964 to 1974, had 'never [been] a great lover of electro-therapy'. He had trained under James Cyriax, a pioneer in manipulation,[48] and felt that treatment for sports injuries should be concerned with good manual techniques and the management of the injury's natural progress. Pilgrim also felt that too many trainers viewed ultra-sound machines and heat lamps as a panacea for all football injuries,[49] something that perhaps reflected a more general misplaced optimism in 'progress' and modernity in the post-war era. New techniques did continue to coexist with older practices such as the tradition where players, whatever the injury, had to attend a club's treatment room on Sunday mornings, mainly because 'something must be seen to be done'.[50]

After the war there was a gradual if uneven incorporation of professional medical practices in football through the growing employment of qualified physiotherapists. With its recognition by the state under the Professions Supplementary to Medicine Act of 1960,[51] physiotherapy had not only gained more credibility but it also gave further impetus in football to professionalize the marginalized role – in medical terms – of the football trainer. Moreover, through the growth in alternative medicine and growing criticism of the medical profession and biomedicine, there was a move towards greater consumer choice in medicine as people, including footballers, became more discerning and critical of the treatment they received.[52] Ironically, by the early 1990s there was a move by alternative and unorthodox practitioners themselves towards professionalization and this allowed alternative medicine to initiate a process of 'exclusionary closure'.[53]

The FA had actually started courses for trainers in the 1930s, although attendance was not compulsory.[54] By 1961–2, while 32 club trainers had attended the trainers' course, 11 others had not.[55] In 1958, in an attempt to improve the standard of care for footballers, the FA had decided to offer – rather than make compulsory – a three-year course leading to an 'FA Certificate in the Treatment of Injuries'.[56] It was hoped that the certificate would be recognized as a minimum qualification for trainers and 32 candidates enrolled on the three-year course in that year.[57] However, clubs fiercely protected their independence and did not want to appoint from a limited number of candidates imposed on them.[58] Personal contacts within football remained the main method of appointment for trainers.

Physiotherapy itself had been subject to an increasing professionalization through the formation of clinical interest groups. One of the earliest groups was the Committee for Research into the Treatment of Athletic Injuries, set up in 1949. The interest group, however, had little success in its aim of encouraging sports teams to employ only chartered physiotherapists. By 1979 there was a total of 14 clinical groups within the CSP, rising to 25 ten years later. One of them, the Association of Chartered Physiotherapists in Sports Medicine (ACPSM) was formed in 1973 and viewed itself as being in direct competition with football trainers. In 1979 it had 275 members and a year earlier it had secured a place on the committee of BASM. In 1980 ACPSM members, in the style of a professional organization trying to establish a monopoly, campaigned to protect its title in the face of unqualified rivals like the 'sponge-and-bucket' men of the football world 'who were physiotherapists to the press'. The membership of the ACPSM had risen to 630 by 1989, highlighting how sports medicine was more generally becoming a growth area.[59]

Some of the severest critics of non-chartered practitioners were actually chartered physiotherapists working in the game.[60] In 1982 Vernon Edwards, then doctor to the England football team, also commented,

> The key person is the physio, but many have very little training … I get anxious when non-qualified people dish out drugs like sweets to deal with aches and pains. It's amazing how few teams have anyone even trained in first aid. Injuries are sometimes treated by someone totally unqualified.[61]

This suggested that in spite of the change towards a more professional approach, football's amateur and voluntary traditions continued to linger. An FA medical committee, for example, had not been formally established until 1983, and even then its role was limited. Practical realities also meant that many in football considered those with experience of treating footballers' injuries were just as suitably qualified as chartered physiotherapists. In addition, like football club doctors (see Chapter 3) the pool of chartered physiotherapists with an expertise in sports medicine was limited. It probably meant that some 'old-style' trainers had more knowledge when it came to treating particular football injuries. Furthermore, it was argued within the football world that GPs did not have the experience of the bone and muscle injuries suffered in football and that the treatment they usually offered – strap it up and rest it for several days or weeks – did not match the demands of a professional sport in which clubs wanted players back playing as soon as possible.[62]

Clubs, therefore, were still reluctant to surrender control over whom they could employ. Even in 2001 Alan Hodson, the head of the FA's Medical Education Centre, admitted that the FA had no control over who football clubs could employ.[63] As a result, the appointment of physiotherapists during this period continued to be through football's 'old boy network' and often in the gift of the manager.[64] While football club physiotherapists had professionalized the role, working conditions probably remained unattractive to women who made up the vast majority of chartered physiotherapists.[65] Amanda Johnson was one of the earliest female chartered physiotherapists to work in professional football when she was recruited by Bury in 1989.[66] For male or female physiotherapists alike the job could be difficult. Johnson identified:

> the virtual seven day week isolation from August to the end of May, the isolation from other professionals, the lack of appreciation and the fact that you are at the whim of a manager whose mood depends on the team's last performance. There is also the danger that, in the eyes of your fellow professionals, your job is of little importance in the real world and that your career is put on hold whilst you are employed by the club.[67]

In addition, because of the volatile nature of football, reflected by an increase in managerial turnover, the physiotherapist's job also became more insecure. Laurie Brown was sacked in 1981 because Manchester United's new manager, Ron Atkinson, wanted to bring in his own staff. This was becoming increasingly common and Brown's successor was actually less qualified than he had been.[68] With the establishment of its Medical Education Centre in 1989, however, the FA's approach began to take a more professional approach. By 2001–2002 the Premiership and Football League demanded that all newly appointed senior physiotherapists had to be chartered. From 2003–2004 they were also required to hold the FA's post-graduate diploma in sports medicine.[69]

Sports medicine practices

In addition to medics attached to sporting organizations, such as trainers and physiotherapists, a variety of practitioners offered specialist expertise, knowledge and services regarding athletes' injuries. It also highlighted the holistic nature of sports medicine because anyone with an appropriate medical qualification – what constituted appropriate was sometimes debatable – could claim an expertise in sports medicine.

The treatment of injuries and the services required naturally varied according to the severity of the injury. While in football much of this treatment was given in-house through the trainer, clubs did call on other services, such as ambulances and hospitals, when they were needed. As far as operations were concerned, there was initially limited expertise or knowledge of injuries commonly sustained by footballers, in particular, cartilage operations, and perhaps just as important, post-operative care. The first known cartilage operation, or meniscectomy, had been performed in 1883.[70] Even up to the 1930s it was one that footballers were loathe to undergo as it could signal the end of their careers.[71] Some surgeons advertised themselves as specialists in football injuries. It was claimed that J. Ward, who practiced in both Bolton and Manchester, was 'England's greatest bloodless surgeon' and had cured footballers of loose cartilage and fluid on the knee, conditions that other doctors had pronounced incurable.[72] By the 1930s West Bromwich Albion sent their players for cartilage operations to a Newcastle surgeon, a Mr. Stewart, 'an authority on knee troubles'.[73] An American pioneer was Robert Hyland. Hyland acted as the team doctor for baseball's St. Louis Browns between 1914 and 1950 on a voluntary basis. He had trained as a surgeon and through his reputation athletes from all around the country, including Ty Cobb and Babe Ruth, visited his clinic.[74]

Probably the earliest example of a sports injuries clinic, which offered athletes specialist treatment for sports injuries, was John Allison's 'Footballers' Hospital'. Initially a hydropathic baths, it was based at Matlock House, Hyde Road in Manchester.[75] Allison was a director of Manchester City and a Liberal councillor. For around twenty years, from the mid 1890s, many football clubs as well as Northern Union rugby clubs sent their players there for the treatment of leg and knee injuries. In general the image of hospitals had been changing from the mid-nineteenth century. A rise in outpatient demand saw a growth in hospital services outside the voluntary sector with more specialist hospitals created. Allison's hospital was part of this trend and surgery was part of the service, although the hospital was mainly used for rehabilitation purposes.[76] The resident surgeon at Matlock House was Walter Whitehead, who it was claimed had performed hundreds of operations on footballers, including those on cartilages. He also helped to devise machines to expedite recovery.[77] The hospital at one stage employed several nurses along with a retired Army surgeon, John J O'Reilly. Matlock House closed down after the First World War and there was no replacement.[78] Of course, many of the sporting injuries and conditions that were treated were relatively unremarkable in a medical sense. However, medics offered not only expertise for certain injuries that athletes suffered regularly, such as hamstring strains and cartilage problems, but also specific rehabilitation programmes as well as a more urgent service that the demands of sport dictated.

In England some athletes began to seek expertise about their injuries from football trainers who at least had experience in dealing with them. During the war Charlton Athletic's trainer, Jimmy Trotter, was able to use the club's electrical equipment to treat private patients.[79] Because of his and Arsenal's reputation Tom Whittaker had also run an informal sports injury clinic at their Highbury ground. Some of his patients were the tennis players Fred Perry and Bunny Austin, and Whittaker was actually the trainer for the victorious 1936 Davis Cup team. He also treated celebrities and public figures as well as other famous sportsmen. These included the cricketers Jack Hobbs and Douglas Jardine and the jockey Steve Donoghue.[80]

Following the Footballers' Hospital, the next clinic that gained a reputation for treating sports-specific injuries was the Park Street Orthopaedic Clinic in London, which opened in 1936. It was headed by Morgan Smart and Bill (William Eldon) Tucker (1903–91), a former England rugby international forward. Tucker was later its director until 1980 when he retired and a founding member of BASM, and in 1955 he was co-opted on to the BASM executive.[81] It was said that, based on his experiences as a rugby player, he wanted to offer a medical service to sportsmen in addition to regular patients. His most famous patient was Denis Compton. Compton, who suffered from a persistent knee injury, was England's premier batsman in the early post-war era and had also played football for Arsenal. Tucker regularly treated the knee before removing the knee-cap altogether in 1955, enabling Compton to continue his cricketing career.[82] Tucker also made himself available at weekends, which was invaluable to elite athletes. On one occasion, after he was called away from a Saturday dinner party, Tucker reset the dislocated shoulder of a jockey, Gay Kindersley, who he had previously operated on.[83] Tucker specialized in manipulation. In 1968 the cricketer Tom Cartwright was a patient whose reach, it was claimed, increased three inches following a Tucker massage. On his later visits Tucker gave him butazolidin tablets, which were usually administered to horses, to aid recovery.[84]

The establishment of Tucker's clinic had coincided with a struggle within medicine between orthopaedics and physical medicine and the perceived unorthodox practice of osteopathy over professional status and medical autonomy. Osteopathy, it was claimed, was a holistic system of manipulation but because its treatments were similar it brought it into direct competition with these orthodox specialisms. Orthopaedics had rapidly gained respectability after World War One (see Chapter 3) while physical medicine had been tainted by a perceived association with non-medically trained bone-setters, although its marginal status was bolstered through its growing popularity. Unlike other medical groups, osteopaths did not seek medical patronage and were seen as a threat. There was a backlash in the medical press. It was claimed that osteopathy was not scientific and it was eventually denied state recognition.[85] In 1963 BASM strongly disapproved of the Golder's Green Athletics Clinic because osteopaths – who were not accepted as BASM members – practiced there.[86]

Athletes were prepared to criss-cross the medical divide to find the treatment that they felt was best for them. From the 1960s footballers were becoming increasingly critical of the medical treatment they received and with the greater scepticism of medicine generally, they began to seek second opinions, including osteopaths. When he was at Manchester United, Denis Law had a long-running knee injury and in 1967 he decided to see an osteopath, which did not go down well with the club doctor and physiotherapist. However, Law found the osteopath's advice and treatment better than at United.[87] Law, because he was a superstar and confident of his own status, was able to ignore the club's medical advice and use other treatments without any fear of recrimination; players not as valuable and those not as experienced would have – and continue to – faced a different dilemma.[88]

Whereas for much of the twentieth century, osteopathy was a marginal practice in the UK, in the US it had been recognized as a medical specialty since 1953. As a form of healing it shares similarities with chiropractic approaches, which are based on the idea that manipulation of the spine can relieve pressure on the nerves and thereby alleviate illness and pain. However, tensions have arisen over the status of chiropractors in American sport. In 1990 there were about 25,000 chiropractors in the States (in Britain there were just 350) compared to nearly 600,000 medical doctors (M.D.). Despite being licensed to practice in all fifty states, the American Medical Association (AMA) campaigned vehemently against chiropractors. Again showing how orthodox profession was keen to protect its turf, in 1963 the AMA's Committee on Quackery described chiropractic as an 'unscientific cult' and eight years later the committee's main mission was to eliminate it.[89] One particularly popular chiropractor, Dr. Leroy Perry, found himself ostracized from American sports teams as a consequence of his profession. His (satisfied) customers included athletes such as Alberto Juantoreno, Henry Rono and Dwight Stones as well as footballers, tennis players and baseball players. Despite a petition signed by several hundred American athletes and coaches before the 1976 Olympics requesting Perry's inclusion on the US Olympic Sports Medicine Committee, it was refused. A similar motion was rejected before the 1980 Olympics. Perry had attended the Montreal Games as a physician for another team and in spite of warnings by their own national medical staff, American athletes continued to visit Perry. Just as noteworthy as the tensions between orthodox and alternative practices was the reliance of athletes on Perry. A hurdler, Dedy Cooper said:

> Everybody talks about Dr. Perry. *Everybody.* The first thing athletes ask at a meet is, 'Is Dr. Perry here?' If he's not some won't compete. Other doctors tell you, 'Rest.' Dr Perry fixes you up; he teaches you how to take care of yourself. We want him.[90]

This rather embellished statement reflected how many athletes were and are still very superstitious. What athletes deem to work they usually keep on repeating. To a certain extent it betrays the underlying anxieties of athletes to stay healthy in an environment that revolves around short-termism.

Similarly, because he wanted to see his own specialist, during the 1982 Spain World Cup, England captain Kevin Keegan secretly flew to Hamburg for treatment on a back injury from Jürgen Rehwinkel. Initially, the manager, Ron Greenwood and the team doctor, Vernon Edwards, had refused but Keegan eventually flew to West Germany for treatment that allowed him to (briefly) participate in the tournament.[91]

Some forms of treatment have been perhaps more alternative than others. When he was England coach, Glen Hoddle used the services of a faith healer, Eileen Drewery. With headlines such as 'Voodoo Woman', it created a stir as well as cynicism in the media. Hoddle, for whom faith became an important part of his life because of Drewery, had frequently visited her from the age of 18. She had healed a hamstring injury, he claimed, and other subsequent injuries with her techniques of the laying of her hands on the head and 'other special centres of the body' together with the use of 'absent prayer'. Hoddle claimed that she cured his father of arthritis of the back after just one session and Richard Green, who was told his football career was over, was playing ten years after Drewery treated his back injury. Hoddle had been keen for his England players to see Drewery, and in the lead-up to the 1998 World Cup three quarters of England's players visited her (Hoddle believed that his biggest regret for England's World Cup exit was not getting Drewery out to France from the start). He claimed not to put any pressure on the players and that some flew from the north of England and abroad to see her. That players visited Drewery again partly reflects the anxieties of athletes over the fear of injuries and the need for them to be healed quickly, although to what extent those who did were there to please the coach is difficult to gauge. Many who visited Drewery were willing to 'give it a go'. Tony Adams had suffered from a long-term ankle problem and had visited a number of medics. On his visit, Adams said, 'I was open-minded about it, believing in taking help wherever I could get it, and was willing for it to work.'[92] Drewery's involvement with England ended following Hoddle's sacking in 1998.

Some athletes have also resorted to homeopathic medicine, which continues to be opposed by elements of the medical profession. One doctor who has built his reputation on this practice has been Hans-Wilhelm Müller-Wohlfahrt. Müller-Wohlfahrt has been the club doctor at Bayern Munich but other athletes he has treated include Roger Black, Paula Radcliffe and Usain Bolt. At one stage in his career the golfer, Jose Maria Olazabal, suffered from rheumatoid arthritis in his feet and was barely able to walk. But following treatment from Müller-Wohlfahrt he won the US Masters again in 1999. Reflecting popular discourse, some of his methods have been deemed controversial. It is claimed that he has used 'calves blood' as well as a substance called Hylart that has been extracted from the crest of cockerels, which is said to lubricate knee injuries.[93] Reaction to his methods in Britain were mixed. They were criticized by BASEM while one physiotherapist condemned his treatments as 'highly questionable on moral and ethical grounds'. Terry Moule – an osteopath ironically – added that there were questions over its long-term side-effects. However, Malcolm Brown, the then medical director of UK Athletics, was more relaxed and claimed that Müller-Wohlfahrt was 'not a crank'. His treatments were actually not dissimilar to the anti-ageing treatments that had been administered in the form of injections of foetal animal cells into the buttocks of celebrities by beauty therapists at Clinique La Prairie in Montreaux since the 1930s. Despite criticism athletes used him because, as Colin Jackson has argued, 'Athletes are not like normal people. Their bodies don't function in normal ways. So normal medicine is not always the answer'.[94]

Similarly, in 2009 it was sensationally reported that Liverpool had sent two of its players to Marijana Kovacevic, a 'mystery horse placenta healer' in

Serbia with the blessing of the club doctor. Footballers from all over Europe had visited her on the basis of recommendations of other players. Her treatment involved using fluids derived from horse placentas and electrolysis to rub on to the afflicted part of the body; in the case of Arsenal's Robin Van Persie, it was ruptured ankle ligaments. She had become so famous in Serbia that she was signed up by a football agency, no doubt so that the agency's injured players could be sent to her for treatment. In a short critique that echoed on-going debates between orthodox and alternative medicine, the *Independent's* health editor, Jeremy Laurance, argued that Kovacevic's treatment represented 'the triumph of faith over reason, the power of belief over evidence'. In other words, it had the effect of a placebo. Because the treatment would not do any harm – or anything – Laurance believed that team doctors would be unconcerned.[95]

For major operations on joints, however, athletes have stuck firmly to biomedicine. Previously football clubs would use their network of consultants or local hospitals. Through their London connections, Arsenal, in the inter-war years could call on specialist orthopaedic surgeons, although other less wealthy clubs would rely on local hospitals. But with the increase in sport's commercialization, some surgeons gained first, a reputation, and then developed a specialty in operating on athletes. One such knee surgeon has been the American, Richard Steadman from Vail, Colorado. His sports medicine background had originally been in skiing and he claimed to have performed surgery on every US skier to win an Olympic medal between 1978 and 2002. He pioneered 'the microfracture technique' for knee surgery and his reputation has crossed the Atlantic for clients to include players from the National Football League and footballers in Europe. It has been estimated that Steadman earns approximately $5 million per year. In comparison, sports surgery in Britain remains a fledgling industry with a top surgeon earning about £200,000.[96]

Sports medicine practitioners and ethical dilemmas

One key area that has distinguished sports medicine from 'normal' medical practices has revolved around the fitness of injured athletes. Any relationship between doctor (or other health professional) and patient has been normally underpinned by three fundamental assumptions. First, the doctor's skill is used exclusively on behalf of the patient; second, the doctor is not acting as an agent on behalf of anybody else whose interests may conflict with those of the patient; and third, the doctor may be trusted with private or intimate information which she/he will treat confidentially and not divulge to others.[97] Because of the nature of sporting competition, authority over when an athlete should return to the field of play – both before and during the contest – has revealed acute ethical dilemmas between sports medics, management, coaches and players due to conflicts of interest and loyalty.

Any discussion of ethics within sports medicine needs to be seen in the context of a progressively more assertive medical profession, which has laid claim to making moral judgements based on their social and professional status. Rather than a neutrally conceived set of morals, the original intention of a code of ethics was political: to separate orthodox medicine from alternative practitioners.[98] On one hand, Victorian doctors were part of 'gentlemanly medicine', which promoted the values of the social elite; on the other, alternative practitioners were labelled charlatans.[99] For ethics particular to sports medicine, Waddington has provided a useful framework based on key areas of practice from his case study of professional football in England. The first one revolves around questions of informed consent. The second one is over 'return to play decisions' following injury and associated quality of care issues. The final area concerns issues relating to medical confidentiality.[100]

In American football the potential conflict of loyalty of the team doctor has been brought in to sharper focus due to the brutality of the sport as well as its more commercial nature. In his sensationalized account of his time as a doctor at the Los Angeles Raiders (1983–89), Robert Huizenga was critical of the chief team physician, Robert Rosenfeld. Huizenga has suggested that Rosenfeld was acting more on behalf of the wishes of the owner – the megalomaniacal Al Davis – rather than for the health of the players. On occasions when Huizenga felt that players needed further examination before going back on the field to play because of a danger of paralysis, Rosenfeld had said to the player, 'You're okay, it's just a bruise.'[101] Interestingly, in 1979 a legal representative for the NFL Player's Association remarked that of the 67 NFL injury grievance cases he had handled the team doctor had been a witness for the club and in opposition to the player in every single one. Where did the doctors' loyalty lie? Dr Bruce Ogilvie, who had worked as a consultant for a number of teams, commented:

> It must be one of the most difficult of all medical roles. You can't be a team physician without becoming a red-hot jock yourself. I know for myself. My heart, soul and identification are with these players. The doctor is no different from me in that regard. But that places him in a very difficult position. He has to make judgements on readiness to play, medical treatment, diagnoses in situations of high stress – going down to the wire for the playoffs, going for the championship. In these situations you can't help but be torn.[102]

In American sport more generally the role of the team physician was seen by some doctors as a way to advertise their services in private practice. An orthopaedist was generally the chief team doctor and he could use his position to obtain almost unlimited referrals of joint or muscle problems. In the 1990s orthopaedic operations averaged around $3–4,000.[103] Moreover, during the 1990s doctors began to pay NFL teams and other sports franchises to work as team physician because it acted as a form of advertising for their main work. In 1989 the Jewett Orthopaedic Group had supplied the newly formed NBA franchise, Orlando Magic, with team physicians and in return received arena advertising. The Jewett Group argued that, 'In this [medical] market, there are a lot of orthopaedic surgeons. A lot of them would be willing to be sponsors … We want the world to know that we do take care of the team.' In 1995 there was a bidding competition to act as the 'official health-care provider' for the Jacksonville Jaguars. For the successful medical group it entailed purchasing luxury executive boxes, advertisements in programmes and donating medical supplies at a cost of around $1 million.[104] The advertising of these medical wares highlighted more generally how American medicine was more market led when compared to Britain.

Ethical dilemmas have not been absent in English association football either. Medical tensions were brought into sharper focus during the second half of the twentieth century when the manager became a more powerful and dominant figure within clubs.[105] While a number of football doctors have remarked that they have enjoyed good relations with the managers they have worked with, they were also aware that the manager could over-rule their opinion concerning the management of players' injuries.[106] The pressure of games could also influence the judgment of managers over injured players. In 1961, during the half-time interval of one game, the Wolves centre-forward, Ted Farmer, discovered that he was urinating blood after being elbowed in the stomach. Despite an examination by the club doctor the Wolves manager, Stan Cullis, forced Farmer to play on. Cullis told the doctor, very forcefully, 'Wait 'til it comes through his backside before you take him off.' The doctor did not intervene any further.[107] Because they have been players themselves, managers think they know the mentality of players and that injuries or 'knocks' are not as serious as players think. Underpinning this idea is that players have to demonstrate a 'good attitude'.[108] When he was club physician at Leeds United (1961–75), Ian Adams resigned on four separate occasions because of arguments with the manager, Don Revie, over the fitness of players, i.e., Revie played them against Adams' advice.[109] Referring to modern sports medicine, Adams has said,

> I wouldn't like to be a full-time [football club] doctor … I would be very loathe to … because your family depends on your employment, and I wouldn't like to have to depend upon the hysteria and stuff that's associated with the football club and possibly the change of manager.[110]

The employment status of the trainer further compounded the power of managers over these 'return to play decisions'. Trainers at English clubs have traditionally been unqualified to work in the NHS (see above) and have been dependent on football and managers as their only source of employment. As a result, a trainer, under pressure because of his employment situation, may have been forced to submit to a manager's demands over when to allow a player recovering from injury to be available for selection. With the increasing number of chartered physiotherapists working in football clubs there has been greater potential for professional autonomy: if they left football at least they were qualified to work outside the game. However, working in football has also presented a challenge to a chartered physiotherapist's clinical autonomy because managers have still wanted some influence over decisions about the fitness of players.[111] 'That is the job' was the opinion of Norman Pilgrim, physiotherapist at Coventry City (1964–76). 'The job is standing up to managers; it's a big part of the job. I know people who are technically good at it but their managers just over-rule them all the time.' Pilgrim claimed he did not mind that side of the job, although managers and coaches at other clubs bullied physiotherapists into making the decisions they wanted.[112] One chartered physiotherapist, who worked for a First Division club in the 1980s and 1990s, has described how his manager would not even allow him on to the pitch until a senior coach, acting for the manager, had assessed the injury of the player. Another chartered physiotherapist at a First Division club in the 1980s stated that, although he and the club doctor agreed on most things concerning player fitness, the manager always wanted 'star' players to perform.[113] When he was at Manchester United, on occasions Laurie Brown, ingeniously, put injured players in plaster as this sight would immediately dissuade the manager from being able to question his opinion. At other times he discovered that managers and players sought a second opinion on his diagnoses without informing him.[114]

Bloodgate

On 12 April 2009 the European Rugby Cup quarter-final between Harelquins and Leinster produced one of the most notorious examples of how sport, medicine and ethics do not mix. What was to become known as 'Bloodgate' led not only to a two-year suspension of the Harlequins' physiotherapist and a General Medical Council (GMC) enquiry into the club doctor's conduct but the club's director of rugby, Dean Richards, would receive a three-year ban from the game and the player involved, Tom Williams, was suspended from rugby for one year (reduced to four months on appeal).

During the game Harelquins had been losing and wanted to put on a specialist goal-kicker with only a few minutes to go. However, they had used up all their substitutions and could not replace anyone unless a player had a blood injury. Thus, Williams was pressurized by Richards to fabricate one. During a break in play he was given a blood capsule by the physiotherapist, Steph Brennan – under Richards' instruction – and bit on it to look as if it had been a blood injury i.e., they tried to cheat Leinster out of the game. Williams said that he felt under pressure from Richards who he claimed as coach was a very authoritarian figure. It was later revealed that Harelquins had used this tactic on four previous occasions. The capsules had been purchased from a joke shop to be used for this particular purpose. On this occasion their opponents became suspicious and another match official also claimed it was fake blood. Williams in desperation then asked the club doctor, Wendy Chapman, to cut his lip with a scalpel for evidence of real blood. For Chapman this went against her medical principles as a doctor her job was to heal not inflict injures.[115]

Williams later signed a prepared statement from Richards about the incident and lied to the European Rugby Cup's disciplinary committee when called as a witness (at the first disciplinary committee meeting Williams had been represented by the club's legal team rather than independent lawyers). There were further consequences. Williams intended to appeal against his original ban but was pressurized by the club to only partly disclose so as to limit the damage. The club subsequently admitted that it had breached its duty of care to Williams and offered him financial inducements for his co-operation. Following the resignation of Dean Richards just before the appeal, however, Williams fully disclosed the evidence.[116]

What were the consequences for Harelquins' medical staff? Chapman, an accident and emergency consultant, also lied to the hearing about her role. She had initially gone with the club's view of events and said that Williams' injury was genuine. She was suspended by the GMC, which described her actions as 'dishonest, likely to bring the profession into disrepute and wholly unacceptable'. The GMC though later allowed her to practice medicine again. For physiotherapist Steph Brennan the consequences were similarly problematic. He had been due to work with the England team but was banned from rugby for two years and so was unable to take up the post. The following year Brennan was struck off by the Health Professions Council for misconduct but won an appeal and instead received a five-year caution.[117]

However, the incident further highlighted how in sport situations can arise where medical practitioners can be placed in difficult situations that clash with the 'normal' doctor-patient relationship. Instead, this episode highlighted sport's peculiar relationship with medicine. Following the incident James Robson, the Scotland doctor who had accompanied five Lions tours, continued to claim that, 'The overwhelming majority of medical people involved in the care of sports people are underpaid and overworked, they are there for the love of it.'[118] Moreover, it also reflected the whole idea of the professional athlete as someone who is essentially 'unhealthy' because of the stresses placed on their bodies, and that this also has had implications for the working practices of medics.

The patient's view

Much of the history of medicine has been written from the perspective of medicine. How have athletes – as patients – reacted to the medical care they have received? This brief section provides some insights into the motivations of athletes as 'abnormal' patients. Paula Radcliffe, for example, has claimed that her pain threshold has been higher than her husband allowing her to endure more pain in some of her treatment with her physical therapist Gerard Hartmann. He used very deep and penetrative tissue work and massage to stimulate quicker recovery of the injured area. But as Radcliffe stated, 'his patient must be able to withstand a reasonable level of pain'. Her husband, Gary Lough, could not. On one occasion when he watched on while Radcliffe was undergoing intensive treatment, he had to leave due to the distress it was causing her. She said, 'The pain was as bad as anything I had ever experienced when working with Gerard, but I welcomed it.'[119]

Of course, context again is instructive, especially for footballers. How often footballers have played when injured has differed from player to player and has perhaps been because of their own perceptions of what constituted an injury. Players have had other motivations for playing through injury, such as wanting to take part in an important game. There were other concerns for some. One player once hid an injury because he feared losing his place in the team; another said that he did not want to let his teammates down. Similar sentiments were also expressed by players in the NFL. The main reason though for playing with an injury was financial. A soccer player from the 1960s and 1970s remarked that the 'money in our day was not like today. With a little bonus and appearance money, it was nice to see it in your wages at the end of the month'.

From a small survey of former players covering the period from the 1940s to the 1980s, it seems that most former players were relatively happy with the treatment they received, although this raises questions over the perceptions they had of the treatment they expected and with what they were able to compare it. Some players were more critical. One player from the early post-war years has described how he sustained an injury during a game but after being 'strapped-up' he played on as no substitutes were then allowed.[120] The strapping was left on even when he had a bath and was not removed until the following morning. It also took his skin off as the trainer had used the wrong side of the tape. The injury was subsequently diagnosed as damage to a cruciate ligament. Someone who played in the 1980s for lower league clubs was critical of the post-operation care he received following an ankle operation and felt this was due to the physiotherapist who was 'inadequately qualified'. A goalkeeper who played during the 1960s and 1970s for clubs throughout the league, though fortunate enough not to sustain any serious injuries, commented that 'physiotherapy didn't seem that sophisticated and attention to injuries on the field seemed clumsy at times – magic sponge and strong smelling salts seemed the answer to most problems!' One player from a top club in the 1970s and 1980s 'felt [that the] medical side was always lacking; physios were lacking knowledge and expertise'.

One particular treatment continues to prove controversial. Cortisone was part of the post-war pharmacological revolution. This particular 'wonder drug' acted as an anti-inflammatory treatment and was primarily used for rheumatoid arthritis. By the 1950s football clubs were using it to alleviate the injuries of players. Cortisone has the effect of disguising pain for three to four hours, and when injected it was converted into cortisol and influences the nutrition and growth of connective tissues. Its use on players though has varied from doctor to doctor with some refusing outright to inject. In the 1960s their use had been more liberal. Denis Law claimed that at Manchester United he and other players regularly received injections to mask the pain in the short-term; there was little consideration of the long-term consequences.[121] Similarly, Ian St. John was placed in a similar situation when he was at Liverpool.[122] A greater awareness has developed amongst athletes over the consequences of using cortisone. However, as Martin Roderick has outlined, the dilemmas that doctors and players have faced over the use of cortisone and other anti-inflammatories has continued into the twentieth-first century.[123]

Legal implications

Because of the sums involved, issues regarding the law and insurance have become more complex for practitioners. One post-war development that did indicate greater interest by football clubs in insurance and legal matters was medical examination of transferred players. These began in Britain during the 1960s although European clubs had introduced them before then. 'Medicals' were a consequence of the rise in transfer fees following the abolition of the maximum wage and more complex insurance arrangements. Although now normal, they are not compulsory nor has there been an established protocol for them or any uniformity between clubs.[124]

Medical examinations for college footballers with intentions of playing in the NFL have taken place at the annual week-long Scouting Combine since the 1982. The Combine includes physical as well as medical evaluations as the main objective is for the team's many coaches and medical staff to sift out the best prospects in preparation for the NFL Draft. Physical tests include a 40-yard dash and bench press repetitions. However, evaluating the health of players has proved problematic, giving a new twist to the doctor-patient relationship. During his interviews of players Robert Huizenga found that players would categorically deny anything was wrong with them. Whereas patients would usually come to his practice and spell out the seriousness of their complaint, at the Combine the patients said nothing and he had to figure out who was lying.[125]

There is no such equivalent in English soccer and perhaps reflects a more scientific tradition within American sport where greater emphasis is placed on statistics. Early medicals in English soccer were routine affairs but gradually became more sophisticated through the use of MRI scans. A doctor and/or physiotherapist would usually ask the player of any past history of injuries, although unsurprisingly players would sometimes keep information from them as it could prevent the transfer. One of the most famous transfer cancellations because of a player failing a medical was that of Asa Hartford's proposed move from West Bromwich Albion to Leeds United in 1971 for a potential club record fee of £177,000.[126] It had been found that Hartford had a small hole in his heart, and it was felt by the Leeds medical team that he may have been susceptible to heart failure due to the stress of playing.[127]

The collapse of Ruud van Nistelrooy's transfer from the Dutch club PSV Eindhoven to Manchester United in 2000 highlighted the new financial risks involved in large transfers. The fee had been £18.5 million, then a British record, but was cancelled because of doubts raised over his knee after his medical. Armed with this knowledge, United's insurers had refused to underwrite a policy unless the club agreed to a clause ruling out seeking compensation for any injury resulting from his weakened knee. As a public limited company with shareholders to satisfy, as well as the prospect of paying van Nistelrooy £42,000 per week without playing, the club did not want to take the risk and called off the deal.[128]

One outcome of these increasingly complex relationships has been legal action brought against sports medics and clubs by footballers who feel that they received poor treatment which has led to medical complications. In 1998 the former Sunderland player Keiron Brady sued the club on the grounds of medical negligence. He had argued that the club had failed to take appropriate action when he reported pain in his right leg despite his complaints in training. Later he was diagnosed with a rare medical condition, a blockage of the popliteal artery in his right leg, which eventually curtailed his playing career.[129] In this case, however, the club was found not to have breached its duty of care to the player.[130]

In American sport legal actions regarding medical care have had a longer history and more expensive outcomes. The first athlete to sue the medical staff of a team was Dick Butkus in 1974. He successfully sued the doctors of the Chicago Bears over repeated injections of cortisone and other drugs to his knees and was awarded $600,000.[131] After his playing career ended in 1987 Kenny Easley sued the Seattle Seahawks' trainer and team doctors for what he said was an overuse of Advil that exacerbated his kidney disease and led to total kidney failure. The case was settled out of court. In 2002 Jeff Novak was awarded $5.35 million for malpractice against Stephen Lucie, a former team doctor of the Jacksonville Jaguars. But instead of the club the player sued the doctor's employers, Jacksonville Orthopaedic Institute, who had been hired by the Jaguars.[132] In addition, there is the potential ticking time bomb for sport in general of the disabling impact of injuries later in life and the financial consequences that this may bring through further legal action. When in 1995 Marty Barrett, then of the Boston Red Sox sued the team physician, Arthur

Pappas, over the treatment he had received, the question of the allegiance of the doctor to the team or to the health of the athlete was brought into even more sharper focus: Pappas, uniquely amongst team doctors, was also an owner of the club.[133] In 1995 his four per cent stake was estimated to be worth $10 million.[134]

For doctors the increase in sport's commercialization has had ramifications for their legal and insurance status. In 2003 Canadian sports doctors had their insurance cover removed by the Canadian Medical Protection Association because the financial risks they were now undertaking were too great. It left doctors exposed to litigation for misdiagnosis from entire teams of athletes who were on potentially multi-million dollar contracts.[135] Similarly, in Britain the Medical Protection Society refused to offer indemnity to any doctors employed by Premier League clubs from April 2008. Members of the Medical Defence Union though did continue to receive an individual professional indemnity insurance covering medical negligence to a limit of £10 million for every claim.[136]

Conclusion

Getting an athlete fit for competition continues to be the nub of the relationship between sport and medicine. Yet this relationship has also been subject to a wider context. Not only has the science changed in the treatment of injuries but this has also been set alongside a change in the nature of sport, especially the growth of commercialization and competition. Whilst there has been change there has also been continuity in the sense that athletes continue to want to compete when injured or it may be more correct to state that they are always injured in some form such are the demands that elite sport places on the body. Hence participation remains a process of 'body management', albeit a unique one with regard to sport.

Footballers in England have been considered assets since the legalization of professionalism in 1885. Because clubs recognized their economic value they employed trainers to maintain fitness and treat common injuries as well as establish links with local hospitals and surgeons. However, this investment gradually increased with the game's changing economic context. With the establishment of the Premier League in 1992, there was an exponential rise in the medical facilities and back-up at top football clubs. Whereas in 1992 a top-level football club may have had a part-time doctor, a physiotherapist who was a 'mate' of the manager, supported by one or two assistants, fifteen years on this situation had changed radically. In 2005 Arsenal, for example, had a medical team of eight excluding doctors. These included fitness coaches, masseurs and four physiotherapists. All held professional qualifications in the field of sport and exercise medicine and can also be seen in light of an on-going process of excluding and marginalising alternative and unorthodox practices.

However, criticism by players of the treatment they have received has continued. Although there has been a greater investment in medical care, there has been an increase in the expectations of the players themselves who are probably better educated in terms of what they know about injuries, the limits of their bodies and just health matters more generally. Commercialization has also increased the independence of top players and loosened their reliance on and ties to clubs. Even in the lower leagues many players (clandestinely) seek second opinions on injuries and their treatment.[137] At the centre of this tension has been the manager or head coach. Sport's unique demands have placed extra pressure on medical practitioners – and has been seen with 'Bloodgate' – can affect their judgement in making decisions contrary to established medical practice.

7

Medicine, Sport and the Female Body

Introduction

In 2007, tucked away in the *Daily Telegraph's* sports round, it was reported that the Indian middle-distance runner, Santhi Soundarajan, was in hospital following a suicide attempt. The previous year she had been stripped of the silver medal she won in the 800 metres at the Asian Games. The reason: she had failed a gender test.[1] It is not known if the two events were linked but two years later the issue of gender testing would be given greater prominence following the victory of the South African Caster Semenya in the women's 800 metres at the 2009 World Athletics Championships in Berlin. As questions were raised over the exact status of her sex, people asked whether it was 'fair' that she should be competing against other female athletes. It is ironic, as Vanessa Heggie has pointed out, that whereas there are probably hundreds of genetic variations that lead to 'unfair' advantages in sport, 'only those associated with gender are used to exclude or disqualify athletes'.[2] While the subject of gender testing is a relatively extreme example which has recurred intermittently throughout the twentieth century, it has reflected not only how the bodies of women continued to be politicized within sport but also that the relationship between female athletes and medicine continued to perpetuate wider discourses regarding the role of women in society.

Jennifer Hargreaves has argued that 'the whole of the history of modern sports has been based on gender divisions'[3] with the presence of women in sport traditionally not only marginal but also marginalized. As Osborne and Skillen have pointed out with regard to sport, 'no realm of social or cultural life is exclusively the property of any given group, but is merely appropriated and in turn constructed as such'.[4] While feminist scholarship has emphasized the 'experience' and changing 'meanings' of leisure in the life-cycle of women,[5] the aim here is to establish how the relationship between women, sport and medicine has been shaped through the prevailing social and medical discourses that this relationship has engendered.

Throughout the twentieth century though there was a significant growth in women's sport and participation generally. At the Olympics, for example, whereas there were no female competitors in 1896, by 2008 they made up 42 per cent of the 11,196 athletes. However, this growth has also reflected contradictory aspects. While there has been rising participation rates mirrored by greater liberalization of women's rights, the growth of women's sport has continued to reinforce gender stereotypes and dominant discourses, which has been mirrored in the representation of female athletes in the media.[6] In sports like gymnastics and figure-skating, for example, an emphasis has been placed on so-called feminine attributes while through their coverage some areas of the media have sexualized female athletes, such as during the Wimbledon tennis championships.

There has never been a consensus over the ideology of female sport. Because sport, especially at elite level, has been about excess it has been more commonly associated with notions of masculinity. As a consequence, images and perceptions of female athletes overstraining have conflicted with prevailing ideals of femininity. Zweiniger-Bargielowska has argued how through sport, physical culture and the life reform movement, the rise of modern female and male bodies was part of a trend towards greater equality between the sexes during the period 1880–1939. Yet this only went so far because the modern woman was still ultimately seen as the 'race mother'. As a consequence,

> the female ideal of a normal body was grounded in long-established notions of femininity, competitive sport remained controversial, and women's pursuit of excessive slimness was widely condemned in the 1930s because these practices were thought to threaten reproductive capacity.[7]

In the British military, however, the ideology of service sport was 'apparently transferred wholesale from the men's services to the women's'. In the 1950s Brigadier Barclay of the Army Physical Training Corps listed among the benefits of physical training for women 'health, morale, contentment, physical efficiency, team spirit and the "psychological outlook"'. Barclay subsequently claimed that 'women who have no aptitude for sport are unsuitable as Leaders'.[8] By contrast, the 2008 edition of the *Diagnostic and Statistical Manual*, published by the American Psychiatric Association, identified an 'intense desire to participate in the games and pastimes of the other sex' as one of the five criteria that psychiatrists may draw on 'to diagnose gender identity disorder in childhood'.[9] Of course this begs the question how do you decide what are the games of the other sex?

Early women's sport and medical theories

Women's sport was not exclusive to the late twentieth century. Foot-races – or smock races, so termed because there was a prize of a dress – between girls and women at village fairs had been common since the seventeenth century.[10] Some women even took up pugilism while the benefits of exercise had also been promoted by Mary Wollstonecraft in her 1792 tract, *A Vindication of the Rights of Woman*.[11] By the end of the nineteenth century the nature of women's sport had changed. First, women's sport as well as many other leisure activities were mainly restricted to the middle classes as up to 1914 the harsh realities of working-class life meant that most women could only snatch a few moments of respite from their arduous daily routines.[12] The administration of women's sport and its attendant values concerning the perceptions of women more generally can be seen in this middle-class context. Second, the nature of women's sporting activity provided fertile debating ground for doctors that revolved around both contemporary medical theories, especially eugenics, and attitudes towards the role of women in Victorian society. A social ideology and practice emerged that preferred to separate rather than mix the functions of the sexes. It was assumed that a women's role was suited to domestic and childrearing duties, whereas men, reinforced by notions of masculinity, were supposedly endowed with greater intelligence and muscular strength more suitable to the sphere of work and competitive sport, symbolizing a modern industrial society.[13]

Importantly, medical theories, particularly the 'vitalistic' theory, contended that the human body contained only a limited, unrenewable amount of energy. As a result, women had to conserve their energy for their essential purpose in life i.e., to bear children.[14] The establishment of gynaecology as a specialist branch of medicine in the nineteenth century was important in shaping medical attitudes towards female athletes because (male) physicians were considered experts on the subject of the female body.[15] Patricia Vertinsky has argued that the late nineteenth century woman was seen as 'eternally wounded' because medical practitioners viewed menstruation as pathological. As a result, women were viewed as chronically weak with only finite amounts of both mental and physical energy due to their menstrual cycle, and energy, therefore, had to be conserved for childbirth.[16] In 1904 the *Practitioner* reported that some gynaecologists and obstetricians had argued that exercise, despite its attempts to produce 'a more vigorous race' and 'advanced muscular development', would make labour more difficult. Physically active British women were compared to oriental women who led 'indolent lives' but who, apparently, had an easy time in labour.[17]

In a social context 'Women were obliged to show restraint, be refined and respectable and confirm at all times the "ladylike" modes of behaviour prescribed for them.'[18] They were also looked upon as 'physically limited', something that the scientific and medical establishments helped to institutionalize. In 1887, for example, the chairman of the BMA proposed that,

> In the interests of social progress, national efficiency and the progressive improvement of the human race, women should be denied education and other activities which would cause overstrain and inability to produce healthy offspring.[19]

In addition, Greg Moon has argued that,

> Doctors continued to view female athletes as women first and sportswomen second, which contributed to the myth of female frailty and made it particularly resistant to change. Early athletes had to fight against the consensus of medical opinion, which still dictated that intense physical activity would harm their potential for reproduction.[20]

However, Moon perhaps overstates the emphasis of the 'consensus'. No doubt this was the dominant idea but like other theories medical ones are always in flux. In particular, with the growing idea that the body was akin to a machine and needed some form of maintenance, doctors began to realize that exercise for women was beneficial to their health. During the late nineteenth century, through their sheer visibility, fit, physically active women challenged the discourse of the 'eternally wounded woman'.[21] During the 1890 to 1914 period physical culture was increasingly thought to promote femininity amongst British women.[22] Most importantly was the growing realization that physical fitness was essential to women, especially those from the upper and middle classes, to produce healthy babies. Due to eugenic-based fears and the strictures of Social Darwinism, physical fitness was now seen as increasingly important to increase fertility levels amongst upper- and middle-class females to both maintain national efficiency as well as preventing too great an imbalance between the numbers of the middle and working classes.[23] How vigorous though and what form this exercise should take continued to be part of the debate. While the need for exercise was accepted, competitive and physical contact sports were condemned. In 1904 it was reported in the *Practitioner* that some gynaecologists and obstetricians felt that 'a moderate amount of exercise tends to promote health in all directions, while undue indulgence in athletics is bad for both man and women'. It was then suggested that regarding the dangers of athleticism in the case of women, practitioners should 'point out the risks in no uncertain language'.[24] One of the fiercest contemporary critics against women's sports was actually a female doctor, Arabella Kenealy. She argued that the development of a woman's muscular structure through sport would jeopardize her brain and reproductive organs[25] and in her *Feminism and Sex Extinction* (1920), she outlined the sterilising influences of competitive games.[26]

Doctors were not just guided by medical knowledge. According to Allen Guttmann the opinions of doctors were also based on their cultural preference for 'refined women', part of what Catherine Horwood has termed a 'patriarchal prudery'.[27] Doctors were sincere in their judgement and when it was realized that an inactive life for women was unhealthy they responded by advocating moderate exercise.[28] Adolphe Abrahams, one of the most outspoken doctors on the pros and cons of women's sport, followed this line of argument. While not completely discouraging girls and women from undertaking exercise, his views were typical of patriarchal attitudes towards women. In 1928, in conjunction with his brother, Harold, they stated that, although they were in favour of exercise for women, they were opposed to any 'severe competition' or 'violent exercise' for girls, women and 'potential mothers'. It was felt that 'woman with her more sensitive nervous organization is much more susceptible to strain than is man'.[29] As late as 1956 Adolphe Abrahams still felt that the exercises of women should help towards 'a better capacity to bear the burdens of womanhood and possible maternity'.[30] As a consequence of medical opinion, women were steered towards certain sports and activities that were deemed feminine and were also moderate. In general vigorous sports were deemed masculine.

The majority of women's modern sports in the nineteenth century developed through the growing female education system plus specialist colleges of physical education for middle-class females. At first the Ling system of gymnastics was promoted as a suitable activity for young women. In 1887 a Swedish woman, Martina Bergman-Österberg, had launched her own college at Dartford in which girls practiced the Ling system. Later, girls also played competitive sports like hockey, cricket, tennis and netball.[31] These were felt to be suitable sports, involving less physical contact compared to the football codes.[32] The first set of rules for netball had been published in 1901; the game had been originally devised by female students at Bergman-Österberg's Physical Training College in Hampstead. Although the American sport of basketball had been introduced into England in the 1890s, it was considered to be too physical for young women and netball was invented as an alternative.[33] In 1894 the *British Medical Journal* had published an article condemning women who played football, stating that, 'We can in no way sanction the reckless exposure to violence, of organs which the common experience of women had led them in every way to protect'.[34]

The major sports that both men and women competed in were golf and lawn tennis. Tennis was originally seen as a social pastime for the middle classes where future partners could meet – a function that continued well into the 20th century. Due to its popularity, the first ladies' singles championship at Wimbledon was introduced in 1884. By 1890 there were 30 ladies' golf clubs and in 1893 the first Ladies' Amateur Golf Championship was played. Hockey was also a popular sport and in 1895 the All-England Women's Hockey Association was formed. In 1911 300 clubs and around 10,000 players were affiliated to the association.[35] Their involvement in the Olympic Games, however, was strictly limited. Women first competed in the 1900 Paris games but they only numbered six and were restricted to tennis.[36] In 1912 women were permitted to compete in swimming, although this was only one event, the 100 metres freestyle. A Greek woman, Melpomene, had actually run in the 1896 marathon despite being refused permission; women's track and field athletics was not seen in the Olympic arena until 1928.[37]

Women and sport in the inter-war years

For British women and sport the inter-war period, as Jennifer Hargreaves has argued, was a time of 'tremendous unevenness and contrasts' and 'spawned new values and practices *and* held on to old ones'.[38] Women in general were becoming more assertive. The First World War had proved an important watershed in the lives of women. Many women during the war had been thrown into previously male-only roles and by 1918 over one million women were working in munitions factories (although most returned to a life of domesticity). In that same year women finally received the vote. In addition, from the 1920s popular culture became increasingly commercialized, stimulating the growth of sports and hence, women's participation.

Many sports continued to be specific to upper-class and middle-class women with certain activities such as climbing, sailing and skiing, only available to these groups. However, there was beginning to be a wider acceptance of women's sport. In 1921, for example, the conference of the Medical Officers of Schools of Association had rejected the view that athletics and gymnastics were bad for the health of girls.[39] Through an expanding physical education curriculum, middle-class girls now enjoyed games like hockey, lacrosse, netball, cricket, tennis and rounders. Working-class girls in contrast were mainly restricted to drill at school and exposed to very little physical recreation once they had left education and started a family.[40]

Nevertheless, during the 1920s 'a changing cultural image of femininity … began to subvert the old idea that athleticism was desexing women'.[41] This transformation was highlighted by a number of sportswomen who came to international prominence, including the American, Mildred Didrikson. An all-rounder, she excelled at high school in team sports like baseball and basketball. At the 1932 Olympics she won two track and field gold medals before turning to professional golf and winning 17 tournaments in a row in 1946.[42] Another American, Gertrude Ederle, became the first woman to swim the English Channel in 1926. The aviators Amelia Earhart and Amy Johnson were able to match and surpass the achievements of men in their field. The most famous female athlete of the 1920s was the tennis player Suzanne Lenglen from France, who, it was claimed, was a bigger draw than her male equivalent, Bill Tilden.[43] Fanny Blankers-Koen later gained notoriety when she won four gold medals at the 1948 Olympics. Women's football also enjoyed a brief period of popularity during and just after the First World War. On Boxing Day 1921 a crowd of 53,000 watched a game at Everton FC's Goodison Park between two women's teams, Dick, Kerr from Preston and St. Helens. It was one of a number of matches organized to raise funds for ex-servicemen and other war-time causes. In that same year, however, the Football Association banned women from playing on the grounds of clubs affiliated to the governing body. Part of the reason given by the FA Council was that it felt 'that the game of football is quite unsuitable for females and ought not to be encouraged'.[44]

From the inter-war period the fashion for physical culture developed greater momentum.[45] In light of debates over the fitness of the nation, for example, one of the original aims of the Women's Amateur Athletic Association (WAAA) had been 'to improve the physique and physical efficiency of the nation'.[46] This was also the era of the 'body beautiful', exemplified by the establishment of physical culture movements throughout Europe and North America. Although originally designed for men, the Health and Strength League opened up its membership to women in 1919. Its magazine, *Health and Strength* regularly extolled women athletes and female physical culture, and also defended women's expanded employment opportunities. With membership at over 100,000 in 1931, a 'Health and Strength' annual display that included physical excellence competitions for men and women was the highlight of the league's activities from the late 1920s.[47] The Women's League of Health and Beauty was founded in 1930 and by 1939 had a membership of 166,000. Rather than competitive sport, it emphasized a clean and healthy lifestyle and put on mass exercise demonstrations based on the nationalist Sokol Movement in Czechoslovakia. It also promoted its own ideals of femininity like healthy motherhood through the 'free' use of the body through exercises and display.[48] During the 1930s the state, in preparation for war, also concerned itself with improving the health of women through the National Fitness Campaign.[49]

With the increase in participation of women, some authors began to give advice on the training methods for elite female athletes. Many of the recommendations advocated a more moderate approach. Although this would perhaps be expected in light of the prevailing medical opinion, Moon has argued that training advice for men was also moderate in tone and the earliest books on athletics for women made recommendations that were similar to those for men. One such publication was F.A.M. Webster's *Athletics of Today for Women* (1930), which recommended a lesser degree of intensity of training for women.[50]

Women's sporting activities, however, were inextricably linked to their life-cycle with the stage of youth – between leaving school and marriage – the pre-eminent period of sport for women.[51] Girls were advised to reduce their levels of physical exertion once they experienced the onset of puberty and this could have had a bearing on the scope and nature of future female sporting activities. Even Webster, an advocate of women's athletics, argued that during the ages between fourteen and eighteen, the athletic activities of girl should be watched and closely regulated as, it was stated, this was the most important period in female life.[52] But the advice of moderation was not just due to the perceived threat to a woman's reproductive function but also reflected notions of femininity. In 1938 Douglas Lowe, 800m Olympic champion in 1928 and 1932, advised that it would be safer for women 'to concentrate on style and grace … and only compete with moderation' as 'they will retain their femininity'.[53]

In addition to the idea of constitutional overstrain and its supposed effects on reproduction, much stress was placed in the literature on women's nerves and emotions. Charles Heald, for example, felt that a woman's recovery from injury would take longer than a man's because 'women were more liable than men to nervous instability'.[54] At the 1936 Olympics it was reported that female athletes were unhappy with their accommodation. The IOC official report stated that it wasn't due to any deficiencies in the hotel 'but merely to the fact that after long and intense training, women are very high strung immediately before difficult contests'.[55] In 1955 the Belgian Medical Society of Physical and Sporting Education announced that women should no longer compete in sport. One of the reasons they gave was that women were 'over vulnerable to emotional factors'.[56]

Female athletics and the Olympics

How did these debates play out in the world of women's sport? What impact did they have on its development? Here the example of the relationship between women's athletics, particularly in England, and the Olympics is used to illuminate the answers. First, there was a significant increase in the development of women's athletics in England during these years. In 1921 the Women's Amateur Athletic Association was formed and four years later it had spawned 25,000 members from over 500 clubs.[57] The WAAA had been very conscious of contemporary debates about the effect of sports on female athletes. Due to persistent criticism about the advisability of athletics for women, the WAAA felt that it was essential to provide evidence that the sport was not harming those participating. To achieve this, the WAAA adopted a policy of moderation. It gained the support of many doctors who in turn were supportive of women's involvement. As much as a pragmatic compromise, the WAAA was led by medical opinion. Tug-of-war, for example, was banned by the WAAA because as one of the 'more trying events', it was considered to be a health risk.[58]

Moreover, through its own medical commissions and testing, the WAAA was always careful not to be seen as putting their athletes at physical risk.[59] Testing athletes was an important policy of the WAAA from the 1920s well into the 1960s.[60] Rather than to ascertain sex,[61] these were tests to confirm femininity, or at least its dominant ideal. Supported with the information of the medical examination of female athletes from these trials, it allowed women's athletics to approach the IAAF and argue for the inclusion of certain events. In 1923 a medical commission, composed of two doctors and Sam Mussabini, had looked into the possibilities of including the pole vault and triple jump in the WAAA programme of events. For reasons unknown, however, the events were considered unsuitable. The following winter a medical commission was reconvened in order to judge whether cross-country racing was suitable for women. The panel consisted of several leading doctors including Dr Shirley Smith from the National Heart hospital. Female runners were examined and doctors 'expressed their great surprise at the runners' condition', adding that cross-country 'in moderation and with proper training was suitable for women'. In 1928 more precise scientific tests were conducted regarding 'stride, oxygen in-take, exhaustion and recovery tests after running. As much as athletes' bodies, the WAAA was concerned with perceptions of women's bodies. During its early years, for example, throwing events were performed with both hands with the two results combined for an overall distance, and was designed to prevent uneven body development.[62]

How was women's athletics received by the IOC? As Kevin Wamsley has argued no other institution has provided more opportunities for female athletes to participate in elite sport than the Olympic Games. Yet on the other hand no institution has shaped more the consumption of women's sport. In this sense, an Olympic culture 'actively promoted the feminized athlete, while tolerating but systematically criticizing those who participated in traditional men's events or who did not exude the typically expected feminine physical traits'.[63] While more women began to compete in the Olympics, participation continued to be limited and there was much resistance within the IOC. It was not only dominated by a male social elite but it was also built on the bourgeois values of the English gentleman-amateur. Pierre de Coubertin, the founder of the modern day games, had wanted the games to be male-only and where the rewards for winners would include female applause. De Coubertin felt that athletics made women appear indecent, improper and ugly.[64] In addition, newspaper reports on the Olympics from the 1920s tended to sexualize female athletes, and after 1932 women were channelled into so-called 'feminine' sports like swimming, gymnastics, figure skating and fencing.[65]

Despite the opposition though the number of women in the Olympics did continue to grow. Why did this happen? Why did the IOC, given de Coubertin's position, not block them? Because historians can sometimes be led by their sources the views of important and more high-profile officials, like de Coubertin, can be given greater prominence over lesser figures despite evidence to the contrary. At the early Olympics where women had competed, these had been organized by local committees who had invited them and it was only after 1912 that the IOC took control over the programme. It is difficult to know why these early Olympics permitted their entry. Reasons may have ranged from voyeurism to people on these committees having feminist sympathies. Certainly, the early female Olympic sports – golf, tennis, archery and figure skating – were those popular amongst the middle classes and so had a social acceptability for the gentleman-amateur.[66]

There was a gathering momentum to modernize and include more women in the Olympics. Some of this was a product of growing political pressure within international sports federations whose members sat on the IOC. Swimming was the first to promote women's participation following the formation of the Federation Internationale De Natation (FINA) in 1908. In 1921 Alice Milliat from France pioneered female international competition, founding the Federation Sportive Feminine International (FSFI). In 1922, under the auspices of the FSFI, the first Women's Olympic Games was held in Paris, and between 1921 and 1936 Milliat organized nine international events, under the title of 'Women's World Games'.[67] The success of the FSFI gatherings caused some embarrassment within the IOC. Sigfrid Edstrøm, who was more politically astute than other members, accepted that women's participation was inevitable if the IOC was to promote itself as the leading body of world sport. However, like de Coubertin his successor as IOC President, Baillet-Latour, he did not favour women's participation.[68]

To a certain extent, women's athletics, in their desire to compete at Olympic level, was willing to conform to dominant male ideas of what constituted a female athlete. In 1925 women's athletics became the subject of the IOC's Pedagogic Conference where one of the key speakers was England's Sophie Eliott-Lynn, vice-President of the WAAA. Moon has argued, however, that the overall effect of her paper 'was to hinder the development of athletics on the world stage for several years' and that in general the opinions of the people supporting women's athletics did not differ greatly from the general attitudes of the day.[69] Eliott-Lynn proceeded to highlight the differences between men and women when they participated in sport, and stressed the possible detrimental effects on the female reproductive system by endorsing the concept of constitutional overstrain. Sports usually suitable for men, therefore, should be modified 'so that they cannot in any way injure the woman'.[70]

In addition, the WAAA had supported the limiting of distances to 1,000 metres to fall in line with other European countries by 1925 – and a reduction in weights for throwing events.[71] In practice, 800 metres or 880 yards, was usually the longest track-distance. Even this was too long for some members of the WAAA, including Eliott-Lynn. She felt that running 'in moderation [was] an ideal sport for women' but that 300 yards should be the longest distance allowed until 'time has proved that damage is not done'. The FSFI recommended lighter throwing objects for women and their ruling became standard for female competitions. For instance, in the shot putt the women threw an 8lb shot; the men 16lbs. The WAAA and the FSFI may have been pioneering a new activity for women but partly through Eliott-Lynn's thinking, it allowed every male-administered governing body to justify restricting women's participation in athletics. The governing bodies were determined that any development would remain within accepted boundaries. The hurdles barriers, for example, were restricted to 2 feet 6 inches by the IAAF whereas the WAAF had wanted a height of 3 feet. It was agreed that the primary role of women was motherhood, and this was not to be altered by the emerging sporting opportunities.[72] Women's track and field first entered the Olympics – in limited numbers – in 1928. However, this would have long-term consequences for the FSFI as it was now doomed to a slow suicide due to its efforts to gain admittance to the Olympics.[73] During the Games themselves there was criticism of the 800 metres because it was felt – incorrectly – that some of the women finished in a distressed state. As a consequence, this event was not put back on the programme until 1960.

The British state and the female athletic body

Debates regarding the nature of women's sport now encompassed a wide range of opinion from what might be termed the modern to the more traditional in which motherhood was seen as their key role in society. These debates were illuminated within the National Fitness Council (NFC). The NFC had been formed following the Physical Training and Recreation Act of 1937, which had the overall aim to improve the fitness of the entire British nation. However, the ideal of 'fitness' was not gender neutral with different ideas on how it could be achieved regarding men and women, as well as boys and girls. There was also an eugenicist context to the issue. Although the Eugenics Society worried about the effects of 'vigorous exercise on the female reproductive organs', it was in their interests to promote physical exercise due to mounting evidence that fitter women produced healthier offspring.[74] Between 1938 and 1939 an NFC Medical Sub-Committee on the 'Desirability of Athletics for Women and Girls' was established to investigate that very subject, especially with regard to competitive sport. In particular, this sub-committee revolved around contemporary debates concerning the effect of competitive sport and certain events on a woman's menstrual cycle, and as a consequence her ability to bear children.[75]

The committee was originally set up, ironically, following a request for a grant by the WAAA to the NFC. Instead, an investigation was set up to consider whether athletics could actually be regarded as beneficial exercise for women.[76] The medical sub-committee was then formed with Adolphe Abrahams in the chair.[77] A disagreement over an initial report led to another more extensive and wide-ranging enquiry. While Abrahams chaired it, four out of its five members were women: Muriel Cornell (nee Gunn), the secretary of the WAAA and holder of the British long jump record; Dr Anna Broman of the Women's Medical Association; Phyllis Spafford of the National Playing Fields Association and the Ling Association of Teachers of Swedish Gymnastics; and Dr Lilias Blackett Jeffries, a consultant gynaecologist.

Interestingly, as part of the committee's remit, it was decided that 'any type of violent exercise which might be detrimental to the essential function of women *should not* necessarily be ruled out'.[78] A number of leading figures on women's sport and physical activity were interviewed about their area of expertise. All reflected the largely middle-class make-up of women's sport.[79] Questions revolved around not just any potential ill-effects on menstruation and their ability to reproduce from strenuous exercise and competitive sport but also an athlete's femininity. For example, they were asked, 'Is the athletic girl at least as "feminine" in appearance and temperament as the average of her sex or does she tend towards aggressiveness and masculinity?' All interviewees felt that there were few if any dangers concerning competitive sport and few precautions were taken. Rowers and swimmers, for example, seldom pulled out of races or stopped training during their period. When Doman was asked 'Is there reason to suppose athletic girls suffer more or less at their periods than the average or non-athletic?' she thought that the athletic girls suffered less. When questioned on taking precautions for swimming only the wearing of ear-plugs was suggested. There was though a continuing concern that sportswomen should be seen to be feminine in appearance and style.

In addition, through Cornell the WAAA circulated 600 questionnaires to its members. Questions again focussed on menstruation, the health positives and negatives of athletics as well as the impact of competition on 'nerve strain'. None of the respondents were 'aware of any ill-effects resulting from their athletic activities'. With married women, there was no evidence of relative sterility or complications during pregnancy and parturition due to their participation in athletics.[80] Following those from the world of sport, a number of women from an educational background – and maybe from a self-improvement tradition – were interviewed.[81] Perhaps unsurprisingly, they were more critical and cautious of women's elite sport because educational establishments aimed to produce 'ladies' with refined tastes and manners rather than elite athletes. Although they did not discourage physical training they did make a distinction between this and highly competitive sport.

Some of the evidence seemed contradictory. Miss Foster, for example, argued that under the strain of regular competition, some first-class tennis players became aggressive and hysterical but that this did not necessarily apply to the 'really great tennis players who were exceptional people'. Dr Garrow said that few girls broke down in training and was generally relaxed over the issue of menstruation and sport. However, 'from the aesthetic point of view, she thought that women looked dreadful when taking part in some highly competitive events, and seriously reduced their sex appeal and corresponding opportunities'.[82] The seemingly robust attitudes of these British women towards menstruation were perhaps beginning to ape those in America. Lara Friedenfelds has argued that a new outlook towards menstruation developed during the Progressive era. More women took seriously the health advice from experts and let go of 'old concerns about protecting their bodies during menstruation so they could work and play all month'. Menstruation was managed in a modern and rational way as women now drew upon expert advice, popular education and consumerism.[83]

As a result, there was little evidence to criticize women's sport on the grounds of its threat to their ability to reproduce. Adolphe Abrahams' only response seemed to be exasperation. He commented that the sub-committee 'had endeavoured to obtain adverse criticism on violent exercise for women and girls but up to the present without success'.[84] A fellow member of the medical committee, Kaye le Fleming, then the chair of the council of the BMA, was critical of highly competitive sport's impact on the female form because it caused 'muscular development'.[85] However, in view of the evidence provided it seemed a weak response. The final witnesses called provided completely different views. Cedric Lane Roberts, a leading gynaecologist and an advocate of abortion,[86] on the whole did not disapprove of the principle of highly competitive sport.[87] In contrast to him, a German gynaecologist, Stephan Westmann, was of the opposite opinion. In his book *Sport, Physical Training and Womanhood* (1939), he had argued that the uterus was the most vulnerable and endangered part of the female body, and that excessive physical exercise – although moderate exercise was recommended – would have an inhibiting effect of the development of the pelvis and, as a result, it would cause difficulties in childbirth.[88] But his medical opinion was also conditioned by social and cultural assumptions. He further argued, 'Competitive sports are alien to the characteristics of the female constitution and are useless as well as harmful in relation to the primary task of woman's life, maternity'.[89] He also warned that, 'Every woman should remember that exaggerated sports involve her in the danger of becoming masculine'.[90] Westmann instead recommended eurhythmics and gymnastics for women because they helped prepare them for maternity.[91] He reiterated this point during his interview adding that violent exercise may lead to sterility. He further failed to endear himself to the female members of the committee by arguing that, psychologically, women were trying to compensate for an inferiority complex through competitive sport. Yet Westmann's views were considered extreme, and Abrahams was even a critic.[92] The committee failed to dig up any substantial evidence that competitive and strenuous sport was a danger to women. Cornell subsequently pushed for the medical sanctioning of events such as the long jump and hurdling.[93] However, before any action could be taken, or medical approval given, the war intervened and the National Fitness Council was disbanded.

Women, sport and medicine in the post-war period

In post-war Britain, partly as a result of the 1944 Education Act, which made physical education compulsory for boys and girls at secondary school, there was a surge in interest and participation regarding women's sport.[94] Nevertheless, some doctors continued to see women's sport in terms of its feminine qualities. Adolphe Abrahams, for example, claimed that:

> Feminine accomplishments require grace, lightness, and rhythmicity, and these
> attributes should characterize the exercises towards which there is perhaps an

instinctive impulsion. Golf, lawn tennis, croquet, swimming, archery, fencing are to be favoured. All forms of violent exercise, especially when accompanied by the nervous tension of serious rather than friendly competition, tend to aggressiveness and to disappearance of that softness and ductility some are glad still to identify with womanhood's charm.[95]

However, the medical debate around women's sport was starting to shift. While some continued to argue that menstruation reduced performance by the 1950s, other medical opinion was providing scientific support for women athletes to counter this argument. A report on the 1952 Olympics, *Sports in the Cultural Pattern of the World*, found that sportswomen were stronger and more physiologically able to cope with physical exercise than had previously been thought. It concluded that even competitive exercise did not affect the menstrual cycles of trained athletes.[96]

Moreover, women's athletics found increasing support from men. In 1955, in an article in *Athletics Weekly*, the coach, George Pallett summed up the history of medical opinion regarding women in athletics and dispelled many of the fears about the detrimental effects of athletics on women's bodies, childbirth and menstruation. Also in 1955, Harold Abrahams now took a different position to that of his brother. He challenged the medical profession to produce any real evidence to support the idea that athletics was bad for women. He argued that women had now been competing around the world in sports for many years and that even if hundreds of women had suffered physically or psychologically, all it proved was that competitive sport was not good for some women just as it had not been good for some men.[97]

Despite the opposition of many male doctors, men like Pallett, played an important role in the development of women's sport. In the preface to her book, *Athletics for Women and Girls*, Sophie Eliott Lynn acknowledged the assistance of a number of male athletes and coaches, in particular, Sam Mussabini.[98] In addition, the foreword was written by Lord Desborough, a member of the British Olympic Council while Brigadier-General R.J. Kentish, another member of the BOC, penned an appreciation. Both were founding supporters of the WAAA. At the grass-roots level of local athletics clubs in England male support was widespread. As Lynne Duval states: 'Wherever a club was based and regardless of whether it catered solely for women or not, the influence of men in the development of women's athletics cannot be denied.'[99] This influence could take the form of coach or officials. In addition, it was fathers and brothers who encouraged their daughters and sisters to play sport. The British sprinter, Dorothy Hyman admitted that her father was the driving force behind her athletics career while the father of swimmer Anita Lonsbrough taught her to swim.[100] Both women were from West Yorkshire, allegedly a traditional bastion of masculinity. It perhaps begs the question of how many men actually took seriously the medical warnings about women playing sport.

However, opposition to women's sport was still deep rooted at the higher echelons of the IOC and IAAF. Avery Brundage, IOC President between 1952 and 1972, was still of the view that women should conform to a certain feminine type, and that they should compete in sports like swimming and gymnastics. However, he was against them competing in masculine events like the shot putt, which was not introduced into the Olympics until 1948.[101] Similar views were expressed by IOC representative, Dr Messerli. He was an historian of the IOC and founder of the Swiss Olympic Committee. In 1952, writing in the *Olympic Bulletin*, he felt that although women's sport was making steady progress there should still be restrictions. It was a view based on both the perception of a woman's role in society and medical opinion that warned against strenuous exercise.

> We are of the opinion, that these restrictions are all for the good, seeing that woman has a noble task in life namely to give birth to healthy children and to bring them up in the best conditions. We must do everything in our power to improve her conditions of living, but on the other hand, we must avoid everything which can be injurious to her health and harm her as a potential mother.[102]

These views were justified for the restriction of women's participation in a number of Olympic events. After the 1936 games certain track and field athletic events – middle and long-distance races plus the triple and high jumps – had been deemed 'unsuitable' for women. Messerli had actually dismissed the reports that women athletes had finished in a distressed state after the 800 metres at the Amsterdam games but instead stated that there was nothing wrong with them, 'they burst into tears, thus betraying their disappointment at having lost the race, a very feminine trait'.[103] He also felt that it was right to exclude women from some skiing events like jumping and Nordic cross-country races as well as long-distance swimming races. Moreover, the exclusion and inclusion of some events was based on notions of femininity. Regarding water polo, for example, 'only men can practice this rough sport' while it was felt that figure skating 'is eminently suited to women' (see below for a critique of this perception).[104] In addition, Messerli disapproved strongly of women's boxing or wrestling. After attending the women's wrestling championships he said that 'I can safely say that I never saw anything more grotesque or less womanly'. He also noted that in 1928 'it seemed to us that some women competitors running the 800 metres were handicapped by too full a bosom'.[105]

Sport, the Cold War and gender testing

Women's sport took on a greater significance in light of the Cold War. The entry of the USSR into the Olympics for the first time in 1952 and its rivalry with the USA for supremacy in the medals table meant that a gold medal won by a woman was as good as that won by a man and Soviet bloc female athletes were more successful than their men. However, their success brought both suspicion and criticism in the West and ultimately ushered in the widespread implementation of sex/gender testing.[106] As Heggie has pointed out, testing for the sex of athletes gives an insight into social attitudes towards gender and in particular 'how the co-option of science in sport … can act to essentialize social categories', when in fact matters of gender are more complicated than a strict male-female divide.[107]

Concerns over the 'true' gender of female athletes were not new. In the 1920s Mary Weston won a number of WAAA throwing titles then in 1934 had a sex change operation. The Czech, Zdenek Koubek, won female athletics titles during the 1930s before in 1936 requesting that the state should recognize him as a man. At the 1936 Olympics questions were raised over the 'masculine' physique of Helen Stephens, the winner of the women's 100 metres. She was subsequently 'tested' and 'passed'. Dora Ratjen, who won a silver medal in the women's high jump at the same Games, was actually called Heinrich and was a case of 'gender uncertainty'. The IAAF introduced a form of sex testing in 1946, which required female athletes at the London Olympics two years later to bring a medical certificate to confirm their sex.[108]

Debates over the 'correct' gender of athletes gained momentum during the Cold War and were reflected in the Western media. Wiederkehr has argued that press coverage showed 'a clear tendency to juxtapose attractive females from the West with ugly and virilised sportswomen from the Soviet bloc'.[109] As a consequence, there was a persistent questioning of the femininity of female athletes from Eastern Europe and their record-breaking performances. In 1968 the German sports physician and former athlete, Ingrid Bausenwein, claimed that five out of eleven track and field female world recordholders were 'not really women'. The achievements of the Press sisters, Tamara and Irina, were given particular attention – they were called the Press brothers.[110]

Sex testing, or at least the calls for it, also needs to be set in the context of debates over cheating due to contemporary anxieties over doping and altitude during this period. In 1967 the newly formed IOC Medical Commission prescribed procedures for drugs and sex testing.[111] Sex tests had been first introduced at the European Athletic Championships in 1966 at which the Press sisters withdrew. These were physical examinations which female athletes found degrading. Mary Peters, Olympic Pentathlon champion in 1972, described it as 'a grope'.[112] Following a series of examinations the Polish athlete, Ewa Klobukowska, then world record holder for the 100 metres, failed the test. In 1970 the IAAF removed her name from the record books. Two years later the IOC introduced a more 'scientific' examination – the Barr body test. It was a sex chromatin or buccal smear test that involved the screening of epithelial cells scraped from inside of the cheek. The cells are then stained to reveal the presence or absence of the Barr body i.e., cellular artefacts. This is caused by the inactivation of one of the two X chromosomes in female cells. Male cells do not show this Barr body as they only have one active X chromosome. The chromosome constitution for a female would be XX, while for a man it would be XY.[113]

Between 1972 and 1990 it was estimated that one in 504 female athletes failed the gender verification test. However, it was also found to be an unjust process because of the number of genetic disorders that could interfere with sex development. This could lead to paradoxical findings between the anatomical sex (which is determined by the type of sex chromosome contributed by the father and forms the social and legal sex of a person) and the chromosomal sex. Thus, some individuals with an apparently normal male chromosome constitution develop to adulthood as girls i.e., XY females.[114] Tests on female athletes were not restricted to finding out their gender. Again, reflecting dominant ideas about the perceived frailty of women's bodies, the WAAA, following the death of Lillian Board from cancer, introduced a (voluntary) scheme for all athletes to allay fears that her disease had been the product of the effects of hard training.[115] In addition to gender testing, the case of Renee Richards further illuminated the physiological debates taking place regarding women's bodies. Richards had a sex change operation in 1975. She was formerly known as Richard Raskin who had been a useful junior tennis player in America. In 1976 Richards made a return to tennis playing on the women's circuit. She refused to take the test but was admitted entry to the 1977 US Open because a Supreme Court judge ruled that there was overwhelming evidence that she was a female. Richards reached the last eight of the tournament but retired soon after.[116]

During the 1980s, after failing the Barr body test, a Spanish athlete, Maria Martinez-Patino, successfully challenged its suitability, backed by human rights activists. While the testing for sex was not too problematic, it was ruled that using the test to judge sporting ability was inappropriate. This led first to the IAAF in 1992 and then the IOC to dispense with the test, and by 2000, despite a brief return to physical examination, sex testing had ended.[117] However, the controversy over Caster Semenya in 2009 would re-ignite these debates and anxieties over an issue that sport – because of the idea that it is based on and perpetuates clear gender divisions – has found difficult in coming to terms with.

Women, sport and the second wave of feminism

Despite the technical and scientific driven disputes over the 'correct' gender of athletes, from the 1960s there was a significant growth in females participating in sport. This was not confined to elite sport but also at the recreational level, especially in the United States. In the 1960s the emergence of identity politics in which feminism and women's liberation had been in the vanguard led to women and girls adopting new lifestyles, including a growing invasion of traditional male activities like sport. Of great symbolic importance was the victory of Billie Jean King over Bobby Riggs in tennis's so-called Battle of the Sexes in 1973. In America this process was reinforced through Title IX of the Education Amendments Act of 1972. It legalized parity between the genders in educational opportunities, including sport, and led to the rise in female educational, recreational and professional competition. Between 1973 and 1998 the number of women engaged in American intercollegiate sport increased by 112 per cent while the rate for men decreased by 11 per cent.[118]

These developments, along with persistent gender inequalities, had initially been highlighted following the 1967 Boston Marathon. Despite being banned, women had reputedly been running marathons at least since the 1896 Olympics. In 1967, however, it was widely publicized that two women, Millie Sampson and more notoriously Kathrine Switzer, had competed in and completed the Boston race. It had been thought within medical circles that a marathon would be harmful to the health of females. Medical opinion though took a significant turn. In 1979 the ACSM, in its first major declaration, stated that 'there exists no conclusive scientific or medical evidence that long-distance running is contraindicated for the healthy, trained female athlete'.[119] Ernst van Aaken, a German coach, actually promoted long-distance running for women. In the face of opposition he had used women and children in experiments to demonstrate that endurance training was not dangerous and concluded that women were better suited to it than men.[120] However, as Jutel has pointed out, changing attitudes towards women's long-distance running were as much the result of reassuring the public that running did not upset traditional gender roles and values as it was about medical opinion.[121] Nevertheless, due to the growing popularity of jogging generally and the improving standards in the event, the women's marathon was included in the Olympic programme in 1984.

In England opportunities were generally restricted for women compared to developments in the States. The 1975 Sex Discrimination Act outlawed the inequality of opportunity and access on grounds of gender but it did not apply to private sports clubs, such as the Marylebone Cricket Club, which could maintain their single sex status. However, the rise in the number of sports centres during the 1970s increased the opportunities for women to play sport, although participation here was largely restricted to the middle classes. The Women's Football Association though was recognized by the Football Association in 1972, fifty years after women's football had been banned from the grounds of clubs affiliated to the FA. More girls began to play the game but when to draw a line between differences between boys and girls had become a matter of legal debate for sporting organizations. In 1978 Theresa Bennett, a twelve year-old girl from Nottinghamshire, took the FA to court under section 44 of the Sex Discrimination Act for refusing to allow her to play for a boys team of the same age. At the time girls under twelve were banned from playing with boys. The FA argued – and was supported by the Women's

FA – that the average woman would be disadvantaged on account of physical strength and stamina compared to the average man. Bennett won her case but lost on appeal.[122] The FA continued to argue that after a certain age there could be 'unacceptable risk of injury to girls'. This decision had been taken on the advice of experts in child development. The ruling was based on the age where puberty would alter the strength and other physical characteristics that differentiate males from females. It was further argued that the muscle strength and power differentials between boys and girls, compounded by different rates of physical development, could lead to these unacceptable risks.[123]

The modern female athlete?

To what extent has this greater liberalization changed women's sport? At the level of pure numbers, there was an exponential increase in the number of female competitors at Summer Olympics. In 1968 they made up 14 per cent of total athletes; by 1996 this had increased to 34 per cent; and by 2008 the percentage was 42 per cent. More sports accepted women but even here dominant ideas about women shaped the nature of their acceptance. Furthermore, due to the growing influence of television, notions of femininity were reinforced through the popularity of 'traditional' female sports.

Some sports like rowing, which first admitted women at the 1976 Games, and were male-dominated, continued to resist female entry on both ideological and political grounds. For women's rowing it had been the initial influence of the Soviet Union that expedited its entry into the Games, reflecting a wider policy concerning women's sport in the Eastern bloc whose governments targeted female athletes for success at international level. According to Schweinbenz, there was a disregard for medical and aesthetic dogma in Eastern European countries in the pursuit of Olympic medals; and in women's sports they were easier to obtain because the standard in depth was not as great as in men's competitions. By contrast, it was expected of female athletes in the West that they remained attractive, did not appear masculine in appearance and retained their femininity.[124]

To a certain extent, these ideas began to break down in the West late in the twentieth century. With a greater emphasis placed on national sporting prestige, women's sport was taken more seriously, certainly at Olympic level. Tennis was also successful from a commercial viewpoint largely due to the efforts of Billy Jean King. However, the development of individual women's sports also needs to be seen in their own particular context. Up until the 1920s, for example, figure skating was a mixed-sex sport in Britain. From the inter-war period it became increasingly feminized and hence segregated. The women were more innovative and reached greater technical levels than the men, while the success and subsequent celebrity status of Sonja Henie meant women's figure skating events were more popular.[125]

Similarly, gymnastics has traditionally represented divisions based on perceptions of masculinity and femininity.[126] In competition these differences have been illustrated through the different apparatus they use. Yet within the sport gender differences have become more complicated as the sport became more competitive. Following the 1972 Olympics and the feats of Olga Korbut, for example, there was much criticism that female gymnasts had been turned into pixies and acrobats. It signalled a significant body change in female gymnasts from previous Olympics. In 1968 Vera Caslavska, the Czech gymnast, won four gold medals and two silvers. Her performances represented a 'demonstration of a mature gymnastics body performing graceful ballet-type routines and typified the model of mature femininity in this sport'.[127] In this period female gymnasts were largely judged on their 'harmonious flexibility and feminine grace', which was founded predominantly on ballet and artistic skills. However, these qualities were soon replaced with ones that were a product of the Soviet Union's sports policy. The Soviet Union led (or forced, along with other Eastern bloc countries) a move towards innovation in female gymnastics. Ironically, this entailed copying men's gymnastics that consisted of more aerial and tumbling elements. For female gymnastics, therefore, to perform these new acrobatic moves the gymnasts needed to be young girls. Not only could undeveloped female bodies perform the same elements as male gymnasts but it was also thought that young girls were not as fearful of performing riskier routines, such as back flips on the beam.[128]

The change in the nature of the sport was further confirmed with the emergence of Romania's Nadia Comaneci at the Montreal Games. In 1976 female US gymnasts were, on average, seventeen and a half years old, stood 5ft 3in and weighed 106 pounds. By 1992 these averages were sixteen years old, 4ft 9in and 83 pounds.[129] It was perhaps ironic that as the bodies of women's gymnastics began to transform in to the shape of little girls, this was partly a product of traditional masculine values. Not only had they borrowed techniques from the men's code but female gymnasts also now developed traditional masculine traits as they trained harder and were now subject to more danger. Just before the 1980 Olympics the Soviet gymnast Yelena Mukhina suffered a debilitating neck injury, which ultimately caused her death in 2006 while Julissa Gomez died in 1991 three years after an accident on the vault apparatus.[130] Moreover, female gymnasts competed through the pain barrier on many occasions and now required strapping on their feet due to the stresses put on them. At the 1996 Games the American Kerri Strug forced herself to take a vault despite a severe injury in order to ensure that the US team won the gold.[131] These developments also brought suggestions that gymnastics – as well as other sports involving young girls like tennis and ice-skating – is a form of child abuse and where athletes are not only bullied by their coaches but they are also subjected to the 'pushy parent' syndrome.[132] In 1995 Joan Ryan stated: 'There simply is no safety net protecting these children. Not the parents, the coaches or the federations.'[133]

Within female gymnastics the changing shape of their bodies due to the pressures of training and the changing regulations of the sport has given rise to eating disorders such as anorexia nervosa and bulimia (conditions which have also been found in female distance runners, figure skaters and ballet dancers).[134] In 1994 the American gymnast Christy Henrich died aged twenty-two after spending six years battling against anorexia. During an international event when she was fifteen years old, a judge had told her that to make the US Olympic team she had to lose weight.[135] Numerous other elite American gymnasts suffered from eating disorders, a number of whom were coached by Bela Karolyi, the former coach of Nadia Comaneci. It became a worldwide issue. In 1995 a former gymnast at the Australian Institute of Sport (AIS) lodged a lawsuit against the AIS, claiming that the Institute's training methods caused her to suffer from anorexia nervosa.[136] In response, in 1997 the International Gymnastics Federation raised the age limit for women to sixteen from fifteen for entry into the Olympics.[137] Moreover, in 2004 British Gymnastics launched a Child Protection Policy in line with the NSPCC's Child Protection in Sport Unit, which reflected increasing public concerns regarding female gymnasts as well as children. Interestingly, there currently seems to be a drift back towards more mature female gymnasts, reflected in the success of Chellsie Memmel and Britain's Beth Tweddle.

In addition to eating disorders, another condition that has been identified specific to female athletes has been the Female Athlete Triad. It was first identified in 1992 and is defined by a combination of disordered eating and heavy training leading to amenorrhea and eventually osteoporosis. It is most common in endurance sports such as running and swimming and those like figure skating, diving, and gymnastics in which appearance is deemed important. Delays in the menstrual cycle of young female athletes because they were underweight became common. Olga Korbut was nineteen at puberty while US Olympic gymnast, Kathy Johnson, did not have her first menstrual period until she was twenty-five. As a consequence, low estrogen levels can diminish bone mineral density and hence lead to osteoporosis.[138] To what extent has the attention been given to this injury/condition reflected older anxieties and patriarchal sensibilities that woman are 'different'? While it could be argued that the focus within the sports medicine press has overshadowed other 'normal' sporting injuries, the female athlete triad does have serious implications. Whether this had any impact on the participation of women in sport and other physical activities is difficult to judge.

Conclusion

In 2005 the last bastion of male sport was penetrated with the announcement that women's boxing was to be included in the 2012 Olympic Games; it had been the only Olympic sport in which women were not represented.[139] Of all sports boxing was the one where for many men 'it just wasn't right' for women to participate. Beyond the rather clichéd reasons of 'a woman's place' etc., most were unable to articulate a coherent response. In crude terms, boxing was perceived to be the epitome of masculinity while fighting was the antithesis of what was considered to be ladylike. The debate over women's boxing continues to echo what Osborne and Skillen have argued, that 'the body has been revealed as a critical site upon which understandings of women's experience have been inscribed'.[140] These understandings though have been social and cultural as much as medical assumptions regarding women's sport. The idea of 'gendered participation' has been based upon prevailing ideas of sex differences, which medical rhetoric has underpinned; and which, in turn, has underpinned medical rhetoric. As a consequence, 'sport remains one of the most resilient bastions of male power and gendered participation'.[141]

What has this meant for women's sport or to be less gender specific, women in sport? Jennifer Hargreaves has argued that with the expansion in the number of women playing sport there has been a blurring of traditional ideas of masculinity and femininity. Moreover, there has been a greater acceptance and evidence of women competing on equal terms in some sports, especially those that place an emphasis on endurance in which women may actually have a physiological advantage. Even in the 1960s British cyclist Beryl Burton held the world record for a twelve-hour time trial in competition with men.[142]

Yet these ultra-distance events are not 'sexy' at this current time if measured in terms of popularity such as television viewing figures. Instead, it is sports that place a higher value on the modern attributes of speed and power that attract most attention in terms of commercial value and it is these sports where differences between the sexes are more pronounced from a physiological perspective. However, as Mary Louise Adams has pointed out with reference to her work on ice-skating, that because the social organization of gender is historically and culturally contingent the 'games and pastimes of the other sex in one era might at another time be the games and pastimes of one's own'.[143] Due to changing ideas of masculinity and femininity, sports in the future may hold different meanings for their audience and place less emphasis on speed and power and more on qualities such as endurance and artistry. Of course, it is difficult to predict the future and it should also be pointed out that many women enjoy participating in and watching traditional masculine sports. Moreover, to what extent has the reality of women's sport reflected these wider perceptions? It has been difficult to assess the impact of these debates on women themselves and their attitude to sport. Joyce Kay has criticized work on the history of women's sport for overly concentrating on the negative aspects. Looking at Britain, she argues that instead, women mostly just 'got on with the job' and paid little attention to the attitudes and opinions of other parties.[144]

8

Boxing

A Medical History

Introduction

In 1991 Michael Watson was stopped in the last round of his contest with Chris Eubank. He later collapsed and was rushed to hospital where he underwent lengthy brain surgery. The fight had been broadcast live and had earlier been the focus of much media hyperbole. As Watson's condition deteriorated it became clear that he was to suffer from the consequences of long-term brain damage. It re-ignited the debate over the ethical nature of boxing and whether the sport should be banned. A few months afterwards a bill to ban the sport was brought before the House of Lords. Although this was defeated, consequences of the Watson-Eubank fight and the Benn-McClellan fight four years later would have important consequences for boxing. In 1999 Watson, now severely disabled, successfully sued the professional sport's governing body, the British Boxing Board of Control (BBBC),[1] for a breach of their duty of care, and received £1 million. Following similar criticisms of the sport during the twentieth century, boxing responded by tightening up its medical regulations. Not only was this for the benefit for the safety of the boxers, however, but also to protect the public image of the sport.

This high profile case highlighted many of the medical issues concerning the relationship between sport and medicine. A case study of boxing in general, and the issue of punch-drunkenness and injuries to the head in particular, pulls together many of the different themes of this book. This includes developments within medicine generally, duty of care, the changing medical provisions of sport, legal aspects and injuries. The focus is essentially on Britain. Other countries have engaged in similar debates but it is Britain where they have been most illuminating. America has lacked a national boxing body while elsewhere the sport did not have the popularity it enjoyed in Britain and the US.

The essence of boxing's relationship with the medical profession has revolved around debates over the morality of the sport. These debates have been embedded in two opposing ethical stances.[2] The first stresses the principle of 'individual autonomy'. In other words, those who freely choose to box know the potential injury and damage they can inflict on opponents and also be inflicted upon themselves, thus they should be granted the right to do so; and others have no right to prevent such freedom of choice. The second stance, and one largely associated with the medical profession, has been based on the idea of 'paternalism': whereas in other sports injuries are accidental, it is the specific aim of boxers to injure and harm their opponents. Such damage, it is argued, is morally objectionable in a civilized society.[3] Of course, notions of a 'civilized society' and 'civilization' are themselves social and cultural constructions, which owe much to the emergence of an English national character in the early nineteenth century built on Burkean conservative values.[4] Moreover, rather than the sport being subjected to a 'civilizing process' in the era since the prize-fighting era, as Sheard has argued,[5] boxing during the twentieth century, at its core, was and remains inherently violent. Instead, this chapter builds on other work by Sheard as well as Welshman that has analysed the relationship between boxing and the medical profession.[6]

Here, medical intervention in boxing and the accompanying debates are analyzed through three overlapping processes. First, the relationship between boxing and medicine owed much to voluntarism with both doctors giving up their free time to supervise boxing promotions as well as highlighting sport's place more generally within civil society i.e., free from government intervention. Second, and most significantly, as part of the emergence of a social democratic ethos and the pervasiveness of welfarism during the twentieth century, the medical profession held a more prominent and visible role in society. Third, boxing's survival has been partly a product of consumerist tendencies which have placed an emphasis on the freedom to choose.

The ethos of boxing and its early history

Boxing, or as it was more commonly known prizefighting, had largely been an illegal activity since the 1700s and its history of the sport has been bound up with its fluctuating legal status over the last 250 years. Initially, boxing contests had been banned largely on the grounds of public order and from 1800 nearly all fights took place in the countryside to frustrate attempts by local magistrates to suppress them.[7] Early in the nineteenth century, prizefighting had been run largely by 'the Fancy', a group of leisured gentlemen who regularly placed wagers on sporting contests, especially in prizefighting and pedestrianism. However, their influence, along with the sport's reputation due to its association with gambling and corruption, waned from the 1820s with the emergence of the moral reform movement and the sport only survived at a subterranean level.[8]

Importantly, for its future survival during the nineteenth and for most of the twentieth century, boxing was part of the curriculum at public schools. Students were inculcated with a sense that boxing was the noble art that had character-building qualities. It was vital to the virility of the British male race and supposedly imbued the principle of fair play. Boxing was inscribed with English virtues. In 1864 it was described as a manly exercise in which fists were regarded as natural weapons. It was said that 'All Englishmen, and therefore, all English boys, are proud of their natural weapon and compare it with the knife, the loaded stick, the knuckleduster and the pistol of other nations'. By contrast, the French system of fighting, Savate was described as contemptible as it was the 'execrable French custom of striking upwards with the knee when at close quarters'. Instead, emphasis was placed on the 'principle of fair play and justice' which is 'strongly developed in an English breast' and where 'no unfair advantage is allowed to either side, no striking upon the vital parts of the body is permitted, and the use of the foot, tooth, or nail is forbidden under the severest penalties'.[9]

The idea of boxing as the noble art that had character-building qualities was still prevalent when medical arguments began to challenge the sport's legality. In the columns of the medical journals, doctors who had boxed at school countered the medical arguments of colleagues. One letter in the *British Medical Journal* in 1955 acknowledged the dangers of the sport but still felt that,

> from the experience of some ten years of active participation, and many more years of interest, that boxing is sufficiently worth while as a virile character sport to justify our taking every precaution to ensure its continuation under conditions of reasonable prudency.[10]

One of the opponents to the first motion calling for the abolition of boxing at the British Medical Association's AGM in 1960 stressed boxing's 'character building' qualities, and concluded by saying 'What would Sir Francis Drake have thought of this motion?'[11]

Boxing and the medical profession

Doctors were often split on the dangers of boxing, partly on cultural grounds. While those who disliked the sport were part of a tradition of self-improvement and rational recreation, other doctors became supporters of the sport after enjoying a public school education in which boxing was part of the curriculum.[12] Lew Blonstein, who was the long-time medical officer for the Amateur Boxing Association (ABA), had first boxed at a club affiliated to the London Federation of Working Boys Clubs in Aldgate when he was eleven. Boxing was introduced into his school when he was in the sixth form and he continued fighting at University College London when a medical student during the 1920s. He fought in inter-hospital matches against other students from Guy's and St. Bartholomew's. Medical students continued to fight in the United Hospital Championship up to at least the 1960s.[13] Given his background, it is perhaps unsurprising that of all the defenders of boxing in light of the increasing attacks on it, Blonstein's voice was the loudest. Blonstein's counterpart in the professional game for many years was John Graham. Although he did not box at school he had whilst serving in the army during the First World War. He continued his interest after the war by training in a gym whilst undertaking his medical studies in Manchester.[14]

That doctors were aware of the damage blows to the head could cause had not been restricted to the twentieth century. However, there was only a limited understanding of how the brain worked in the medical world. Neurology was still an embryonic specialty by the late nineteenth century. It had largely evolved out of psychiatry. Nerve doctors, as neurologists were called, were mainly concerned with organic diseases whereas psychiatrists treated the functional disorders of nervous patients, especially after the Great War.[15] Research on reflexes, however, had led to a number of conditions being attributed to neurological diseases. Strokes, for example, had been diagnosed in 1658 while Parkinson's disease was first recognized as a clinical condition attributed to some form of damage to the brain in 1817. In 1906 Alois Alzheimer outlined the clinical and neuropathological evidence for the disease that would carry his name. Because of the ignorance of how the brain worked, brain surgery on living patients was mostly guesswork. For hundreds of years no one had dared to operate on the brain. The work of two Englishmen, John Hughlings Jackson and David Ferrier, on epilepsy in the late nineteenth century, led to a more confident mapping of locating tumours and mapping the brain generally. Another Englishman, Victor Horsley, later became the world's first specialist neurosurgeon.[16] As a result, without the knowledge that boxing could produce significant brain damage, doctors were able to pursue their interest in boxing. And even when this medical knowledge came to light, a culture of resistance had been built up within a significant section of the medical profession. Due to the enthusiasm of some doctors for the sport, it allowed boxing to call on their support, thus giving it some credibility.

In light of the lack of medical knowledge, the medical profession was not that interested in boxing in the early twentieth century. Instead, it had previously turned its attention to the physical dangers of football (see Chapter 2). An early mention of boxing as a hazard to health had appeared in the *Lancet* in September 1893 under the heading of 'Revival of Prize-fighting: Serious Results'. Little was known of the medical effects of boxing and any objections were usually on moral and social grounds. One letter to the *Lancet* in 1901 had hoped that the medical profession would throw some light 'on what appears to be a ghastly mystery in the matter of these last three deaths ... under apparently the safest of conditions'.[17] In 1913 the *Encyclopedia of Sport* had made an indirect reference to brain damage but rather than through repeated blows to the skull, the focus was on punches to the jaw and how this force transmits through to the brain.[18]

The modernization of boxing

During the late nineteenth century, similar to other sports, boxing was 'modernized'. Rather than make the sport safer, it would both change the nature of boxers' injuries and ultimately lead to the condition of punch-drunkenness. The modernization of sport has exhibited a number of features such as codification, national and global competitions and the establishment of a governing body. Boxing's status as a major sport had partly been saved through the publication of the Marquis of Queensbury Rules in 1867. The rules included the introduction of a specified number of three-minute rounds with one minute between each round; previously prizefights only ended when one of the combatants retired, i.e., it was a test of endurance. Importantly, whereas prizefights were bareknuckle affairs, in the amateur game the use of gloves, or 'mufflers' as they were known, was made mandatory. Holding and wrestling moves were also now outlawed. The new rules enabled boxing to shake off the mud – and blood – from its boots of the spectacle of bareknuckle pugilism and gave the sport more respectability as well as to express its manly qualities where only the use of fists was allowed. The rules' main purpose was to essentially create a new sport: amateur boxing. Like other sports during this period, amateurism enabled it to distance itself from the sordidness of professionalism.[19] As a result, amateur boxing took place in the public schools, the universities, the armed forces as well as the medical schools. The Amateur Boxing Association, newly formed in 1880, adopted the Queensbury rules.[20]

Boxing's legal status had been given greater credibility by the 1882 *R v Coney* case because an important distinction was made between a prizefight and a sparring match – with gloves – over the issue of consent. It was judged, and presumed, that a boxing contest was like a sparring match and, therefore, legal because it was not the intention of the boxers to fight until one of them was exhausted.[21] As Gunn and Ormerod have argued, 'the questionable legality of boxing as we now know it came about by default rather than design'. Indeed, boxing in England has never been declared legal. Rather its legality was largely due to the fact that it was not prizefighting. It was not until the infamous 1995 case of *R v Brown* that the question over consent in boxing arose again. Here, certain acts of sado-masochism had been declared illegal despite consent being given by the participating adults. As a consequence, boxing's legality was brought into question, although not challenged.[22]

Another key event in boxing's modernization was the establishment of the National Sporting Club (NSC) in 1891, which acted as a *de facto* governing body for the professional branch of the sport.[23] It was a commercial venture and because of the game's reputation the NSC strove to make itself and the sport respectable. Contests took place in near silence with the audience dressed in dinner jackets. Its membership and administrators comprised members of society's elite including royalty.[24] The NSC also adopted the Queensbury rules, as well as adding some of its own. These stipulated a maximum number of fifteen rounds (twenty for championship contests) and a scoring system was put in place with contests decided by the referee and judges. In the case of a knock down the boxer had to get up within ten seconds or would lose the contest.

Nevertheless, following the deaths of some boxers during fights at the NSC, there were a number of legal challenges to the sport around the turn of the twentieth century.[25] The case that had the most far-reaching consequences followed the death of Murray Livingstone in 1901, an American who used the name Billy Smith. It also led to the state of boxing being raised in the House of Commons where a Mr Tennant asked the Home Secretary if he could 'abolish this institution'.[26] Charges of manslaughter were brought against the NSC and its management and the opponent of Livingstone, Jack Roberts. The prosecution argued that the contest was really a prizefight and therefore unlawful while the defence maintained that it was one of skill.[27] The jury agreed with the defence; the contest had been a boxing match not a prizefight.[28] Following this trial the reputation of boxing grew as the case had legitimized the NSC rules and inadvertently popularized the sport. Except for one case in Birmingham in 1911,[29] the legality of boxing has not been challenged since in a British court of law.

Boxing in other countries was also under threat from the law. In 1912, across the Channel, the regulations for future boxing contests in France had to be submitted to the Prefect of Police before the sport could continue.[30] Boxing on the other side of the Atlantic was continually under legal scrutiny. Canada had banned prizefighting in 1881, although boxing clubs continued.[31] Boxing in America, or more specifically, New York, was legalized and then criminalized on a regular basis up to 1920. In 1896, for example, the sport was legalized in the state under the Horton Law only to be repealed four years later. Boxing was again legalized in 1911 but again declared illegal in 1917. Finally in 1920, under the Walker Law, the sport's legality was firmly established and as a consequence laid the foundations for New York's position as the centre of world boxing for the next fifty years.[32]

Medical concerns over boxing were not absent at this stage. Doctors attended fights at the NSC and they gave the boxers a pre-fight examination. In 1911 the medical officer of the NSC was Dr Collins; the ABA's medical officer was a Dr Allport.[33] Gloves had to be a minimum of six ounces, a measure designed to make the sport safer while some types of punches were outlawed including the kidney punch, hitting with the elbow and a head butt. Boxers also had to hit with the knuckle part of the glove. Not only was this the only method from which to score points but hitting with an open glove was illegal. They were also not allowed to wear rings on their fingers and the boards of the floor of the ring were padded. Following the death of Michael Riley in 1900 contests were reduced from twenty rounds to fifteen, except for championship fights.[34]

The role of the referee was also important. His authority in the ring was all-powerful, even at the expense of medical advice. Because the emphasis was initially placed on the sporting aspect of the contest rather than the welfare of the boxers, the referee's duty lay with the spectators to ensure that boxers were not only fighting fairly but also not feigning injury.[35] Compared to the bloody violence of prizefighting, boxing was now, to use a medical metaphor, more 'clinical'. Rather than fights, the modern boxing contest made boxers concentrate on targeting specific areas of the body, in this case, any part of the front or sides of the head or body above the belt.

Despite the establishment of professional boxing in Britain on a firmer footing, the governance of the sport came under increasing pressure from promoters. The NSC could only hold 1,200 spectators, which limited both its commercial potential and influence.[36] In 1909, to maintain its pre-eminence, the NSC had brought in eight different weight classes and instituted the Lord Lonsdale Championship Belts. In 1929, partly to dilute the influence of promoters as well as regulate the sport more firmly at the professional level, the British Boxing Board of Control (BBBC) was formed. It became responsible for awarding licences to promoters, managers, boxers, referees, masters of ceremonies, ringmasters, trainers and seconds alike.[37]

The culture of boxing

Future medical debates were significant given boxing's place in British society. In terms of popularity, up to 1939, boxing was second only to football amongst the working classes. A boxing boom took place during the inter-war years, and there were about 5,000 registered professionals. The sport's influence was also felt throughout the upper echelons of society. At top public schools, such as Rugby, Repton, Eton and Charterhouse, boxing remained part of the curriculum.[38] Organized boxing in the army had begun in the mid-1880s and in 1891 the Public Schools Championships had started, under the control of the Army. A schools championship, now under the umbrella of the ABA, began in 1921. In the next year the London Schools ABA was established. Following the Second World War a national body, a Schools ABA, was formed and in 1953 the total nationwide entry for the national schools championship was 53,000.[39]

A change in fighting style due to the sport's commercialization had important medical consequences. In the early twentieth century British, small hall crowds had appreciated defensive skills based on the straight left – left jab – which generally encouraged skill and discouraged sluggers.[40] By the 1930s, however, there was a shift towards a more aggressive, American style. As they were putting on the shows, promoters preferred fighters, known as 'promoters' men', who would go 'toe to toe'. At the same time they left themselves open to more punishment and, as result, the possibility of some form of brain damage.

The nature of boxing's relationship with medicine was also shaped by the struggle for control of boxing between the BBBC and the promoters. The treatment of boxers by managers and promoters alike could be exploitative and there was little emphasis placed on their welfare.[41] During the inter-war period boxers in the preliminary contests at shows, which could last up to ten rounds, were obliged to pay what was known as 'seconds' money; boxers called it 'blood money'. Out of the few shillings they earned, boxers, instead of the promoters, were forced into giving the house seconds a cut. If they did not pay up they were unlikely to get further work.[42] The sport was largely based on casualized labour and with the aim of improving conditions and pay, the National Union of Boxers was formed in 1934. At first it was more interested in the fighters' financial welfare than their health but by 1939 medical provision had risen to the top of its agenda.[43]

What medical regulation existed in boxing up to 1939 was not particularly comprehensive. In 1942, when an amateur, Randolph Turpin fought and lost a fight only a few hours after been (accidentally) hit on the head by a brick on a building site. He later felt groggy and was sick for hours afterwards. This had not been noticed before the contest.[44] John Graham described how after one fight he complained to the referee that he should have stopped it earlier to prevent the beaten boxer from taking too much punishment. The referee simply replied, 'But he wasn't out, doctor.' Furthermore, before Graham could reach the badly defeated boxer he had been thrown over the shoulder of a 'burly second like a bag of oats'. An hour afterwards Graham was putting stitches into the boxer's eyebrow but was arguing with the trainer who said, 'What it wants doctor is antipholgistine'; a preparation that quickly stops the bleeding but leaves the eyebrow scarred and puffed up and more likely to bleed the next time there is contact on the scar.[45] The future world light-heavyweight champion, Freddie Mills, had his first fight in 1936. It's likely that he wore a pair of ordinary shorts and plimsolls. Boxers then were able to turn up at a tournament and hope to get a fight. He would be told to see the doctor and pay the Inspector 5 shillings. There was no real medical or a trial to see if he could look after himself.[46] It was not all that uncommon for a boxer to have two bouts on one evening. On one occasion, in 1936, Mills fought the same opponent twice in the same night, knocking him out twice in the first round. In the first fight the crowd had taken the view that the count had been too quick by the referee.[47]

During the first half of the twentieth century fighters fought a huge number of contests. Jimmy Wilde, for example, the Welsh flyweight world champion from 1916 to 1920, had 145 professional fights and more than 800 overall. Len Harvey, the leading middleweight of the inter-war years had 412 contests while Jack Matthews, the 'Fighting Barber' from Stoke (and father of Stanley) fought in 350 bouts.[48] Many contests were catch-weight with lighter fighters allowed to box heavier ones.[49] There was also no mandatory rest period between fights and boxers also took fights at short notice. Freddie Mills, for example, met Bruce Woodcock only twenty-one days after a very tough fight against Gus Lesnevich.[50] Furthermore, boxing booths were totally unregulated. Gordon Cook, a former lightweight champion of Wales, was a chronic gambler who was still boxing in the fairground booths at the age of forty-two in the 1930s. He had a glass eye, which he would keep in a handkerchief during the bout, using a towel as cover to slip it back at the end. Few in the crowd seem to have noticed.[51] Furthermore, there were murmurs that powerful promoters could influence the opinions of doctors. Ray Clarke who went on to become the Board's general secretary claimed that, 'In those days [before 1950] the Board's chief medical officer was Phil Kaplin and he was [Jack] Solomons' man. If Solomons wanted it, he would OK it: "He's fit to fight."'[52]

The punch drunk boxer

During the thirties a greater awareness emerged of boxing's long-term medical consequences in the form of punch-drunkenness. Because of how boxing had developed as a sport this disease was a peculiarly modern one. The figure of the punch-drunk boxer, if not the medical condition, had been well-known in boxing circles. The phrase is probably American in origin and was used in a boxing context in American newspapers in 1913 and 1914.[53] Terms like 'punchy' and 'groggy', which were alcohol related, were also used to describe some former fighters who it was felt were a bit 'slow' and had fought too many fights. By 1937 the American doctor, J.A. Millspaugh, had coined the medical term 'dementia pugilistica' for 'punch drunk'.

The image of punch-drunk boxers was becoming more widely disseminated within popular culture such as in Ernest Hemingway's 1926 short essay, 'The Battler'.[54] An American comedian and impressionist from the 40s and 50s, Red Skelton, created 'Cauliflower McPugg', a former 'punchy' boxer. The play, and later a film, The Square Ring (1953), looked at the seedier side of the professional game and also featured a punch-drunk boxer who was exploited by promoters, giving 'an ironic twist to the claim of professional boxing to regard itself as a noble art'.[55]

One of the seminal moments that reflected a shift in medicine's relationship with boxing was the publication of an article 'Punch Drunk' by Harrison Martland in 1928. For the first time a link between boxing and brain injury, based on the opinion of 'shrewd laymen' including a fight promoter, was made in a medical journal.[56] Other articles on the neurological symptoms of boxing followed. In 1937 C.E. Winterstein's 'Head Injuries Attributable to Boxing' was published in the Lancet. Like Martland, he concluded that a cause of punch-drunkenness was simply 'continued hammering' and that the symptoms did not increase after a boxer stopped fighting.[57] Four years later, Ernst Jokl published *The Medical Aspect of Boxing* in which for the first time the sport's abolition was advocated.[58]

This growing awareness in medical circles had coincided with a greater concern for the welfare of boxers within some boxing circles. In 1933 the American-based National Boxing Association had discussed a proposal for boxers to wear leather helmets (a forerunner of headguards) to prevent them from getting 'punch-drunk'. Although the editor of the sport's trade journal in Britain, *Boxing*, called it a stunt, he admitted that there may be something in it. He added that, 'I could name many boxers who have been "punch-drunk" – who have become nervous and physical wrecks – and that is not the thing we want in boxing'.[59] In the same issue there was criticism of how the sport was organized to the detriment of boxers, particularly how some licensed managers operated. The editor alleged that they were 'nothing but parasites' whose only qualification was a term of imprisonment. He added that these managers had ruined the careers of many boxers because their only thought was how much money they could make out of a boxer before he was too punch-drunk to fight any more. He would then be discarded to make way for another 'deluded youngster'.[60]

Professional boxing was also gaining a seedy reputation amongst the popular press and the phrase 'punch-drunk' began to take on libellous connotations. In 1939, for example, the boxing manager, Ted Broadribb, had successfully sued the *Sunday Dispatch*, which claimed that he was punch-drunk.[61] Another trial was held following an article that appeared in the *Daily Mirror* in 1938 titled, 'So this is boxing', which featured 'the scandal of punch-drunk boxers'.[62] It was claimed that one young fighter, managed by his father, had become punch-drunk because he had had too many contests against experienced fighters early in his career. They sued the paper.[63] During the trial the BBBC's secretary, Charles Donmall had said that to claim a boxer was punch-drunk meant that 'he was so helpless and so battered to pieces that it was impossible for him ever to engage in a professional boxing contest again'.[64] The plaintiff argued that if a fighter was deemed to be punch-drunk no promoter would sign him for a contest. The father and son won the case.[65]

Debates concerning the punch-drunk boxer also tapped into contemporary anxieties about inter-war society, in particular the popular memory of shell-shocked soldiers as wretched figures whose symptoms included stumbling gaits, tics, tremors and shakes.[66] In the boxing and daily press there were a number of references to boxers 'who have become nervous and physical wrecks'.[67] In addition, punch drunkenness mirrored contemporary perceptions in relation to mental disability and pointed to debates concerning mental deficiency and citizenship.[68] Negative eugenics – obsessed with the idea of social degeneration – had long been pre-occupied by the threat posed with the mentally ill.[69] Moreover, social degenerates as well as the feeble-minded were associated with the working class, and it was this class that dominated boxing.

Boxing, welfarism and politics

The twenty-five year period from 1945 set the tone for boxing's relationship with medicine for the rest of the century. The medical evidence about the health risks of boxing and especially punch-drunkenness began to mount in the medical journals while new medical technology was able to highlight the health risks that boxers took both long-term and short-term. The language also changed. It became more medicalized. Punch-drunk was replaced by 'traumatic encephalopathy' and 'chronic concussion'. Through the expansion of television the dangers of boxing were now beamed into the living rooms of the public, none more so when Benny Paret died following a live fight with Emile Griffith in New York in 1962. These developments were set against the creation of a welfare state in Britain that had promoted a greater sense of social democracy.[70] It not only invoked a 'cradle to grave' culture but there was more emphasis on health and safety in the workplace, albeit mainly in nationalized industries.[71] Moreover, a campaign to abolish the sport was headed by the MP Edith Summerskill. Boxing now became a political issue and the sport's authorities responded to the growing criticism by initiating a culture of safety, something highlighted by the BBBC appointing Colonel John Graham as its Chief Medical Officer in 1946.

Because of a rise in the number of reported deaths in the ring, a greater awareness of the perceived need for safer boxing also developed amongst the popular press. Between 1926 and 1951 thirteen fighters had died as a result of injuries inflicted in British rings, including two after the war. In 1951 the sports columnist for the *Empire News*, Harold Mayes, had investigated the causes of 'Deaths in the Ring'.[72] He followed this up with a series of articles advocating some safety measures. These included giving all boxers a log-book and suspending a fighter for six months after he had been knocked-out. He also suggested that the ideal boxing referee would be a 'medical man'.[73]

Interestingly, it was the amateur game that had initiated a greater drive towards boxing safety. In 1949 the Amateur European Boxing Association held a meeting on the question of traumatic encephalopathy.[74] The following year it introduced a raft of safety measures that were adopted by a newly-formed medical commission of amateur boxing's international governing body, the International Association for Amateur Boxing (AIBA). These included boxers not being able to fight after being knocked out and being banned for one year if they had been knocked out three times in a row. In addition, boxers under seventeen would not be able to compete in international events. The medical commission was also to compile a database of the physical state of international amateur boxers.[75] Medical controls were also tightened up at the Olympic boxing tournament. Previously, there had been a 'box-off' for the bronze medal between the losing semi-finalists. These box-offs last took place at the 1948 Olympics. In 1955 it was decided that for 1956 the losing semi-finalists would share bronze medals.[76] Two years later the AIBA suggested that the number of bouts at Olympic tournaments should be reduced as too many were thought to be a danger to boxers.[77]

In 1950 boxing authorities in all parts of the world were tightening up existing regulations. In the USSR the Committee for Physical Culture and Sport declared that a man would be declared the loser if he was knocked down three times in the same round. In addition, a boxer injured during a contest could now be removed on the decision of a doctor or a chief judge.[78] However, not everyone was completely in favour of these moves, highlighting not only the cultural resistance to medicine's increasing influence on the sport but also that boxing was a commercial venture. The editor of *Boxing News* felt that the sport as a spectacle had suffered because of the emphasis now placed on shorter bouts. He believed that British professional boxers no longer had the reserves of stamina or were able to stand 'the wear and tear of a marathon contest'.[79] Commenting on the AIBA's medical commission recommendations of 1950, *Boxing News* was broadly in agreement but it warned 'they have to realize that boxing is a tough sport and must remain so. The boxers must be cared for – but not molly-coddled'.[80]

In 1951 the London ABA also introduced a medical welfare scheme, subsequently adopted by the national body and set-up by Lew Blonstein. On joining a club every boy was examined by its medical officer as well as having a chest x-ray or an electrocardiogram. Boys with a squint were not accepted. In addition, the boy was given a log-book that stated that he was fit to box. It had to be produced at every contest and in it was recorded any injury received in a bout by the medical officer present and his recommended time of rest.[81]

Following the initiatives of the amateur authorities the BBBC established a medical sub-committee in 1950, headed by John Graham. From the start, eliminating punch-drunk fighters was its main aim, and one of the committee's first moves was to change the term punch-drunk to 'chronic concussion'.[82] Other medical controls included the appointment of medical officers, plus a deputy to each of the BBBC's eight regional areas. Now every applicant for a boxer's licence was subject to a medical examination by a registered doctor before he could embark on a professional career. At first there was no neurological examination, although there was a psychological test that included questions on the boxer's recent memory and whether there had been evidence of a change in character.[83]

Of course, these initiatives were prescriptive and to what extent examinations were comprehensive is unclear. One boxer, both professional and amateur, from the late 1950s has claimed that although he needed a medical certificate to gain a licence all this necessitated was a visit to his local GP. Furthermore, there was no medical exam involved, he was automatically upgraded from amateur to professional. Examination before an amateur fight took place two to three hours before the contest, and took about five minutes. In this time the doctor examined a boxer's blood pressure, made him 'cough', tested the bones, breathing plus the eyes and ears.[84] The British heavyweight, Henry Cooper, described a similar pre-fight test where a doctor would grip a boxer's hand to discover if anything was broken. He was then checked for a hernia or a rupture. The boxer also had to bend down with his feet together and his eyes closed. It was felt that there would be something seriously wrong if the boxer fell over.[85]

Without the technology it was difficult to detect brain injury and because of the absence of any treatment for the condition, emphasis was placed on prevention. The role of the referee was also brought into sharper focus. Under the new medical sub-committee, the area medical officers lectured all licensed referees on the medical aspects of boxing with particular reference to chronic concussion. They were instructed – although this was left open to interpretation – that they must not allow a boxer to take unnecessary punishment and 'under no circumstances allow a defenceless boxer to be struck'. If a referee ignored these instructions it could result in a suspension or losing his licence.[86]

The medical profession's growing criticism of boxing

It could be argued that these measures were partly in response to doctors' growing attention to boxing's medical aspects during the 1950s. By the end of the decade the weight of medical evidence regarding the dangers of boxing had grown to such an extent that in 1959 the *Lancet* called for the sport's abolition. Significantly, it stressed the moral aspect of their decision by stating that 'as doctors we have a clear duty' to campaign for its abolition.[87] A year later an (unsuccessful) motion was put forward at the BMA's AGM calling for the abolition of boxing for the first time.[88]

When concerns had first been raised about the benefits of the sport, emphasis had been placed on safety rather than abolition. In 1954 and 1955 articles, written by Blonstein and Graham on the medical aspects of their sport, had appeared in the *British Medical Journal* (*BMJ*).[89] Both Blonstein and Graham admitted that the sport was dangerous but that they had taken the necessary steps to prevent punch-drunkenness in boxers and that, anyway, more deaths and injuries took place in other sports. This response was one that would echo throughout the rest of the twentieth century. In an editorial, showing more sympathy with the amateurs, it was hoped that the controlling body of professional boxing would listen to the words of its medical advisers.[90]

Increasingly, through articles and letters in the medical journals, there were growing criticisms of the sport's dangers. In 1957 the *British Medical Journal* had published four papers in one issue on the subject, recognizing that 'boxing is by no means the innocuous sport that some suppose it to be is apparent from the attention paid in recent years to the injuries sustained in the ring by both amateurs and professionals'.[91] The articles included one by MacDonald Critchley, described as a world famous neurosurgeon, who wrote dispassionately about the growing evidence that punch-drunkenness was a serious cause of progressive physical and mental deterioration in professional boxers.[92] Blonstein had again contributed an article defending amateur boxing asserting that he had never observed the punch-drunk syndrome in any fighter from their ranks.[93] In summarising the articles, the accompanying editorial felt that, 'Many will feel that the benefits derived from boxing outweigh its dangers'. However, it also warned that 'this opinion will be hard to sustain unless every reasonable step is taken to minimize the risks of permanent injury'. Although not damming of the sport, the article suggested the weight of evidence was becoming increasingly influential in informing medical opinion on the subject.[94]

Advances in medical science, particularly knowledge of the workings of the brain, gradually helped to change the nature of the boxing debate. In 1929 a German psychiatrist, Hans Berger, had invented the electroencephalogram (EEG), which could record electrical currents generated on the brain. Professor Douglas Gordon was another pioneer in the use of ultrasonics in the diagnosis of brain injury. In 1947 he set up the first EEG clinic in London.[95] By 1957 an English physician, William Grey Walter, had developed an EEG topography, which helped to locate the origins of an epileptic fit within the brain. Arguments over the effectiveness of the EEG for mapping any brain injuries of boxers continued throughout the 1950s.[96] By 1957 the *BMJ* felt that serial EEG recordings could be of value in detecting early evidence of cerebral damage.[97]

Edith Summerskill and the campaign to abolish boxing

At the same time that the boxing authorities were taking greater responsibility for their fighters and the awareness of the medical profession regarding the sport's dangers was increasing, the Labour MP, Edith Summerskill launched a campaign to ban the sport. Summerskill herself epitomized post-war social democracy. A qualified doctor, she was a socialist, a modernizer and a feminist who was particularly interested in family planning and was a supporter of Marie Stopes; and like Stopes she was also a eugenicist. Her views on boxing partly reflected a wider paternalistic impulse within the Labour Party to 'improve' the population's leisure habits. In reality little reform took place, mainly because the majority of Labour voters preferred popular cultural tastes.[98]

Why did she want to ban boxing? Penny Summerfield has argued that her opposition should be seen in a Cold War context. Summerskill felt that boxing glamourized violence, and that instead young men should be taught to 'hate violence and control their aggressive instincts in the interests of world peace'.[99]

Her argument against boxing also combined medical reason with morality. In 1950 she had described one particular fight as a 'degrading exhibition', and later, boxing as 'appealing to sadistic impulses and the lowest and crudest passions in man'.[100] In 1956 she wrote *The Ignoble Art*, which again invoked medicine with a high moral tone and was replete with social democratic sensibilities.[101]

> The fact is that a pleasurable feeling is induced by the sight of one man beating another into insensibility, and this primitive emotion, which in civilised people should be disciplined, is fostered by those responsible for staging these bouts. The brutishness of man is no secret. It is revealed every day in our criminal courts. We have yet to evolve into a higher society.[102]

Summerskill was the public face of the campaign to abolish the sport. This led her to confront the boxing establishment, debating with the promoter, Jack Solomons, on whether professional boxing should be banned.[103] Both in 1953 and 1954 she had opposed amendments to the Budget to reduce Entertainment Duty on boxing. Proponents had argued that unless the duty was cut the sport would not survive; this is exactly what Summerskill had wanted. In 1960, following a debate, she attempted to introduce a bill in the Commons to ban professional boxing but lost the vote 120 to 17. Two years later she introduced a bill in the Lords to prohibit the authorization of boxing matches for profit. This motion also failed but the vote was much closer – 29 to 22 – and it led to the Royal College of Physicians setting up a committee to examine boxing. Its outcome, the Roberts Report (see below), was published in 1969.[104]

Another significant landmark in the boxing debate and its public visibility was a two-day conference at Goldsmith's College on the 'Medical Aspects of Boxing' in 1963 (the papers and the ensuing discussions were published as a book in 1965). Hosted by BASM, it included representatives from the BMA, both the royal colleges of physicians and surgeons, the ministries of Health and Education as well as Blonstein and Graham representing the medical face of the amateur and professional boxing bodies, respectively. Head injuries drew the most attention. The neurosurgeon, McDonald Critchely, drew attention to the punch-drunk syndrome, or as he preferred to call it, 'chronic progressive traumatic encephalopathy', highlighting that it was difficult to diagnose the condition in its early stages.[105] The conference ended with a panel discussion that was chaired by Arthur Porritt and included Edith Summerskill who restated her opposition to the sport.[106]

Criticisms of the sport did not go unheeded. In 1964 the BBBC brought in the 21-day rule; any professional boxer who had been knocked out or if the contest was stopped by the referee would now be automatically suspended for twenty-one days. Previously his licence would have been suspended just until he had been passed fit by the Board doctor, and he might have been back in the ring again after four days. In addition, any boxer would be suspended if a doctor reported him unfit to continue boxing for an undetermined period due to an injury.[107] The new rule had important economic consequences for the sport as it led to a further decline in the number of boxing shows. Promoters were now unable to hire journeymen boxers who fought – and usually lost – on a regular basis. Following the Second World War boxing went into decline and the number of professional fighters fell from about 5,000 in the 1920s and 30s to 1,000 by 1950; in 1971 the figure was 250.[108]

What was the impact of these debates on the general public? Social change was perhaps important here. In the post-war period family life was increasingly centred on children and accompanied with greater anxieties for their safety.[109] Where once parents gave boxing gloves to boys as Christmas presents, now they were more questioning of the sport's merits.[110] In 1954 the National Association of Organisers and Lecturers in Physical Education had met opposition over boxing in schools from parents who were afraid 'that a blow on the head would affect a boy's mental powers'.[111] In 1960 a Mr Casson wrote to the Medical Research Council asking for their advice on the dangers of boxing. His eight-year-old boy wanted to take up the sport but he wanted to know what the doctors thought of the sport before he agreed.[112] Boxing was also removed from the curriculum of most schools – state and private. In 1966 the Inner London Education Authority advised its schools to remove boxing from their curriculum.[113]

Britain's private schools were another barometer as the sport, like fagging, the cane and cold baths, had largely disappeared by the mid-1980s. Rather than the headmasters of whom some still believed that the sport was replete with manly, character-building qualities, the parents – who paid the fees – forced the issue. The increasingly professionalized middle classes now placed a greater emphasis on educational achievement than social values and no longer accepted the traditional view of the benefits of boxing. Eton gave up boxing in the mid-1970s and instead offered the pupils judo to work off their aggression. Boxing at Marlborough had been banned in the mid-1960s. The school's medical officer and its authorities had decided it was too dangerous.[114] Charterhouse was amongst the first to ban the sport in 1957. This had largely been through the efforts of the school doctor, Dr Waycott, who was described as young, intelligent and holding 'mildly progressive views'. In addition to boxing, he had wanted to ban nude bathing, early morning school and corporal punishment. It was only the latter that was not repealed.[115]

The Roberts Report

The publication of the Roberts Report in 1969, in light of Edith Summerskill's campaign, was an important moment in boxing's relationship with medicine.[116] The final report conclusively made the link, for the first time, between the length of a boxer's career and the number of bouts (referred to as 'occupational exposure') he fought with the severity of 'traumatic encephalopathy', i.e., neurological damage suffered.[117] A random sample of professional boxers had been taken from a population of 16,781 registered with the BBBC between 1929 and 1955 and who had been a professional for at least three years. Within the sample of 250 it was found that 37 suffered from chronic brain damage.[118]

'Roberts' was part of significant on-going changes in medicine and public health in post-war Britain. Virginia Berridge has argued that the publication in 1962 of the Royal College of Physicians report on smoking had been a key stage on 'the road to the new modernized and mediatized medicine and public health'. The report on smoking signified 'a new willingness on the part of medicine to speak to the public and to use the media to do so'. This new media-friendly approach contrasted significantly with its previous secretive approach to public matters. In addition, the report also marked a paradigm shift with the growing acceptability of the epidemiological mode of investigation – mainly on chronic diseases – rather than the biomedical, laboratory-based model. The smoking report was not only an important catalyst for evidence-based medicine but the ensuing debate highlighted how publicity on medical issues would now have the authority of the profession behind it.[119]

While systematic in its research and findings, the Roberts Report, mainly a medical history of the sport during the inter-war period, was relatively sympathetic to boxing. 'Roberts', acknowledging the greater medical controls imposed by the sport's authorities since 1945, stated that, 'Medical supervision of the sport was not a prominent feature of professional boxing before the war as it became soon after and has become, increasingly since'.[120] In addition, most of the fighters who had been afflicted by traumatic encephalopathy had fought before the war: the younger the fighter, the less chance of brain injury. This was something that the BBBC was quick to point out, predicting that in five years a report would produce dramatically different results.[121] Furthermore, despite pressure from Summerskill and Lord Platt, a former president of the Royal College of Physicians, the government considered that the sport, highlighting its quasi-legal status, was 'adequately controlled by the authorities' and did not 'intend to introduce statutory limitations or measures to prohibit professional boxing'.[122] However, the overall findings of the report were largely lost in the confirmation of the link between boxing and chronic brain damage. Instead, despite the improvements in medical care, 'Roberts' had confirmed boxing's inherent dangers.

The BMA and the campaign to ban boxing

The Roberts Report also changed the nature of the medical debate. Ever since, boxing has had to defend and justify itself in light of growing medical evidence. The attitude of the boxing authorities shifted from one of denial to a need to manage the sport's dangers. The medical profession became more assertive and more confident in its public pronouncements through its new relationship with the media, and in 1982 the British Medical Association finally called for the sport's abolition.[123]

In 1982 it was estimated that since 1945 at least 336 boxers worldwide had died from injuries sustained in the ring, of which nine had been in Britain.[124] Despite a rise in professional British boxers from 250 in 1971 to 480 in 1980, this still represented a picture of a sport in decline.[125] Numbers within the amateur ranks also fell. In 1979 there had been 44,850 registered amateurs on the ABA's books; this had dropped to 30,540 by 1987.[126] By 1984 there was little dispute about boxing's dangers and the BBBC's chief medical officer, Dr Adrian Whiteson, in response to the BMA's stance, accepted this. In an open letter, he emphasized the board's 'philosophy on the medical protection of boxers'. He continued, 'As Chief Medical Officer my approach has always been that preventive controls are the key to making a physically hazardous sport as safe as possible'. He then tellingly invoked the claim that boxing was about freedom of choice. With the banning of boxing unlikely, what was now most important was the sport's medical management rather than if it was dangerous or not.[127]

Boxing had come under further scrutiny following the deaths of a number of high-profile boxers and criticism of the sport in the media. In 1978 the Italian Angelo Jacopucci went into a coma and died of a celebral haemorrhage after being 'battered to defeat' by the British fighter, Alan Minter. Subsequently, three people were charged with his manslaughter in an Italian court – the referee, the ringside doctor and Jacopucci's manager. All were later acquitted.[128] In New York, boxing was briefly suspended in 1979 following the death of Willie Classen. An inquiry by the State senate was held, indicating the importance the authorities were giving the matter. Boxing resumed a few weeks later following neurological training courses for physicians and referees alike.[129] In 1982, however, the South Korean, Duk Koo Kim died after lapsing into a coma following his US-wide televised world title fight against Ray Mancini.[130] The fatality that received most publicity in Britain was that of the Welsh bantamweight, Johnny Owen, in September 1980. A blood clot developed on his brain after being knocked out by Lupe Pintor and in the motion of falling his head struck the floor heavily.[131] Young Ali from Nigeria died after being knocked-out by Barry McGuigan in 1982.

The spectacle of boxing was also beginning to be seen by some boxing supporters as barbaric and uncivilized. Following what was called a 'one-sided pummelling' of Randall Cobb by Larry Holmes for 15 rounds, Howard Cosell, America's best known sports commentator, vowed that the sight was so sickening he would never report on another boxing match.[132] The fight that aroused the most controversy was Muhammad Ali's defeat against Larry Holmes in 1980. It was shown around the world and it was widely believed that Ali took too much punishment. Ali was later diagnosed with Parkinson's disease. Similarly, the former World heavyweight champion, Joe Louis, was portrayed by television as a 'shambling hulk' in his declining years.[133] In 1980 *The Times'* boxing correspondent, Srikumar Sen, a former Oxford boxing blue, had urged the BBBC to oppose Ali continuing his career after the Holmes fight against the British heavyweight, John L Gardener. He also opposed the fight between Sugar Ray Leonard and the British boxer, Maurice Hope, on the grounds that Hope had 'a good chance of being seriously injured'.[134] During the contest Hope was duly knocked out and lay on the canvas unconscious for almost 10 minutes, his body shaking in convulsive shudders. It prompted another attempt to ban the sport in Parliament: the bill failed by 77 votes to 47 to gain a second reading in the Lords. It had been moved by Lord Grfye who felt that, 'The perpetration of violence was evil' and that 'Anything [that] encouraged or glorified it damaged the fabric of civilised society'.[135]

The research of Roberts was built upon by further work, especially J. Corsellis, a neurologist who examined the brains of fifteen former boxers in 1973. From this study, symptoms of 'progressive neurological deterioration' became apparent and proved that chronic concussion was a much more insidious process than had been first thought. Some fighters had begun to deteriorate mentally while still boxing. With others the process had been slower and could take ten to twenty years after retirement until the condition was noticed. This could then lead to the onset of cerebellar ataxia, slurring dysarthia, confusion and intolerance to alcohol. The personality could also deteriorate along with violent behaviour and rage reactions with symptoms of Parkinson's disease also appearing. Several had ended up in psychiatric institutions. Of the two world champions in the study, one died severely demented in a psychiatric hospital; the other died a vagrant and also seriously mentally deranged. The cardinal point of the study was that the brain could not withstand the repeated trauma that apparently even relatively light blows to the head could induce.[136]

While boxing and its dangers were now a frequent topic in the mainstream medical journals, it is interesting that the subject was hardly broached in sports medicine's main journal, the *British Journal of Sports Medicine*. In a letter to the journal, for example, one prominent BASM member, Rex Salisbury Woods, also the honorary medical officer for Cambridge University boxing club, bemoaned the constant attacks on boxing during this period for making the sport less popular, especially in schools.[137] In 1991, the year of the Watson-Eubank fight, there were no articles on boxing. The BASM position had been spelt out in an editorial of the journal in 1983. It asserted that the medical risks of amateur boxing were few, and made the point that even professional boxing was now more strictly controlled than it had been twenty years previously.[138] Another editorial in 1986 had complained that while there were plenty of column inches on injuries sustained in boxing, there were relatively few reports devoted 'to favourable influence of sport on health and well-being'.[139]

Nevertheless, a global consensus emerged over the dangers of boxing. Because, by the early 1970s it was perceived as 'the world's most comprehensive modern welfare state',[140] it was perhaps unsurprising that professional boxing was banned in Sweden in 1969. It was banned in Norway in 1982 although amateur boxing still continued in both countries.[141] By 1984 there had also been calls for an outright ban on boxing by the medical associations of Britain, Canada, America and Australia as well as the World Medical Association.[142] In 1980 the Canadian government had set up a task force to inquire into the dangers of the sport following the deaths of two professional boxers in Canadian rings.[143] In 1983 a ban on boxing was called for by the *Journal of the American Medical Association* after the publication of new research that claimed chronic brain damage was common amongst boxers.[144] However, a report by the association's Council on Scientific Affairs concluded that 'the sport does not seem any more dangerous than other sports presently accepted by society'.[145]

Following its decision to campaign to abolish the sport, the BMA's board of science and education commissioned a report, in co-operation with the ABA (although not the BBBC). Its subsequent publication in 1984 concluded that brain damage was a likely consequence of either amateur or professional boxing and that even one punch could cause permanent brain damage. In addition, because of new x-ray scanning techniques the damage associated with the 'punch-drunk' syndrome was now detectable before the clinical signs – slurred speech, staggering movements, poor co-ordination and memory loss.[146] In the same year the BMA voted to stage a campaign against the sport 'to influence public opinion to ultimately ban boxing' – both professional and amateur.[147]

Reaction to the BMA's report varied. Despite an editorial headline, 'The noble art of brain damage', *The Times* said in 1984, that any banning of boxing would be an 'unwarranted interference with individual liberty'.[148] Unsurprisingly, following its co-operation, the ABA was unhappy about the report and felt that the BMA had hijacked the debate for its own political ends.[149] The BBBC had anticipated the report's outcome and refused to co-operate. The board's chief medical officer, Dr Adrian Whiteson, not only emphasized the freedom of choice argument but that boxing was safer than sports like rugby union and rugby league. It was pointed out that between 1969 and 1981 480 people had died in sport in Britain: two had been professional boxers and three amateurs.[150] Moreover, it was argued that if boxing was banned it would create other problems i.e., it would 'go underground', and it was better for boxing to be properly controlled.[151] Nevertheless, in what can be described as something of a public relations exercise, following the report the board introduced CT scans for new professionals who had had a vast number of amateur fights.[152]

Medical arguments against boxing had been enhanced by scientific advances in the examination of the brain, in particular, Computerized Axial Tomography

(CAT or CT) scans that had been invented by the British engineer, Godfrey Hounsfield in 1967. It transmitted fine x-rays through the patient to produce detailed cross-sections, which were computer processed, creating a 3-D picture revealing pathologies in the brain of various kinds. Unlike other tests such as the EEG, the new techniques revealed the extent of brain damage before there was any outward or visible evidence of deterioration.[153] Due to the improvements in brain scanning techniques, it was reported that a manager, Burt McCarthy, had cut his links with one of his boxers, David Pearce, because of a possibility of neurological problems.[154]

During the 1980s the IOC continued to closely monitor the debates over boxing and set up medical commissions in 1983 and 1990. In 1984 the AIBA made headguards compulsory at the Olympics tournament.[155] The English amateur boxing authorities also tightened up their regulations. By 1990 any amateur boxer over thirty was medically re-examined every year until he was thirty-five when he had to retire; before thirty he only had to be examined at five-year intervals. A boxer knocked out or where the referee had stopped the contest, the rest period was a minimum of 28 days. If he was knocked-out again within 84 days, he wouldn't be allowed to fight for at least another 84 days.[156]

In the professional game perhaps the most significant development was the reduction of title fights – World, European and British – from 15 rounds to 12 rounds from 1983.[157] In addition, each doctor on the BBBC medical panel now had to be trained in the management of the unconscious patient.[158] No tournament was allowed to take place without two doctors in attendance and they needed to have 'a working knowledge of sports medicine and trauma management'. Certain medical facilities had to be on site and an ambulance on standby. A local hospital had to be advised that a tournament was taking place, although the need for a neurological unit to deal with head injuries was not compulsory at this stage.[159]

Boxing on the ropes

Boxing injuries and deaths remained an ever-present danger. Between 1993 and 1996 six boxers had been seriously injured in the ring and two had died. Based on research between 1974 and 1998, it was indicated that, on a worldwide basis, an average of five fighters died each year. A significant number of injuries occurred during title fights when boxers were physically in peak condition, which increased the potential of serious injury.[160] Compared to other sports, however, boxing remained relatively safe. According to figures from the Office of Population Censuses, between 1986 and 1992 there was one death in boxing in England and Wales compared with 412 deaths in water sports.[161]

The campaign to ban boxing perhaps reached its peak in the mid-1990s. It had been given greater credence due to the injuries received by Michael Watson and Gerald McClellan in their contests with Chris Eubank and Nigel Benn in 1991 and 1995, respectively. Both fighters were left severely impaired following the fights. In April 1994 the British boxer, Bradley Stone, died from severe brain damage following his contest against Richie Wenton, and the next year James Murray also died in the ring.[162] In 1995 the death of Murray had prompted another attempt to ban the sport through Parliamentary legislation. Like the other four since 1981 the bill was defeated.[163] The *Guardian* newspaper had long campaigned for the abolition of the sport and in the aftermath of the Benn-McClellan contest, an editorial stated that, 'Boxing remains a brutal sport that degrades not just the combatants but the spectators too. A civilised society would insist it was stopped'.[164]

Although this was familiar stuff from the abolitionists, predictions of the sport's demise were now also being made amongst boxing aficionados. After the death of James Murray, John Morris, the secretary of the BBBC, remarked that, 'We are responding to the biggest crisis there has ever been in boxing'.[165] Similarly, in the wake of Murray's death, Harry Mullan, who had been editor of *Boxing News* for the previous eighteen years, expressed doubts that the sport could continue. He said, 'I think anyone with half a conscience or a heart or an ounce of compassion has to wonder what he's doing in boxing'. Despite his long association with the sport, Mullan felt that 'the negatives are beginning to outweigh the pluses I'm afraid. These tragedies are happening far more frequently than they were when I came into boxing. I'm sure there must be more than coincidence behind that'.[166] In October 1995 John Rodda, the *Guardian*'s boxing correspondent, retired after forty-nine years of reporting on the sport. This had been three weeks after James Murray's death on which he had written that 'the drip, drip, drip on my conscience has taken me close to the point where I believe it [boxing] should be banned', and describing boxing as 'the noble art (that) now seems little more than a bloody way of making money'.[167] Even the promoter, Frank Warren, whose livelihood was dependent on the sport, said in the same month, 'I've spent a long time defending boxing and trying to justify it and I'm not doing that any more'.[168]

In addition to concerns over boxing's safety, many commentators felt that the spectacle of boxing was becoming tasteless and tacky (although boxing had always had a reputation for seediness).[169] These criticisms were mainly a product of its relationship with television, which largely financed the sport. Both the Watson and McClellan fights had been subject to much hyperbole and media coverage; thirteen million watched the Benn-McClellan fight.[170] Another consequence of television's growing influence was the proliferation – the alphabet soup – of governing bodies, detracting from boxing's credibility as a sport. By 1999 there were thirteen such organizations – WBC, WBA, WBO, IBF etc. Unlike other governing bodies, like motor racing's FIA and the Jockey

Club, it meant that boxing was unable to centralize data on injuries and hence, formulate a strategy for their prevention and treatment.[171] In an attempt to improve the sport's image in Britain, professional boxers formed themselves into a union, the Professional Boxers' Association in 1992. It represented around 300 of Britain's 650 professional fighters and it made improving medical regulations and campaigning for better insurance and pension conditions its prime objectives.[172] In 1994 the union brought out its own safety code for boxing.[173]

The British Medical Association maintained their publicity drive against boxing with the publication of *The Boxing Debate* in 1993. A new priority was a ban on under-16s boxing. The report also claimed that advances in brain scanning had improved the accuracy of tests on boxers, and had revealed damage not previously traced.[174] In addition, there was a more populist approach to its campaign. In 1996 it launched a sixty-second anti-boxing advert that was screened in cinemas. The commercial featured two conkers banging against each other, which eventually turned into human brains.[175] The BMA's language also became more emotive and populist. 'Chronic concussion' was replaced with 'brain damage'. One doctor compared a violent punch with an effect similar to a 'blancmange being whisked around in a wood box. It scrambles the brain'.[176] A punch from a heavyweight boxer, it was estimated, was like being hit with a 6kg mallet at 20mph. Another BMA claim was that every time a boxer was hit with a hard punch to the head he could lose up to 20,000 brain cells.[177]

Medical control, however, was also being shaped by the changing nature of the sport. To appeal to television audiences, fighters with an all-action style were sought while boxers took advantage of developments in sports science, such as nutrition, which enabled them to train longer and hence, give and take more punishment. More boxers introduced weight-training into their training schedules (see Chapter 4). In addition, although gloves had got heavier to cushion blows, the bandaging of hands formed a padding that meant a boxer could hit to the head with full force without taking much risk of injuring his hands, thus increasing the chances of inflicting brain damage.[178]

Medical bureaucracy was further increased in the immediate aftermath of the Watson-Eubank fight. It had been found that proper resuscitation procedures had not been in place and that the ringside doctor was not an expert in resuscitation. If these measures had been in place, Watson may not have suffered from long-term brain damage. Moreover, Watson was not stretchered off until fourteen minutes after the end of the fight and it was another fourteen minutes before he received resuscitation at the nearest hospital.[179] The BBBC, in conjunction with the Minister for Sport, announced eight new safety measures. In particular, there had to be an ambulance standing by with paramedics who could take a boxer to a pre-advised neurosurgical unit at a nearby hospital and full, adequate resuscitation equipment had to be available at the ringside, supervised by fully trained staff.[180] Significantly, these were mandatory regulations and legally formalized boxing's relationship with medicine because now boxing shows could not go ahead if these measures were not in place. Despite these measures being in place for the Benn-McClellan fight though it did not prevent McClellan suffering from brain damage.[181]

Even before the McClellan and Murray fights, the BBBC had commissioned a report by an independent medical panel in 1994.[182] Recommendations included the suspension period for boxers knocked out or stopped to be extended from 28 to 45 days nor to spar for 28 days. In addition, the referee was permitted to consult a ringside doctor who, between rounds, could alert referees to problems. Traditionally, the referee had been the sole arbiter in this area. The report's most significant recommendation though was that all professional boxers should undergo a Magnetic Resonance Imaging (MRI) scan – an upgrade on CAT scans in detecting brain damage. MRI scans were made compulsory in 1997.[183]

In addition to MRI scans and medical care during fights, more attention was devoted to the preparation of boxers, especially with regard to the effects of dehydration through weight loss. Following a successful operation on Paul Ingle in 2000, it was stated that he was the fourteenth boxer to require an emergency procedure after a contest in a British ring since 1986, and in all but one, weight loss was a factor.[184] This had been a problem, or even a tradition, long associated with the sport where fighters would deprive themselves of liquids in order to make the weight. Some fighters used laxatives, diuretics, saunas and starvation diets to shed excess pounds in a hurry. Following the weigh-in their weights could balloon up to over a stone. Fighting in the nine stones featherweight division, for example, Ingle's weight was up to twelve stones during contests.[185] It was believed that there may have been a link between rapid weight reduction and the loss of cerebral spinal fluid, the fluid in which the brain is suspended, and hence a factor in some boxers developing blood clots on their brains and thus requiring surgery after fights.[186]

In 2001 the BBBC introduced regulations where before all championship contests, boxers had to be weighed when a fight was announced or a contract signed. There was to be a second weight check three days before the weigh-in, which was to take place between 24 and 36 hours before the fight. In addition, all boxers were subject to random weight checks to ensure any weight loss was gradual and not likely to cause dehydration. There was to be a greater emphasis on education with more scrutiny of training techniques. In addition, every trainer had to keep a training diary for all boxers, detailing fitness and training programmes, records of sparring and regular monitoring of weight before and after every session. All trainers and seconds were to undergo compulsory courses in techniques of weight reduction as well as diet and nutrition. However, the PBA's chairman, Barry McGuigan called these measures 'old-fashioned'.[187] By 2006 a 'check weigh-in' had been introduced for title fights to take place three days beforehand in which boxers had to be within three per cent of the weight limit.

Conclusion

While boxing has survived, despite the overwhelming medical evidence that has proved its dangers, the sport remains one punch away from crisis i.e., a death in the ring. Ironically, the sport's survival depends on a close relationship with medicine. So close, that possibly the most effective way for doctors to stop professional boxing would be to withdraw their labour. As professional boxing promotions legally require the presence of doctors, their absence would make it impossible for the event to take place.[188]

The relationship has not been an amicable one. Rather the medical profession has attempted to impose its will and influence on the sport, both in a medical and ethical sense. Boxing's resistance and survival has been partly based on its autonomy, a product of British sport's voluntary principles. It meant that any interference by the state would be taken reluctantly. Within this struggle, the medical profession's growing influence on boxing's ethical debate mirrored the changing status of doctors during the twentieth century. One member described the BMA as 'the medical adviser to the nation', and felt that it had a duty to persuade fellow citizens to recognize health hazards, something that it had done with campaigns on compulsory seat-belts and the ban on tobacco advertising.[189] The ethos of welfarism that had permeated society was mirrored by the medical profession's greater concern with boxing, backed up with growing medical evidence. Yet the debate over boxing and its ethical nature also harks back to on-going cultural tensions that have revolved around the notion of 'civilization', dating back to the early nineteenth century. The Golden Age of prize-fighting had been brought to an end due to the onset of the moral reform movement and similar ethical and moral arguments were invoked in attempts to abolish the sport, albeit in a different context during the second half of the twentieth century.

By the twenty-first century boxing was undergoing a mini-revival. It perhaps reflected a shift towards more consumerist attitudes in society generally. During the 1990s the consumption of violence showed few signs of abating. Not only did boxing survive but there was also great interest in the, albeit manufactured, World Wrestling Federation. Martial arts retained their popularity whilst other combat sports, such as Total Fighting and Ultimate Fighting, were causing concern amongst the medical profession.[190] Worst of all for many doctors and in the boxing fraternity, women's boxing was made legal in 1998, and was an Olympic sport for the London 2012 games.[191] In 2007 professional boxing was even re-introduced into Sweden after a break of thirty-six years.[192] It is unlikely that boxing in Britain will be banned in the near future – although its legality has yet to be tested in court. It may be that, because of what may be perceived to be suffocating medical regulations, the sport will fade away. The grass roots of the sport could decline due to pressure from the public and parents, in the case of children. However, there still seems to be a market for violent sports and compared to the emergence of new combat sports and the prospect of boxing going underground, the government may actually prefer that boxing remains legal.

Conclusion

In 2009 the city of Leicester hosted the Special Olympics Great Britain (SOGB) National Summer Games. The Special Olympics movement had been founded in America in the 1960s and catered for athletes with learning disabilities. SOGB was formed in 1978. It was part of the British voluntary tradition, which relied on the efforts of its members to run competitions and training programmes for athletes. SOGB embraced a Sport for All philosophy rather than one geared up for elite competition. Events within the games were classified not according to disability as in the Paralympics but on an athlete's ability. SOGB has around 8,500 athletes while in 2008 an estimated 2.25 million athletes worldwide took part in Special Olympics sporting activities. In a number of ways Special Olympics echoes some of the ideas around health that have been associated with sport since the Victorian era. Special Olympics have been hugely beneficial to the lives of the athletes and families involved.[1] The Games themselves carry important wellbeing and health rewards – people with learning disabilities have been amongst the most poverty stricken and least healthy in society – as well as a sense of a positive, collective shared experience during the week. For athletes, training for and then competing at the Games improves fitness levels and wellbeing, and gives them a sense of purpose and confidence: *mens sana in corpore sano*.

The Paralympics have provided a different lens through which to view the development of the relationship between sport and medicine. These had emerged out of the Stoke Mandeville Games, founded in 1948, as part of the rehabilitation – both physical and mental – of injured servicemen from the Second World War.[2] By the mid-1960s the status and meaning of disability had begun to shift with the emergence of identity politics and the demand for greater leisure provision as part of a move to greater social inclusion. Although initially built on the basis of health, disability sport took on a life of its own and became a fixture in the global sporting calendar. In 1988 Seoul hosted the first official Paralympics. In more recent years, especially in Britain, Paralympians have also benefitted from significant state investment and through television coverage have been able to develop their own personalities and celebrity culture similar to able-bodied athletes. Unlike the Special Olympics, the Paralympics are highly competitive and have not been without cheating scandals. For example, some of the Spanish basketball team that won the learning disability category at the 2000 Sydney Paralympics did not have learning disabilities. The Paralympics have also been wrought with issues over the identity of disabled athletes because it has reinforced as well as challenged notions of disability. In particular, the medical categorization of athletes, based on functional difference, has given disability an (unwanted) cultural legitimacy and a sense of stigma because it creates a hierarchy amongst Paralympians.[3]

Further ethical debates not only over the identity of Paralympians but also of able-bodied athletes were raised at the 2011 World Athletics Championship. Oscar Pistorious, the South African 400 metre runner, became the first Paralympian athlete of his type to compete at elite 'able body' level. Pistorious, who had been born without either fibula, used prosthetic limbs – called 'Cheetah blades' – to run.[4] Doubts had previously been raised over the 'legality' of Pistorious's blades. The question was posed whether the technology gave him an unfair advantage. In 2008, following extensive testing and representation before the Court of Arbitration for Sport, he was eligible to qualify for the Olympics.[5]

This brief section on disability sport offers further evidence of the complex and wide-ranging nature of the relationship between sport and medicine. In general, this book has provided a historical overview of a number of the constituent elements present in this relationship since around 1800. The relationship between sport and medicine may not be a symbiotic one but because sport is an activity based on bodily movement – and the association with medicine that this entails – it is unsurprising that this relationship has been continuous since sport emerged as a social and cultural phenomenon. Historical continuities, however, cannot mask the forces of social transformation that have been constantly at work in shaping this relationship. On a broader historiographical point, placing the history of sport and medicine in comparative contexts also reveals how medical practices have differed or converged relative to broader social history of medicine narratives, such as specialization and professionalization. With reference to sport and medicine, three overlapping forces can be identified.

First, there has been the commercial and global expansion of sport, which has provided a demand for medical services and scientific knowledge. Without sport there can be no sports medicine and since the early professional sports and then the growth of international competition stimulated by the so-called Cold War, sports medicine and sports science have become important components in this process.

The second major force at work has been the role of the state. To a certain extent there has been a relatively parallel development in when and how nations have used sport for the purposes of national prestige and to improve the fitness of populations. However, this process in terms of its intensity and the importance bestowed on sport has been subject to each nation's prevailing political culture. At one end of the scale, sport in Britain and America has traditionally been part of a voluntary tradition whereas in the Soviet Union, for example, it was closely controlled by the government. In addition, medical professions have developed along national and political lines, which has conditioned how sports medicine organizations have been funded and ultimately the role they have played.

Finally, the athletic body has evolved alongside changing conceptions of the body's capabilities since around 1800, especially the transition from Galenic to Western medicine. Initially, the classical Greek body was the model but with the expansion in scientific medicine, the bacteriological revolution and the growth of physiology the body was increasingly seen as a machine that no longer had a limited supply of energy. Due to a closer relationship with science, the potential capabilities of the athletic body increased exponentially.

The modern relationship between sport and medicine emerged out of a growth in physical culture from the late eighteenth century. In Europe gymnastics promoted a growing understanding of the body. In addition, as Dorothy Porter has pointed out for the nineteenth century, health had begun to dominate discourses over social welfare.[6] The benefits of sport and exercise increasingly blended with concerns over the health of nations and the emergence of the early welfare state. National fitness became a pre-occupation for major Western countries from the late nineteenth century. A healthy population was required both to meet the demands on the working body that industrialization had brought as well as preparation for war. Mass physical education programmes were products of these concerns.

Modern sport was partly a consequence of the cult of athleticism in British public schools where games were seen as character-building in the process of making men. The expanding middle classes appropriated traditional sports, such as football, pugilism and pedestrianism and increasingly codified them and established governing bodies run by gentleman-amateurs. Importantly, they imbued sport with a set of values, especially amateurism, which became the dominant ideology – although not the only one – of sport for much of the twentieth century. British sports were taken elsewhere and amateurism became the main ideology in international sports federations, including most importantly the IOC. Although it was often a more flexible interpretation of amateurism, it provided a framework which other countries could work within and exploit, especially when it came to the Olympics. As a consequence, amateurism was constantly reinvented until the pressures of commercialization and competition became difficult to resist. But it was also in this context that medicine's relationship with sport was shaped with values that would play a significant role in the ideas underpinning sporting ethics.

Sport itself was an important feature of modern life and reflected the shift from economies fixed on production to ones based on consumption. The masses had more time and money to spend on their leisure. Along with America, Britain also pioneered sports commercialization and professionalization. The notion of the professional athlete who worked regular hours for a regular wage was born. But with this lifestyle came unique working conditions and especially the threat and reality of dealing with injuries.

Moreover, the increasing intensity of competition meant greater resources had to be devoted to the training and preparation of athletes. Early ideas of the athletic body were framed around the methods of early trainers and coaches, which were grounded in their own experiences and empirical observations.

Yet coaches were adaptable and increasingly sought and made use of scientific medicine. To a certain extent, based on research on fatigue in the workplace and on the battlefield, the athletic body was increasingly seen as a machine and athletes could be trained to the point of exhaustion. In this sense, sports medicine served a different purpose to most other forms of medicine because the focus here was on bodies which were healthy rather than those that were ill. It also highlighted how ideas of excess for training not only replaced those of moderation but were also part of the sporting discourse.

It may have initially offended amateur sensibilities in Britain but elsewhere there was a rush to exploit the new possibilities. Germany and America were initially in the vanguard but with the onset of the Cold War after 1945 and national prestige at stake, Eastern European countries were the first to exploit science and medicine on a large scale. With sport an arm of the state, a more organized approach was adopted to training and coaching. Countries adopted different methods that have to a certain extent been dependent on national political culture. For much of the twentieth century, state support was limited for British sport, certainly when compared to the Soviet Union and later even Australia. By the twenty-first century, however, British sport at elite Olympic level was just as integrated into the state. And with its adoption of World Class Performance programmes and Long Term Athletic Development strategies – with its eugenic overtones – there is more than a hint of the old East Germany about this approach. The new British approach was also a by-product of sport's growing global reach and commercial power. Because of its media profile and possibilities for political gain, sport was becoming too important for governments to ignore. Moreover, as some elite sports were incorporated within the state machinery they gravitated towards unwieldy bureaucracies that were subject to targets and a culture of managerialism. It is doubly ironic that modern sport was a Western, bourgeois invention and it was Eastern bloc countries who through their state-run institutes sought initially to 'hot-house' athletes, but it is now Western nations who have begun to ape this approach.

At the same time as sport was increasingly appropriating medical science, the medical profession was developing a greater interest in sport. Much of this early interest was personal as many doctors were keen on sport but alongside this they could also see opportunities in sport's expansion. In the West it mirrored a wider political concern of doctors to exclude so-called alternative practitioners and for doctors to ring-fence their own expertise. The specialization of sports medicine has proved problematic mainly because of the opaque nature of the practice and sports medicine itself was continually re-defined. Elite athletes sought specialists in particular fields rather than sports medics who were often generalists. As sporting competition intensified, athletes and sports bodies gradually looked towards sports scientists for a cutting edge; for elite athletes in particular, sports medicine was seen as the key to recovery from injuries.

What about the doctors? In Britain at least, the medical profession was for much of the twentieth century dominated by men and was essentially middle class and conservative in its outlook. These values manifested themselves in a number of ways and were particularly apparent in the relationship between women and sport. Medical opinion fused with social discourse in shaping the nature of female sporting activity. Yet the medical profession also had to respond to social and political change. During the twentieth century the notion of gentlemanly medicine faded as a meritocratic ethos permeated society. Doctors, however, still looked upon themselves as the medical advisor to the nation, something apparent in their highly public campaign to ban boxing. But this campaign was also noticeable for the high moral tone of the arguments and invocation of the idea of 'civilization'. It also echoed wider debates about leisure in which middle-class reformers have looked on disapprovingly at working-class activities.

Finally, it may be worthwhile reflecting on what the relationship between sport and medicine means and its potential consequences. In a stimulating article, David Runciman posed the question, 'Is the rise of the super-athlete ruining sport?' Because of rapidly advancing technology, there was a fear that sport would lose its appeal. Runciman argued that while athletes aspire to:

> an ideal of natural human excellence ... there is something increasingly unnatural about athletic achievement at the highest level – it is by definition an abnormal accomplishment – and something even more unnatural about the idea that human beings can keep getting faster ad infinitum.[7]

As a consequence, these 'super-athletes' are extending the gap between the elite and recreational athletes at an exponential rate. While it could be argued that this is the point of elite sport, in increasing their remoteness sport begins to look ridiculous. To a certain extent, sport's 'abnormality' reflects wider debates over the nature of medical power and fears over the influence of an authoritarian medical perspective, which has been associated with biomedicine and a collaboration between doctors and the state. In this sense, elite sport due to the growing influence of medicine and science can be seen in these biomedical terms.

Similar sentiments, however, have been expressed about sport's relationship with commerce for over one hundred years and also with the same sense of foreboding. People are often more likely to see crisis in the present. Adam Smith once said that there is a lot of ruin in a country. Perhaps the same could be said of sport. Thus, while sport has devoted more resources to medicine there is perhaps a danger of presentism due to an over emphasis placed on sport's so-called medicalization i.e., the extension of rational, scientific values in medicine to sport. It offers a doomsday scenario, or a moral panic, where athletes become merely extensions of the research of the doctors and scientists who help them.

A recent aspect of this slightly dystopian outcome has been the emergence of new genetic technologies. With the mapping of the human genome, for example, it has been argued that the implementation of genetic testing in sport rather than giving athletes an unfair advantage will instead make all athletes the same. This 'genetic determinism' is based on the idea that certain body types are suited to certain kinds of sports and has been employed in rugby union and tennis.[8] Moreover, Miah has argued that genetic testing along with potentially genetic engineering could have important consequences for the human rights of athletes.[9]

There is more than a hint of nostalgia implicit in the construction of such scenarios. In particular, the shadow of amateurism with its notion of fair play hangs heavy. Amateurs had initially considered training a form of cheating. As Heggie has pointed out, 'there has never been a time when people weren't worried that artificial techniques would ruin sport'.[10] And of course sport itself is an artificial construction which has devised its own rules and codes of behaviour. Moreover, there is always the issue of the athlete – the 'patient' – and agency. Athletes are not passive recipients, and can make their own decisions while environmental factors are also important in contributing to the success of athletes. Even in communist countries, athletes were far from the robots often featured in popular discourse; they took part because they were good at it and enjoyed it.

Finally, it may also be worth posing the question where will it all end? As elite athletes are only separated by tiny margins the use of genetic technologies at an early stage, like other methods used to enhance athletic performance, would be significant. How acceptable this would be to a wider public, which understands sport to be – somewhat erroneously – a level-playing field, is equally questionable. It is perhaps further confirmation that ultimately sport at the elite level is an 'unhealthy' practice.

Notes

Introduction

1 J.G.P. Williams (ed.), *Sports Medicine* (London: Edward Arnold, 1962).

2 J.G.P. Williams, *Medical Aspects of Sport and Physical Fitness* (London: Pergamon Press, 1965), pp. 91–5. Homosexuality was legalized in 1967.

3 James Pipkin, *Sporting Lives: Metaphor and Myth in American Sports Autobiographies* (London: University of Missouri Press, 2008), pp. 44–50.

4 Paula Radcliffe, *Paula: My Story So Far* (London: Simon & Schuster, 2004).

5 Roger Cooter and John Pickstone, 'Introduction' in Roger Cooter and John Pickstone (eds), *Medicine in the Twentieth Century* (Amsterdam: Harwood, 2000), p. xiii.

6 Barbara Keys, *Globalizing Sport: National Rivalry and International Community in the 1930s* (Harvard: Harvard University Press, 2006), p. 9.

7 Richard Holt, *Sport and the British: A Modern History* (Oxford: Oxford University Press, 1989), p. 3.

8 Deborah Brunton, 'Introduction' in Deborah Brunton (ed.), *Medicine Transformed: Health, Disease and Society in Europe, 1800–1930* (Manchester: Manchester University Press, 2004), p. xiii.

9 Cooter and Pickstone, 'Introduction' in Cooter and Pickstone (eds), p. xiv.

10 Patricia Vertinsky, 'What is Sports Medicine?' *Journal of Sport History*, 34:1 (Spring 2007), p. 87.

11 Cooter and Pickstone, 'Introduction' in Cooter and Pickstone (eds), p. xiv.

12 It was originally called the Association Internationale Médico-Sportive (AIMS). In 1933, the name was changed to Fédération Internationale de Médico-Sportive et Scientifique before it adopted its current title in 1934.

13 Vanessa Heggie, 'Specialization without the Hospital: The Case of British Sports Medicine, *Medical History*, 54: (2010), p. 458.

14 Parissa Safai, 'A critical analysis of the development of sport medicine in Canada', *International Review for the Sociology of Sport*, 42 (2007), p. 326.

15 B. Thompson, *et al*, 'Defining the Sports Medicine Specialist in the United Kingdom: A Delphi Study, *British Journal of Sports Medicine (BJSM* hereafter), 38 (2004) 214.

16 Paul McCrory, 'What is sports and exercise medicine?' *BJSM*, 40 (2006) pp. 955–7.

17 See John Welshman, 'Only Connect: The History of Sport, Medicine and Society', *International Journal of the History of Sport (IJHS* hereafter), 15:2 (August 1998), pp. 2–5.

18 John V. Pickstone, 'A brief history of medical history', http://www.history.ac.uk/makinghistory/resources/articles/history; Jeffrey Hill, 'British Sports History: A Post-Modern Future?', *Journal of Sport History*, 23:1 (Spring 1996), pp. 1–19.

19 Jack W. Berryman and Roberta J. Park (eds), *Sport and Exercise Science: Essays in the History of Sports Medicine* (Urbana: University of Illinois Press, 1992).

20 For example, Charles M. Tipton, 'Sports Medicine: A Century of Progress', *Journal of Nutrition*, 127:5 (May 1996), pp. 878s–85s; John D. Massengale and Richard A. Swanson (eds), *The History of Exercise and Sport Science* (New York: Human Kinetics, 1997).

21 Nicholas D. Bourne, 'Fast Science: A History of Training Theory and Methods for Elite Runners Through 1975' (Unpublished PhD Thesis, University of Texas, Austin, 2008).

22 For example, Roberta J Park, 'Physiology and Anatomy are Destiny!?: Brains, Bodies and Exercise in Nineteenth Century American Thought', *Journal of Sport History*, 18:1 (Spring 1991), pp. 31–63; 'Boys' Clubs Are Better Than Policemen's Clubs': Endeavours by Philanthropists, Social Reformers, and Others to Prevent Juvenile Crime, the Late 1800s to 1917, *IJHS*, 24:6 (June 2007), pp. 749–75; 'Physiologists, physicians, and physical educators: Nineteenth century biology and exercise, hygienic and educative', *IJHS*, 24:12 (2007), pp. 1637–73; 'Setting the Scene – Bridging the Gap between Knowledge and Practice: When Americans Really Built Programmes to Foster Healthy Lifestyles, 1918–1940', *IJHS*, 25:11 (2008), pp. 1427–52; 'Sharing, arguing, and seeking recognition: International congresses, meetings, and physical education, 1867–1915', *IJHS*, 25:5 (2008), pp. 519–48. See also Harvey Green, *Fit for America: Health, Fitness, Sport and American Society* (Baltimore: Johns Hopkins University Press, 1986).

23 Patricia Vertinsky, 'Exercise, Physical Capability, and the Eternally Wounded Woman in Late Nineteenth-Century North America' in Berryman and Park (eds), pp. 183–211; 'Making and marking gender: Bodybuilding and the medicalization of the body from one century's end to another', *Sport in Society*, 2:1 (1999), pp. 1–24; 'Body Shapes: The Role of the Medical Establishment in Informing Female Exercise and Physical Education in Nineteenth-Century North America' in J.A. Mangan and Roberta Park (eds), *From 'Fair Sex' to Feminism: Sport and Socialization of Women in the Industrial and Post-industrial Era* (London: Frank Cass, 1987), pp. 256–81.

24 Roberta J. Park, '"Cells or soaring?": Historical reflections on "visions" of body, athletics, and Modern Olympism', *IJHS*, 24:12 (2007), pp. 1701–23; 'Physicians, Scientists, Exercise and Athletics in Britain and America from the 1867 Boat Race to the Four-Minute Mile', *Sport in History*, 31:1 (March 2011), pp. 1–31.

25 Rob Beamish and Ian Ritchie, *Fastest, Highest, Strongest: A critique of high-performance sport* (London: Routledge, 2006); Vanessa Heggie, '"Only the British Appear to be Making a Fuss": The Science of Success and the Myth of Amateurism at the Mexico Olympiad, 1968', *Sport in History*, 28:2 (June 2008), pp. 213–35; Alison Wrynn, 'The Athlete in the Making: The Scientific Study of American Athletic Performance, 1920–1932', *Sport in History*, 30:1 (March 2010), pp. 121–7. For a history of coaching see special edition on 'Coaching Cultures' in *Sport in History*, 30:1 (March 2010).

26 John Hoberman, *Mortal Engines: The Science of Performance and the Dehumanization of Sport* (London: Macmillan, 1992); Ivan Waddington, *Sport, Health and Drugs: A Critical Sociological Perspective* (London: E & FN Spon, 2000), Chapters 6 and 10; Barrie Houlihan, 'Building an international regime to combat doping in sport' in Roger Levermore and Adrian Budd (eds), *Sport and International Relations: An Emerging Relationship* (London: Routledge, 2004).

27 Paul Dimeo, *A History of Drug Use in Sport 1876–1976: Beyond Good and Evil* (London: Routledge, 2007); Thomas Hunt, *Drug Games: The International Olympic Committee and the Politics of Doping, 1960–2008* (Austin: University of Texas Press, 2011). For a variety of approaches to this issue see special edition on Drugs in *Sport in History*, 25:3 (December 2005).

28   Neil Carter, 'Metatarsals and Magic Sponges: English Football and the
     Development of Sports Medicine', *Journal of Sport History*, 34:1 (Spring
     2007), pp. 53–74; 'The Rise and Fall of the Magic Sponge: Medicine and the
     Transformation of the Football Trainer, *Social History of Medicine*, 23:2
     (August 2010), pp. 261–80.
29   For example, S. Loland, B. Skirstad and I. Waddington (eds), *Pain and Injury in
     Sport: Social and Ethical Analysis* (London: Routledge, 2006).
30   Ivan Waddington, 'Jobs for the Boys: A Study of the Employment of Club
     Doctors and Physiotherapists in English Professional Football', *Soccer and
     Society*, 3 (2002), pp. 51–64; Ivan Waddington, Martin Roderick and Graham
     Parker, *Managing Injuries in Professional Football: A Study of the Roles of
     the Club Doctor and Physiotherapist* (Leicester: Leicester University Press,
     1999); I. Waddington, M. Roderick and R. Naik, 'Methods of Appointment and
     Qualifications of Club Doctors and Physiotherapists in English Professional
     Football: Some Problems and Issues', *British Journal of Sports Medicine*, 35
     (2001), p. 48; Dominic Malcolm, 'Sports medicine: A very peculiar practice?
     Doctors and physiotherapists in elite English rugby union' in Loland *et al* (eds),
     Pain and Injury in Sport, pp. 165–81; Dominic Malcolm and Ken Sheard, '"Pain
     in the Assets": The Effects of Commercialization and Professionalization on the
     Management of Injury in English Rugby Union.' *Sociology of Sport Journal*, 19
     (2002), pp. 149–69; Dominic Malcolm Unprofessional Practice? The Status and
     Power of Sport Physicians, *Sociology of Sport Journal*, 23 (2006), pp. 376–95.
31   Ken Sheard, '"Brutal and Degrading": The Medical Profession and Boxing,
     1838–1984', *IJHS*, 15:1 (1998), pp. 74–102; 'Boxing in the Civilizing Process'
     (Unpublished PhD Thesis, Anglia Polytechnic, 1992).
32   Vanessa Heggie, *A History of British Sports Medicine* (Manchester: Manchester
     University Press, 2011), p. 2.
33   Jeffrey Hill, *Sport, Leisure and Culture in Twentieth Century Britain*
     (Basingstoke: Palgrave, 2002), p. 2.
34   Christopher S. Thompson, *The Tour de France: A Cultural History* (Los Angeles:
     University of California Press, 2008), pp. 96–7.
35   Tony Mason and Eliza Riedi, *Sport and the Military: The British Armed Forces
     1880–1960* (Cambridge: Cambridge University Press, 2010), pp. 42–4.
36   Neil Carter, 'From Knox to Dyson: Coaching, Amateurism and British Athletics,
     1912–1947', *Sport in History*, 30:1 (March 2010), pp. 59–60.
37   Richard Holt, 'The Amateur Body and the Middle-class Man: Work, Health
     and Style in Victorian Britain', *Sport in History*, 26:3 (December 2006),
     pp. 358–62.
38   Interview between Geoff Dyson and Tom McNab, c.1968, transcript in possession
     of the author. I am grateful to Tom McNab for access to this interview.
39   Quoted in Tony Mason, *Sport in Britain* (London: Faber and Faber, 1988),
     pp. 113–14.
40   For a discussion of political culture related to professional societies see Harold
     Perkin, *The Third Revolution: Professional Elites in the Modern World*
     (London: Routledge, 1996).
41   For example, see John Hoberman, *Darwin's Athletes: How Sport has Damaged
     Black America and Preserved the Myth of Race* (Boston: Houghton Mifflin,
     1997); Ben Carrington and Ian McDonald (eds), *'Race', Sport and British
     Society* (London: Routledge, 2001); David Wiggins, *Glory Bound: Black
     Athletes in a White America* (Syracuse: Syracuse University Press, 1997); Ian

Brittain, *The Paralympic Games Explained* (London: Routledge, 2010); Julie Anderson, '"Turned into Taxpayers": Paraplegia, Rehabilitation and Sport at Stoke Mandeville, 1944–56', *Journal of Contemporary History*, 38 (2003), pp. 461–75; P. David Howe, 'The tail is wagging the dog: Body culture, classification and the Paralympic movement', *Ethnography*, 9 (2008), pp. 499–517.

42   Dimeo, *Drug Use*.

43   John Welshman, 'Boxing and the historians', *IJHS*, 14:1 (1997), pp. 195–203.

Chapter 1   Sport as Medicine: Ideas of Health, Sport and Exercise

1   Ina Zweiniger-Bargielowska, *Managing the Body: Beauty, Health, and Fitness in Britain, 1880–1939* (Oxford: Oxford University Press), pp. 170–1.

2   Bernard Harris, *The Origins of the British Welfare State: Social Welfare in England and Wales, 1800–1945* (Basingstoke: Palgrave, 2004), p. xi.

3   Klaus Bergoldt, *Wellbeing: A Cultural History of Healthy Living* (translated by Jane Dewhurst) (Cambridge: Polity, 2008), pp. 1–6.

4   *Ibid.*, pp. 55–6.

5   Vivian Nutton, 'Humoralism' in W.F. Bynum and Roy Porter (eds), *Companion Encyclopedia of the History of Medicine, Volume One* (London: Routledge, 1993), p. 281.

6   Roberta Bivins, *Alternative Medicine? A History* (Oxford: Oxford University Press, 2007), p. 12.

7   Human temperaments bear humoural names: choleric, melancholic, sanguine and phlegmatic.

8   Bivins, *Alternative Medicine?*, p. 9.

9   *Ibid.*

10   Jack W. Berryman, 'Exercise and the Medical Tradition from Hippocrates through Antebellum America: A Review Essay' in Berryman and Park (eds), p. 3.

11   For a critique of this period see Peter Dear, *Revolutionizing the Sciences: European Knowledge and its Ambitions, 1500–1700, Second Edition* (Basingstoke: Palgrave Macmillan, 2009).

12   *Ibid.*, Chapters 7 and 8; Bergdolt, *Wellbeing*, p. 202; Roy Porter, *The Greatest Benefit to Mankind: A Medical History of Humanity* (New York: W.W. Norton, 1997), p. 218; Bivins, *Alternative Medicine?*, p. 33.

13   Wolfgang Behringer, 'Arena and Pall Mall: Sport in the Early Modern Period', *German History*, 27:3 (2009), p. 334.

14   Bergdolt, *Wellbeing*, p. 200.

15   *Ibid.*, p. 229.

16   *Ibid.*, pp. 236–7.

17   Harris, *British Welfare State*, pp. 16–19.

18   Dorothy Porter, *Health, Civilization and the State: A history of public health from ancient to modern times* (London: Routledge, 1999), p. 63.

19   Keys, *Globalizing Sport*, pp. 1–16.

20   Porter, *Health, Civilization*, pp. 97–110; Deborah Brunton, 'Dealing with Disease in Populations: Public Health, 1830–1880' in Brunton (ed.), pp. 196–204.

21   Matthew Ramsey, 'Public Health in France' in Dorothy Porter (ed.), *The History of Public Health and the Modern State* (Amsterdam: Rodopi, 1994) pp. 45–118.

22   Paul Weindling, 'From Germ Theory to Social Medicine: Public Health, 1880–1930' in Brunton (ed.), p. 239.

23   See Kay Schiller and Christopher Young, 'The History and Historiography of
      Sport in Germany: Social, Cultural and Political Perspectives', *German History*,
      27:3 (2009), pp. 313–30.
24   Jan Todd, 'The Classical Ideal and its Impact on the Search for Suitable Exercise:
      1774–1830', *Iron Game History*, 2:4 (1992), p. 7.
25   Margaret MacMillan, *Peacemakers: The Paris Conference of 1919 and Its
      Attempt to End War* (London: Hodder, 2001), p. 365.
26   Todd, 'The Classical Ideal', p. 7; Felix Saure, 'Beautiful Bodies, Exercising Warriors
      and Original Peoples: Sports, Greek Antiquity and National Identity from
      Winckelmann to 'Turnvater Jahn', *German History*, 27:3 (2009), pp. 358–73.
27   Saure, 'Beautiful Bodies', pp. 358–73.
28   Christiane Eisenberg, 'Charismatic Nationalist Leader: Turnvater Jahn', *IJHS*,
      13:1 (March 1996), pp. 14–26. A Turnfeste was a very large gymnastic festival
      in which the Turnen performed mass gymnastic exercises along with listening to
      patriotic orations and pledging their allegiance to the Kaiser.
29   Arnd Kruger, 'The role of sport in German international politics, 1918–1945' in
      P. Arnaud and J. Riordan, (eds), *Sport and international politics* (London:
      E. & F.N. Spon, 1998), p. 80; Porter, *Health, Civilization*, p. 304.
30   Porter, *Health, Civilization*, p. 304; Jean Barclay, *In Good Hands: The History
      of the Chartered Society of Physiotherapy 1894–1994* (Oxford: Butterworth
      Heinemann, 1994), pp. 4–5.
31   Holt, *Sport and the British*, pp. 94–5.
32   Eugen Weber, 'Gymnastics and Sports in *Fin-de-Siècle* France', *American
      Historical Review*, 76:1 (February 1971), pp. 70–7.
33   Peter Radford, *The Celebrated Captain Barclay: Sport, Money and Fame in
      Regency Britain* (London: Headline, 2001), pp. 60–8.
34   Todd, 'The Classical Ideal', pp. 8–9.
35   Peter McIntosh, 'Archibald Maclaren', *Dictionary of National Biography*, 2004
      [accessed 18 Nov 2004: http://www.oxforddnb.com/view/article/50298].
36   Frank Galligan, 'The History of Gymnastic Activity in the West Midlands,
      with special reference to Birmingham, from 1865 to 1918: With an analysis
      of military influences, secular and religious innovation and educational
      developments' (Unpublished PhD thesis, Coventry University, 1999), p. 263.
37   Bruce Haley, *The Healthy Body and Victorian Culture* (London: Harvard
      University Press, 1978), p. 3.
38   Haley, *Healthy Body*, pp. 19, 4; Holt, *Sport and the British*, p. 361.
39   Dominic Erdozain, *The Problem of Pleasure: Sport, Recreation and the Crisis of
      Victorian Religion* (Woodbridge: Boydell Press, 2010).
40   Holt, *Sport and the British*, p. 76. Sport in the schools, however, was generally
      organized and ran by the boys.
41   Haley, *Healthy Body*, p. 167.
42   *Times Higher Education*, 26 March 2009, p. 48.
43   Tony Collins, *A Social History of English Rugby Union* (London: Routledge,
      2009), pp. 1–21.
44   Holt, *Sport and the British*, pp. 74–88; Eliza Riedi and Tony Mason, '"Leather"
      and the Fighting Spirit: Sport in the British Army in World War I', *Canadian
      Journal of History*, 41 (2006), p. 496.
45   Patrick F. Devitt, *May the Best Man Win: Sport, Masculinity, and Nationalism
      in Great Britain and the Empire 1880–1935* (Basingstoke: Palgrave, 2004),
      pp. 1–13. Notions of masculinity though differed according to social context.

While the working classes, for example, adopted many of the games of the elites, there was less acceptance of the attendant values associated with the games.

46 Holt, 'The Amateur Body, pp. 352–69.
47 Harris, *British Welfare State*, pp. 104–24.
48 Hill, *Sport, Leisure and Culture*, pp. 165–6.
49 Claire Parker, 'The Rise of Competitive Swimming 1840 to 1878', *The Sports Historian*, 21:2 (November 2001), pp. 54–67.
50 J. Hurt, 'Drill, discipline and the elementary school ethos' in W.P. McCann (ed.), *Popular Education and Socialization in the Nineteenth Century* (London: Methuen, 1977), p. 176; Galligan, 'Gymnastic Activity', pp. 257–74.
51 *Ibid.*, p. 189; Tony Mason, *Association Football and English Society 1863–1915* (Brighton; Harvester Press, 1980), p. 125 n19.
52 John Welshman, 'Physical Education and the School Medical Service in England and Wales, 1907–1939', *Social History of Medicine*, 9:1(1996), pp. 32–4.
53 John Welshman, 'Physical Culture and Sport in Schools in England and Wales, 1900–40', *IJHS*, 15:1 (April 1998), p. 56.
54 Hill, *Sport, Leisure and Culture*, p. 167.
55 Holt, *Sport and the British*, pp. 136–48. For other literature regarding rational recreation see Peter Bailey, *Leisure and Class in Victorian England: Rational recreation and the contest for control, 1830–1885* (London: Methuen, 1987); Dave Russell, *Popular Music in England, 1840–1914: A social history, Second edition* (Manchester: Manchester University Press, 1997), Chapters 2 and 3.
56 Mason, *Association Football*, p. 123 n6.
57 For a detailed study of the origins and motivations of these and similar organizations see John Springhall, *Youth, Empire and Society; British Youth Movements, 1883–1940* (London: Croom Helm, 1977). Tammy Proctor, '(Uni) Forming Youth: Girl Guides and Boy Scouts in Britain, 1908–39', *History Workshop Journal*, 45 (1998), pp. 105–6.
58 Mason, *Association Football*, pp. 82–7; Colm Kerrigan, 'London Schoolboys and Professional Football, 1899–1915, *IJHS*, 11:2 (August 1994), pp. 287–97.
59 Roger Munting, 'The Games Ethic and Industrial Capitalism before 1914: The Provision of Company Sports', *Sport in History*, 23:1 (Summer 2003), pp. 45–63; Kathleen Jones, *The Making of Social Policy in Britain 1830–1990* (London: Athlone, 1994), pp. 42–4.
60 James Moore, 'The Fortunes of Eugenics' in Brunton (ed.), pp. 266–97.
61 Zweiniger-Bargielowska, *Managing the Body*, p. 24.
62 Porter, *Health, Civilization*, pp. 166–73.
63 Jones, *Social Policy*, p. 77.
64 Geoffrey Searle, *The Quest for National Efficiency: A study of British politics and British political thought 1899–1914* (Oxford: Blackwell, 1971), pp. 54–67.
65 Zweiniger-Bargielowska, *Managing the Body*, pp. 72–3; Report of the Inter-Departmental Committee on Physical Deterioration 1903–4.
66 Porter, *Health, Civilization*, p. 147.
67 Porter, *Greatest Benefit*, p. 417.
68 Berryman, 'Exercise', pp. 35–6.
69 Green, *Fit For America*, pp. 6–7.
70 Todd, 'The Classical Ideal', p. 6.

71   Gertrud Pfister, 'The Role of German Turners in American Physical Education', *IJHS*, 26:13 (2009), pp. 1893–1925.

72   Roberta J. Park, 'Physiologists, Physicians, and Physical Educators: Nineteenth-Century Biology and Exercise, Hygienic and Educative' in Berryman and Park (eds), pp. 137–40.

73   Green, *Fit for America*, pp. 182–3.

74   Park, 'Sharing, arguing', pp. 519–48.

75   Porter, *Health, Civilization*, pp. 147–62.

76   Green, *Fit for America*, pp. 219–33.

77   *Ibid.*, pp. 233–40; Michael Oriard, *Reading Football: How the Popular Press Created an American Spectacle* (London: University of North Carolina Press, 1993), pp. 214–15.

78   Porter, *Health, Civilization*, p. 305.

79   Dorothy Porter, 'The Healthy Body' in Cooter and Pickstone (eds), p. 202.

80   Zweiniger-Bargielowska, *Managing the Body*, pp. 1–14.

81   Porter, *Health, Civilization*, p. 306.

82   Eugen Sandow, *Life is Movement: The Physical Reconstruction and Regeneration of the People* (London: National Health Press, 1919), pp. 282–3.

83   Zweiniger-Bargielowska, *Managing the Body*, pp. 36–50.

84   *Ibid.*, pp. 46–50; Hans Bonde, 'I.P. Muller: Danish Apostle of Health', *IJHS*, 8:1 (December 1991), pp. 347–69; I.P. Muller, *My System: 15 Minutes' Exercise a Day for Health's Sake* (London: Link House, 1904).

85   Green, *Fit For America*, pp. 242–50. See also Jan Todd, 'Bernarr Macfadden: Reformer of Feminine Form' in Berryman and Park (eds), pp. 213–32.

86   Mark Dyreson, 'Johnny Weissmuller and the Old Global Capitalism: The Origins of the Federal Blueprint for Selling American Culture to the World, *IJHS*, 25:2 (2008), pp. 268–83.

87   Zweiniger-Bargielowska, *Managing the Body*, pp. 298–9.

88   Ina Zweinigier-Bargielowska, 'Raising a Nation of 'Good Animals': The New Health Society and Health Education Campaigns in Interwar Britain', *Social History of Medicine*, 20:1 (2007), pp. 73–89; Porter, *Health, Civilization*, pp. 303–8.

89   Ina Zweinigier-Bargielowska, 'Building a British Superman: Physical Culture in Interwar Britain', *Journal of Contemporary History*, 41:4 (2006), pp. 596–602.

90   Zweiniger-Bargielowska, *Managing the Body*, pp. 169–74.

91   Porter, *Health, Civilization*, p. 208.

92   Angela Teja, 'Italian sport and international relations under fascism' in Arnaud and Riordan (eds), pp. 147–70.

93   Keys, *Globalizing Sport*, p. 3.

94   *Ibid.*, pp. 158–72; Nikolaus Katzer, 'Soviet physical culture and sport: A European legacy?' in Alan Tomlinson, Christopher Young and Richard Holt (eds), *Sport and the Transformation of Modern Europe: States, media and markets 1950–2010* (London: Routledge, 2011), pp. 18–34.

95   Keys, *Globalizing Sport*, p. 115.

96   Porter, *Health, Civilization*, p. 193.

97   Erik Jensen, *Body By Weimar: Athletes, Gender and German Modernity* (Oxford: Oxford University Press, 2010).

98   Barbara Cole, 'The East German Sports System: Image and Reality (Unpublished PhD: Texas Tech University, 2000), p. 54; Keys, *Globalizing Sport*, p. 125.

99   Keys, *Globalizing Sport*, pp. 125–6.

100   For a similar response amongst other countries in the British Empire see
      Charlotte Macdonald, *Strong, Beautiful, and Modern: National Fitness in
      Britain, New Zealand, Australia and Canada, 1935–1960* (Wellington,
      NZ: Bridget Williams Books, 2011).

101   Zweiniger-Bargielowska, *Managing the Body*, pp. 329–30.

102   Anne Hardy, *Health and Medicine in Britain since 1860* (Basingstoke: Palgrave,
      2001), pp. 77–9.

103   *Ibid.*, p. 108.

104   Stephen G. Jones, 'State Intervention in Sport and Leisure in Britain between the
      Wars', *Journal of Contemporary History*, 22 (1987), p. 167; Hugh Cunningham,
      'Leisure and Culture' in FML Thompson (ed.), *The Cambridge Social History of
      Britain, 1750–1950* (Cambridge: Cambridge University Press, 1990), p. 323.

105   Welshman, 'Physical Education', pp. 40, 64–5; Charles Webster, 'The Health of
      the School Child During the Depression' in N. Parry and D. McNair (eds), *The
      Fitness of the Nation-Physical and Health Education in the Nineteenth and
      Twentieth Centuries: Proceedings of the 1982 Annual Conference of the History of
      Education Society of Great Britain* (History of Education Society, 1983), pp. 73–4.

106   Elsa Davies, 'National Playing Fields Association' in Richard Cox, Grant Jarvie
      and Wray Vamplew (eds), *Encyclopedia of British Sport* (Oxford: ABC-Clio,
      2000), pp. 275–6.

107   It had been originally called the Central Council of Recreative Physical Training
      but this was changed to the Central Council of Physical Recreation in 1944.

108   H. Justin Evans, *Service to Sport: The Story of the CCPR – 1935–1972*
      (London: Pelham, 1974), pp. 31, 39.

109   Zweiniger-Bargielowska, *Managing the Body*, p. 313.

110   Porter, *Health, Civilization*, p. 208.

111   *Ibid.*, pp. 209–11.

112   *Ibid.*, pp. 211–2.

113   Harris, *British Welfare State*, p. 303.

114   *Lancet*, 21 November 1953, pp. 1053–7.

115   Robert Crawford, 'Healthism and the Medicalization of Everyday Life',
      International Journal of Health Services, 10:3 (1980), pp. 365–88.

116   Virginia Berridge, 'Medicine, public health and the media in Britain from
      the nineteen-fifties to the nineteen-seventies', *Historical Research*, 82:216
      (May 2009), p. 361.

117   Virginia Berridge, 'Medicine and the Public: The 1962 Report of the Royal
      College of Physicians and the New Public Health', *Bulletin of the History of
      Medicine*, 81: (2007), pp. 286–311.

118   Virginia Berridge, *Health and Society in Britain since 1939* (Cambridge:
      Cambridge University Press, 1999), p. 88.

119   Zweiniger-Bargielowska, *Managing the Body, passim.*

120   Mike Saks, 'Medicine and the Counter Culture' in Cooter and Pickstone
      (eds), pp. 114–20. Roberta Bivins has argued that cross-cultural or alternative
      medicine never went away and these therapies have their origins in Ancient
      Egypt and Greece. Bivins, *Alternative Medicine?*, p. 171.

121   Nancy Phelan and Michael Volin, *Yoga for Women* (London: Arrow, 1963),
      p. 23; Carey Watt, Book Review of John J. MacAloon (ed.), *Muscular
      Christianity in Colonial and Post-Colonial Worlds* (London: Routledge, 2008),
      IJHS, 26:15 (2009), pp. 2287–8; Bivins, *Alternative Medicine?*, p. 79;
      Zweiniger-Bargielowska, *Managing the Body*, pp. 35–6.

122   Mason, *Sport in Britain*, pp. 83–4.

123 J. Smith Maguire, 'Leisure and the Obligations of Self-Work: An Examination of the Fitness Field', *Leisure Studies*, 27:1 (2008), p. 61; Matthew Frew and David McGillivray, 'Health Clubs and Body Politics: Aesthetics and the Quest for Physical Capital', *Leisure Studies*, 24:2, (2005), pp. 161–2; Roberta Sassatelli, 'The Commercialization of Discipline: Keep-Fit Culture and Its Values', *Journal of Modern Italian Studies*, 5:3 (2000), pp. 396–7.

124 Jutta Braun, 'The People's Sport? Popular Sport and Fans in the Later Years of the German Democratic Republic', *German History*, 27:3 (2009), pp. 414–28.

125 Porter, 'Healthy Body', pp. 212–15.

126 Mick Green, 'Olympic Glory or Grassroots Development?: Sport Policy Priorities in Australia, Canada and the United Kingdom, 1960–2000', *IJHS*, 24:7 (July 2007), p. 930.

127 Penny Tinkler, 'Cause for Concern: young women and leisure, 1930–50', *Women's History Review*, 12:2 (2003), p. 241.

128 Park, 'Setting the Scene', pp. 1427–52.

129 Thomas M. Hunt, 'Countering the Soviet Threat in the Olympic Medals Race: The Amateur Sports Act of 1978 and American Athletics Policy Reform', *IJHS*, 24:6 (June 2007), pp. 798–800.

130 Phil Dine, 'Sport and the State in contemporary France: from la Charte des Sports to decentralisation', *Modern and Contemporary France*, 6:3 (1998), p. 310.

131 For the relationship between sport and the state in the Third Republic (1870–1939) see Richard Holt, 'Sport, the French, and the Third Republic', *Modern and Contemporary France*, 6:3 (1998), pp. 289–99.

132 Lindsay Sarah Krasnoff, 'Resurrecting the nation: The evolution of French sports policy from de Gaulle to Mitterand' in Tomlinson *et al* (eds), pp. 67–82.

133 N. Baker, 'The Amateur Ideal in a Society of Equality: Change and Continuity in post-Second World War British Sport', 1945–48, *IJHS*, 12:1 (April 1995), p. 101.

134 Martin Polley, *Moving the Goalposts: A history of sport and society since 1945* (London: Routledge, 1998), p. 10.

135 Wolfenden Committee on Sport, *Sport and the Community*, London: CCPR, 1960, paragraphs 269–72.

136 For the even greater role of local government in British sport see Barrie Houlihan, *The Government and Politics of Sport* (London: Routledge, 1991), p. 51.

137 Krasnoff, 'Resurrecting the nation', pp. 67–82.

138 Roger Bannister, 'Sport, Physical Recreation, and the National Health', *British Medical Journal* (23 December 1972), p. 712.

139 Richard Holt and Tony Mason, *Sport in Britain 1945–2000* (Oxford: Blackwell, 2000), p. 150. Sport for All was originally a European Commission initiative.

140 Berridge, *Health and Society*, p. 88.

141 Mason, *Sport in Britain*, p. 82. For the role of leisure centres in Northern Ireland see Holt and Mason, *Sport in Britain*, p. 189 n16; Hill, *Sport, Leisure and Culture*, pp. 173–4.

142 Holt and Mason, *Sport in Britain*, p. 166.

143 *Ibid.*, pp. 154–5.

Chapter 2 This Sporting Life: Injuries and Medical Provision

1 Oriard, *Reading Football*, p. 205.

2 John Harding, *Living to Play: From Soccer Slaves to Socceratti – A Social History of the Professionals* (London: Robson, 2003), p. 105.

3 Steve Sturdy, 'The Industrial Body' in Cooter and Pickstone (eds), p. 217.

4 Brad Beaven, *Leisure, citizenship and working-class men in Britain, 1850–1945* (Manchester: Manchester University Press, 2005), Chapter 1.

5 Haley, *Healthy Body*, p. 225.

6 Zweiniger-Bargielowska, *Managing the Body*, pp. 27–8; Andrew August, 'A culture of consolation? Rethinking politics in working-class London, 1870–1914', *Historical Research*, 74:183 (August 2001), pp. 193–217; Stan Shipley, 'Tom Causer of Bermondsey: A Boxer Hero of the 1890s', *History Workshop Journal*, 15 (1983), p. 31.

7 See Steven Fielding, Peter Thompson and Nick Tiratsoo, *'England Arise!' The Labour Party and Popular Politics in 1940s Britain* (Manchester: Manchester University Press, 1995).

8 Muller, *My System*, p. 24.

9 Sandow, *Life is Movement*, pp. 390–2.

10 Collins, *Rugby Union*, p. 19.

11 *Field*, 18 December 1880, p. 920.

12 Tony Collins, *Rugby's Great Split: Class, Culture and the Origins of Rugby League Football* (London: Frank Cass, 1998), p. 129.

13 *Ibid.*, p. 214.

14 For a critical analysis of these injuries see Tony Collins, 'History, Theory and the "Civilizing Process"', *Sport in History*, 25:2 (August 2005), pp. 298–9.

15 Football refers to both the rugby and soccer codes. *Lancet*, 6 January 1894, p. 40; 24 March 1894, pp. 756, 764–7.

16 Collins, 'History, Theory', pp. 298–9.

17 *Lancet*, 16 November 1907, pp. 1402–3.

18 *Lancet*, 19 September 1908, p. 886.

19 James Whorton, '"Athlete's Heart": The Medical Debate Over Athleticism, 1870–1920', *Journal of Sport History*, 9:1 (Spring 1982), pp. 38–9.

20 RH Anglin Whitelocke, *Football Injuries* (London: Medical Officers of Schools Association, 1904).

21 *The Times*, 27 May 1910, p. 10.

22 Collins, *Rugby's Great Split*, p. 124.

23 Green, *Fit For America*, p. 233.

24 See Oriard, *Reading Football*.

25 Steven A. Riess, *Sport in Industrial America 1850–1920* (Wheeling, Il: Harlan Davidson, 1995), p. 116.

26 Roberta Park, '"Mended or Ended?": Football Injuries and the British and American Medical Press', 1870–1910, *IJHS*, 18:2 (June 2001), pp. 110–33.

27 Howard Savage, Harold W. Bentley, John T. McGovern and Dean F. Smiley, *American College Athletics, Bulletin Number 23* (New York: Carnegie Foundation for the Advancement of Teaching, 1929), pp. x–xxi.

28 Savage *et al*, *American College Athletics*, pp. 140–2.

29 *Ibid.*, pp. 144–5.

30 Michael Oriard, *King Football: Sport and Spectacle in the Golden Age of Radio and Newsreels, Movies and Magazines, the Weekly and the Daily Press* (Chapel Hill: North Carolina Press, 2001), p. 173.

31 *Ibid.*, p. 106. For a more recent scandal concerning the sacking of Pennsylvania State University's coach, see *Times Higher Education*, 24 November 2011, pp. 20–1.

32 Richard D. Hawkins and Colin W. Fuller, 'A prospective epidemiological study of injuries in four English professional football clubs', *BJSM*, 33 (1999), pp. 196–203.

33 S. Drawer and C.W. Fuller, 'Propensity for osteoarthritis and lower limb joint pain in retired professional soccer players', *BJSM*, 35 (2001), pp. 402–8. Although the figure is relatively low when considering the high injury levels.

34 Martin Roderick, 'The sociology of pain and injury in sport' in Sigmund Loland, Berit Skirstad and Ivan Waddington, *Pain and Injury in Sport: Social and ethical analysis* (London: Routledge, 2006), pp. 17–33.

35 Tony Collins, *Rugby League in Twentieth Century Britain* (London: Routledge), 2006, pp. 151–3.

36 Holt, *Sport and the British*, p. 173.

37 John Williams, *Red Men* (Edinburgh: Mainstream, 2012).

38 Interview with Ian Adams, 22 August 2005.

39 Malcolm and Sheard, '"Pain in the Assets"', pp. 149–50.

40 Questionnaire survey of footballers. Qualitative data was extracted from the replies of 19 former professional footballers. I am grateful to John Rowlands for his help.

41 *Daily Telegraph* (Sport), 25 June 2009, p. 14.

42 *Field*, 7 July 1883, p. 11.

43 I am grateful to Honor Godfrey at the Wimbledon museum for this information.

44 *The Times*, 30 December 1889, p. 10.

45 Roger Cooter, 'The Moment of the Accident: Culture, Militarism and Modernity in Late-Victorian Britain', in Roger Cooter and Brian Luckin (eds), *Accidents in History: Injuries, Fatalities and Social Relations* (Amsterdam: Rodopi, 1997), pp. 107–9.

46 Hardy, *Health and Medicine*, p. 36.

47 Roderick, 'Pain and injury in sport', pp. 17–33.

48 Beaven, *Leisure, citizenship*, p. 111.

49 Sheard, '"Brutal and Degrading"', p. 78.

50 John A. Williams, 'Winter Sports' in J.R. Armstrong and W.E. Tucker (eds), *Injury in Sport: The Physiology, Prevention and Treatment of Injuries associated with Sport* (London: Staples Press, 1964), pp. 250–1.

51 Harding, *Living to Play*, p. 106. Admittedly, these figures were gathered by a newspaper, and the methodology used is not known. However, they do indicate the accepted nature of injuries in football.

52 Matthew Taylor, *The Leaguers: The Making of Professional Football, 1900–1939* (Liverpool: Liverpool University Press, 2005), p. 155.

53 Charles Buchan, *A Lifetime in Football* (London: Sportsmans Book Club, 1956), p. 71.

54 Tony Mason, *Passion of the People? Football in South America* (London: Verso, 1994), p. 25.

55 Martin Roderick, Ivan Waddington and Graham Parker, 'Playing Hurt: Managing Injuries in English Professional Football', *International Review for the Sociology of Sport*, 35:2 (2000), pp. 165–80.

56 R.D. Hawkins *et al*, 'The association football medical research programme: an audit of injuries in professional football', *BJSM*, 35 (2001), pp. 43–7.

57 Mason and Riedi, *Sport and the Military*, pp. 68–73. See Chapter 2 for more detail on officer sports.

58 Virginia Holgate, *Ginny: An Autobiography* (London: Stanley Paul, 1986), p. 51.

59 Nick Skelton, *Only Falls and Horses* (London: Greenwater, 2001), Chapter 29.

60 Savage *et al*, *American College Athletics*, p. 155.

61 R. Salisbury Woods, 'Disorders and Accidents of Athletes', *Practitioner*, (September 1930), pp. 414–16.

62 *Observer* (Sport), 19 May 2002. Hingis made a brief comeback a few years later.

63 *New York Times* (Sports), 25 May 2006, D1, D6.

64 Marcus Trescothick, *Coming back to me: The Autobiography* (London: Harper, 2008).

65 *Guardian* (G2), 16 April 2001, pp. 2–4.

66 Thompson, *Tour de France*, p. 216.

67 Martin Tolich and Martha Bell, 'The Commodification of Jockeys' Working Bodies: Anorexia or Work Discipline' in Chris McConville (ed.), *A Global Racecourse: Work, Culture and Horse Sports* (Melbourne: Australian Society for Sports History, 2008), pp. 101–13.

68 James Huntington-Whiteley (ed.), *The Book of British Sporting Heroes* (London: National Portrait Gallery, 1998), p. 31.

69 Dick Francis, *Lester: The Official Biography* (London: Michael Joseph, 1986), pp. 71–2.

70 Wray Vamplew, 'Still Crazy after All Those Years: Continuity in a Changing Labour Market for Professional Jockeys' in A. Smith and D. Porter (eds), *Amateurs and Professionals in Post-War British Sport* (London: Frank Cass, 2000), pp. 119–21. A study of the medical treatment received by horses would make an interesting subject but it is beyond the scope of this book.

71 Waddington, *Sport, Health*, pp. 103–4.

72 Harris, *British Welfare State*, Chapter 11; Mike Savage and Andrew Miles, *The Remaking of the British Working Class 1840–1940* (London: Routledge, 1994).

73 Taylor, *The Leaguers*, Chapters 3 and 4.

74 A. Clement Edwards, *The Compensation Act 1906* (London: Chatto and Windus, 1907), pp. 8–10.

75 Taylor, *The Leaguers*, p. 129.

76 Colin Fuller, 'Implications of health and safety legislation for the professional sportsperson', *BJSM*, 29:1 (1995), p. 5.

77 Ronnie Johnston and Arthur McIvor, 'Marginalising the Body at Work? Employers' Occupational Health Strategies and Occupational Medicine in Scotland c.1930–1974', *Social History of Medicine*, 21:1 (April 2008), pp. 127–44.

78 Mason, Association Football, p. 107.

79 Collins, *Great Split*, pp. 126–7.

80 www.coylehamiltonwillis.com/gaa/gaa.htm [accessed 24 September 2005].

81 Taylor, *The Leaguers*, p. 161.

82 Middlesbrough FC Minutes, 19 September 1898.

83 Middlesbrough FC Minutes, 14 November 1898, Middlesbrough turned professional in 1899–1900.

84 Harding, *Living to Play*, pp. 106–7.

85 Wolverhampton Wanderers FC, Rules for players 1914–15. Information provided by Wolverhampton Wanderers FC.

86 Wolverhampton Wanderers Football Club (1923) Ltd., Season 1933–34, Player's Ticket; Hull City AFC, Season 1939–40, Player's Ticket.

87 Collins, *Rugby League*, p. 49.

88 *FA Bulletin*, April 1955, p. 436.

89 Vamplew, 'Still Crazy', pp. 124–5.

90 Ken Foster, 'Developments in Sports Law' in Lincoln Allison (ed.), *The Changing Politics of Sport* (Manchester: Manchester University Press, 1993), pp. 105–24.

91 *Guardian*, 24 February 2004.

92   Hugh Cunningham, *The Invention of Childhood* (London: BBC Books 2006), pp. 211–45.

93   Cooter, 'The Moment of the Accident', pp. 107–9.

94   Frederick O. Mueller and Jerry L. Diehl, 'Annual Survey of Football Injury Research, 1931–2003', National Center for Catastrophic Sport Injury Research, http://www.unc.edu/depts/nccsi/AllSport.htm [accessed 22 October 2004].

95   Amateur Athletic Association Archives, Annual Report 1950.

96   Les Woodland (ed.), *The Yellow Jersey Companion to the Tour de France* (London: Yellow Jersey Press, 2003), p. 119.

97   Pierre de Coubertin, Timoleon J. Philemon, N.G. Politis and Charalmbos Anninos, *The Olympic Games: B.C. 776–A.D. 1896, Second Part, The Olympic Games in 1896* (London: H.G. Grevel, 1897), pp. 86–7.

98   Charles J.P. Lucas, *The Olympic Games 1904* (St. Louis: Woodward and Tiernan, 1905), p. 51; A.J. Ryan, 'History of sports medicine' in A.J. Ryan and F. Allman (eds), *Sports Medicine* (London: Academic Press, 1974), pp. 24–5.

99   British Olympic Council, *The Fourth Olympiad: London 1908* (London: British Olympic Council, 1908), pp. 72–3. The refreshments en route were supplied by Oxo.

100 Stockholm Organising Committee, *The Olympic Games of Stockholm 1912* (Stockholm: Swedish Olympic Committee/Wahlstrom and Widstrand, 1912), p. 1003, 1015.

101 *Ibid.*, pp. 832–42.

102 John Bryant, *The London Marathon: The History of the Greatest Race on Earth* (London: Arrow, 2005), pp. 188–91.

103 See, for example, J.R. Miles, 'The racecourse medical officer', *Journal of the Royal College of General Practitioners*, 19 (1970), p. 228.

104 Timothy Collings and Stuart Sykes, *Jackie Stewart: A Restless Life* (London: Virgin, 2003), pp. 123–42; Sid Watkins, *Life at the Limit: Triumph and Tragedy in Formula One* (London: Pan, 1996), pp. 12–28; *Beyond the Limit* (Basingstoke: Macmillan, 2001), Appendix 2.

105 Personal correspondence with Dr Hugh Seward, chairman of AFLMOA and team doctor for Geelong in Australian Football League.

106 Martin Johnes, '"Heads in the Sand": Football, Politics and Crowd Disasters in Twentieth-Century Britain', *Soccer in Society*, 5:2 (Summer 2004), pp. 135–6.

107 Wray Vamplew, 'Playing with the rules: Influences on the development of regulation in sport', *IJHS*, 24:7 (2007), p. 862; Foster, 'Sporting Law', pp. 105–7.

108 Holt, 'The Amateur Body', pp. 353–62.

109 Collins, *Rugby Union*, pp. 18–19.

110 *Evening News* (Glasgow), 15 October 1931, p. 1; *Daily Record*, 16 October 1931, p. 7; *Sunderland Echo*, 14, 15 February, p. 12, 3 March 1936.

111 *Sunderland Echo*, 3 March 1936.

112 Taylor, *The Leaguers*, pp. 252–5.

113 FA Minutes, Council, 24 April 1936; 4. Minutes of Referees' Committee, 3 April 1936.

114 Personal correspondence with Dr Hugh Seward, chairman of AFLMOA and team doctor for Geelong in AFL.

115 J.B. Byles and Samuel Osborn, 'First Aid', *Encyclopedia of Sport* (London: G.R. Putnam, 1912).

116 Tom McNab, Peter Lovesey and Andrew Huxtable, *An Athletics Compendium: An annotated guide to the UK Literature of Track and Field* (Boston Spa: British Library, 2001), p. xl. Presumably there was a similar impact on the pole vault.

117 Wray Vamplew, 'Still Crazy', p. 124.

118 FA Minutes, Council, 2 March 1936; 4. Minutes of Referees' Committee, 17 February 1936.

119 Williams, 'Winter Sports', pp. 250–1.

120 Patrick Murphy, *'Tiger' Smith of Warwickshire and England* (Guildford: Lutterworth Press, 1981), p. 7.

121 John Arlott, *Fred: Portrait of a Fast Bowler* (London: Coronet, 1971), pp. 17–18.

122 The figures included college and school football as well as the NFL.

123 http://www.unc.edu/depts/nccsi/AllSport.htm [accessed 27 September 2007].

124 John Underwood, 'An Unfolding Tragedy', *Sports Illustrated*, 14 August 1978.

125 *The Times*, 7 December 2011, p. 46.

126 N. Biasca, S Wirth and Y Tegner, 'The avoidability of head and neck injuries in ice hockey: an historical review', *BJSM*, 36:6 (2002), pp. 410–27.

127 K.K. Eaton, 'Motor Racing', *Journal of the Royal College of General Practitioners*, 20 (1970), p. 42.

128 Collins *Rugby Union*, Chapter 4.

129 J.P. Nicholls, P. Coleman and B.T. Williams, *Injuries in sport and exercise: A national study of the epidemiology of exercise-related injury and illness, A Report to the Sports Council* (November 1991); Doris Weightman and RC Browne, 'Injuries in Rugby and Association Football', *BJSM*, 8:4 (December 1974), pp. 183–7; *British Medical Journal (*hereafter, *BMJ),* 18 June 1977, pp. 1556–7.

130 Weightman and Browne, 'Injuries', pp. 183–7.

131 *BMJ*, 18 June 1977, pp. 1556–7. In 1978 it was anticipated that every NFL player would sustain at least one injury during the season. Underwood, 'An Unfolding Tragedy'.

132 John Brooks and Colin Fuller, *England Rugby Injury and Training Audit* (London: Professional Rugby Players' Association, 2005).

133 *Ibid.*

134 Dominic Malcolm, Ken Sheard and Stuart Smith, 'Protected Research: Sports Medicine and Rugby Injuries', *Sport in Society*, 7:1 (2004), pp. 96.

135 Brooks and Fuller, *England Rugby Injury*. For a historical perspective of the development of rugby union's rules see Collins, *Rugby Union*, Chapter 6.

136 Malcolm *et al*, 'Protected Research', p. 96.

137 J.P.R. Williams, *JPR: Given the Breaks: My Life in Rugby* (London: Hodder, 2006), pp. 98–102.

138 *BMJ*, 18 June 1977, pp. 1556–7; 19 August 1995, p. 511; 14 December 1996, p. 1550.

139 J.R. Silver, 'The impact of the 21st century on rugby injuries', *Spinal Cord*, 40 (2002), pp. 552–9; Timothy Noakes and Ismail Jakoet, 'Spinal cord injuries in rugby union players', *BMJ*, 310 (27 May 1995), pp. 1345–6.

140 *Observer*, 3 September 2006.

141 *Guardian*, 6 October 2006. http://www.guardian.co.uk/sport/2006/oct/06/rugbyunion.gdnsport3 [accessed 20 December 2007].

142 *Guardian*, 30 August 2006.

143 *Daily Telegraph* (Sport), 16 January 2008, p. 13.

Chapter 3   Sports Medicine: Pioneers and Specialization

1 Neal Bascomb, *The Perfect Mile: Three Athletes. One Goal. And less than Four Minutes to achieve it* (London: Harper Collins, 2004), pp. 105–6; Richard Lovell, 'Choosing People: An Aspect of the Life of Lord Moran (1882–1977)', *Medical History*, 36: (1992): 442–54.

2 Holt, 'The Amateur Body', pp. 358–62.

3 Collins, *Rugby Union*, p. 108.

4 For close analysis of this process, see Heggie, *British Sports Medicine*, chapters 4–6.

5 Harold Perkin, *The Rise of Professional Society: England Since 1880* (London: Routledge, 1989), pp. 3–4.

6 Joanna Bourke, 'Wartime' in Cooter and Pickstone (eds), p. 591.

7 Deborah Brunton, 'The Emergence of a Modern Profession?' in Brunton (ed.), p. 129.

8 Roger Cooter, 'The meaning of fractures: orthopaedics and the reform of British hospitals in the inter-war period', *Medical History*, 31: (1987) pp. 306–32.

9 Porter, *Greatest Benefit*, pp. 383–4.

10 Heggie, 'Specialization', p. 458.

11 Allan J. Ryan, 'Sports Medicine in the World Today' in Allan J. Ryan and Fred L. Allman Jr. (eds), *Sports Medicine 2nd Edition* (London: Academic Press, 1989), pp. 3, 13.

12 *New York Times*, 21 December 1997.

13 John Bale, 'The Mysterious Professor Jokl' in John Bale, Mette K. Christensen and Gertrud Pfister (eds), *Writing Lives in Sport: Biographies, Life-histories and Methods* (Aarhus: Aarhus University Press, 2004), p. 26.

14 David R. Bassett, 'Scientific contributions of A.V. Hill: exercise physiology pioneer', *Journal of Applied Physiology*, 93 (2002), p. 1567. I am grateful to Julie Anderson for this reference.

15 Brunton, 'Modern Profession?' in Brunton (ed.), p. 120.

16 Mike Saks, *Orthodox and Alternative Medicine: Politics, Professionalization and Health Care* (London: Continuum, 2003), pp. 38–41.

17 Jose Harris, *Private Lives, Public Spirit: Britain 1870–1914* (London: Penguin, 1993), p. 56.

18 Porter, *Greatest Benefit*, p. 628.

19 Brunton, 'Modern Profession', p. 120.

20 Saks, *Orthodox and Alternative Medicine*, p. 3.

21 Mike Saks, 'Introduction' in Mike Saks (ed.), *Alternative Medicine in Britain* (Oxford: Clarendon Press, 1992), pp. 1–21; *Orthodox and Alternative Medicine*.

22 Toby Gelfand, 'The history of the medical profession' in Bynum and Porter (eds), *Volume Two*, p. 1119.

23 Malcolm, 'Unprofessional Practice?', pp. 376–95.

24 Park, '"Cells or Soaring?"', p. 6.

25 Allan J. Ryan, 'Sportsmedicine History', *Physician and Sportsmedicine* (October 1978), pp. 77–8.

26 *Lancet*, 5 October 1912, p. 977; W. Hollmann, 'Sports medicine in the Federal Republic of Germany', *BJSM*, 23:3 (1989), p. 142.

27 Anon., 'Inauguration of sports medicine at the University of Giessen 1920', *International Journal of Sports Medicine*, 23: (2002), pp. s164–5. See also Heggie, *British Sports Medicine*, pp. 185–91.

28 Gigliola Gori, *Italian Fascism and the Female Body: Sport, Submissive Women and Strong Mothers* (London: Routledge, 2004), pp. 75–81; Simon Martin, *Sport Italia: The Italian Love Affair with Sport* (London: I.B. Tauris, 2011), pp. 55–7.

29 Jim Riordan, 'Sports Medicine in the Soviet Union and German Democratic Republic', *Social Science and Medicine*, 25:1 (1987), pp. 19–26.

30 Katzer, 'Soviet physical culture', p. 24.

31 Milton I. Roemer, 'Internationalism in Medicine and Public Health' in Bynum and Porter (eds), pp. 1417–25. Interestingly, one of the great supporters of the League of Nations was Philip Noel Baker who was also a member of the British amateur sporting elite.

32 The physicians included Hüntemuller and Herxheimer from Germany and Bramwell and Ellis from Britain.

33 Amsterdam Olympic Committee, *The Official Report of the IXth Olympiad, Amsterdam 1928* (Amsterdam: Olympic Committee of the Amsterdam Olympic Games, 1928), pp. 950–6.

34 E. Ergen, F. Pigozzi, N. Bachl and H.H. Dickhuth, 'Sports medicine: a European perspective. Historical roots, definitions and scope', *Journal of Sports Medicine and Physical Fitness*, 46: 2 (June 2006), p. 169.

35 Guiseppe La Cava, 'Sports medicine in modern times: A short historical survey', *Journal of Sports Medicine and Physical Fitness*, 13:3 (July-September 1973), pp. 155–8; 'The International Federation for Sports Medicine', *Journal of the American Medical Association*, 162: (17 November 1956), pp. 1109–11.

36 K. Tittel and H.G. Knuttgen, 'The development, objectives and activities of the International Federation of Sports Medicine (FIMS)' in A. Drix, H.G. Knuttgen and K. Tittel (eds), *The Olympic Book of Sports Medicine, Volume 1 of the Encyclopedia of Sports Medicine* (Oxford: International Olympic Committee, 1988), pp. 7–9.

37 Initially, it was called the American Chapter of FIMS but was renamed the American College of Sports Medicine in 1955.

38 Jack Berryman, *Out of Many, One: A History of the American College of Sports Medicine* (Champaign, Ill: Human Kinetics, 1995), Chapters 1–3; Wrynn, 'Athlete in the Making', pp. 124–5.

39 It was soon dissolved due to the war and then reformed in 1949.

40 Alison Wrynn, '"Under the Showers": An Analysis of the Historical Connections between American Athletic Training and Physical Education', *Journal of Sport History*, 34:1 (Spring 2007), pp. 37–51.

41 Peter Sperryn, 'A personal letter from the retiring honorary secretary', *BJSM*, 17:3 (September 1983), p. 217.

42 Elsworth R. Buskirk and Charles M. Tipton, 'Exercise Physiology' in Massengale and Swanson (eds), p. 417.

43 Allan J. Ryan, 'Sports Medicine in the World Today' in Allan J. Ryan and Fred L. Allman (eds), *Sports Medicine* (London: Academic Press, 1974), p. 9.

44 Anon., *Lancet*, 19 November 1960, p. 1144.

45 http://www.acsm.org/AM/Template.cfm?Section=About_ACSM [accessed 10 August 2010].

46 Peter McCrory, 'Warm Up', *BJSM*, 35 (2001), p. 209.

47 L.A. Reynolds and E.M. Tansey, *The Development of Sports Medicine in Twentieth Century Britain* (Transcript of a Witness Seminar) (London: Wellcome Trust, 2009), p. 38. (Hereafter, *Witness Seminar*).

48 Berryman, *Out of Many*, pp. 3–6, 13–14, 23.

49 Fred Mason, 'R. Tait McKenzie's Medical Work and Early Exercise Therapies for People with Disabilities', *Sport History Review*, 39:1 (2008), p. 56; Wrynn, 'The Athlete in the Making', pp. 124–5.

50 John Bale, 'The Mysterious Professor Jokl' in John Bale, Mette K. Christensen, Gertrud Pfister (eds), *Writing Lives in Sport: Biographies, Life-histories and Methods* (Aarhus: Aarhus University Press, 2004), pp. 25–40. (Jokl is pronounced 'Joke-el').

51 Ernst Jokl, *The Medical Aspect of Boxing* (Pretoria: Van Schaik, 1941).

52 Carol Porter McCullough, *The Alexander Technique and the String Pedagogy of Paul Rolland* (Phoenix: Arizona State University Press, 1996).

53 'Dr Ernst F. Jokl, a Pioneer in Sports Medicine, Dies at 90', *New York Times*, 21 December 1997; John Bale, 'Lassitutde and Latitude: Observations on Sport and Environmental Determinism', *International Review for the Sociology of Sport*, 37: (2002), pp. 147–8; Floris Van Der Merwe, 'Ernst Franz Jokl as the Father of Physical Education in South Africa', NASSH Proceedings 1990.

54 Heggie, *British Sports Medicine*, p. 190.

55 Welshman, 'Physical Education', p. 39.

56 Heggie, *British Sports Medicine*, p. 11.

57 *Manchester Guardian*, 2 August 1956, p. 8.

58 BASM AGM, 27 February 1953. The following year BASM was accepted as an associate member of FIMS.

59 Quoted in *Witness Seminar*, p. xxxvi.

60 BASM Executive Committee Minutes, 23 June 1952.

61 Anon., *BASM Bulletin* (1968), pp. 96–104.

62 Adolphe Abrahams, 'Athletics' in Humphrey Rolleston (ed.), *The British Encyclopaedia of Medical Practice: Volume 2* (London: Butterworth, 1936), p. 225; Anon. *Lancet*, 10 April 1937, pp. 899–90.

63 Adolphe Abrahams, *The Human Machine* (London: Penguin, 1956), p. 134.

64 He was also an advisor for the 1981 film, *Chariots of Fire*, about the 1924 Olympics but in the film he was referred to as Tom Watson.

65 Wolfenden Committee on Sport, Draft Report, 8 July 1960.

66 Douglas G.A. Lowe and Arthur E. Porritt, *Athletics* (London: Longmans, 1929), p. 84.

67 Berridge, *Health and Society*, p. 88.

68 Peter Mandler, *The English National Character: The History of an Idea from Edmund Burke to Tony Blair* (New Haven: Yale University Press, 2006), p. 217.

69 Berridge, 'Medicine, public health'.

70 An advisory Sports Council was first established in 1965 and it gained its Royal Charter in 1972 giving it executive powers.

71 Wolfenden Committee on Sport, *Sport and the Community* (London: CCPR, 1960–61), pp. 105–6.

72 See Heggie, 'Only the British', pp. 213–35.

73 For an in-depth analysis of this process, see Heggie, *British Sports Medicine*, Chapter 5.

74 Interview with Ian Adams, 22 August 2005; *Witness Seminar*, 25–30; Anon., *BJSM*, (December 1975); Henry Robson, 'Obituary: William Eldon Tucker', *BJSM*, 25:4 (1991), p. 241.

75 The Institute of Sports Medicine (ISM) was jointly sponsored by BASM, the British Olympic Association and the Physical Education Association. It had initially been founded as a specialist postgraduate medical institution for the promotion of sports medicine knowledge through research and education.

BASM, as a membership organization that aspired to charity status, was unable to establish an academic institute on legal grounds, and it was felt at the time that the ISM would act as BASM's academic arm to give it greater credibility within medicine as a whole.

76   Dan Tunstall-Pedoe, 'Obituary: Dr John G.P. Williams', *BJSM*, 29:4 (1995), pp. 220–2.

77   Heggie, 'Specialization', pp. 461–8.

78   Heggie, *British Sports Medicine*, pp. 148–9.

79   Carter, 'Mixing Business?', pp. 69–91; *Witness Seminar*, p. xxiv, 70 n.186.

80   Tunstall-Pedoe, 'Obituary', pp. 220–2; *Witness Seminar*, pp. 21–2, 25, 128–9.

81   Anon., *BJSM* (September 1978), p. 157.

82   *Witness Seminar*, pp. 128–9.

83   Peter Sperryn, 'Secretary's Column', *BJSM*, 11:2 (June 1977), p. 242.

84   Tunstall-Pedoe, 'Obituary', pp. 220–2.

85   *Witness Seminar*, p. 87.

86   These included the British Institute of Musculoskeletal Medicine (1992), formed from the merger of the Institute of Orthopaedic Medicine and the British Association of Manipulative Medicine (1993).

87   BASM, AGM, 25 May 1977; BASM, AGM, 14 October 1984.

88   BASS combined the Biomechanics Study Group, the British Society of Sports Psychology and the Society of Sports Sciences. In 1993, it was renamed the British Association of Sport and Exercise Sciences.

89   *Witness Seminar*, p. 74 n.195.

90   *Ibid., passim*.

91   Henry Robson, 'Editorial', *BJSM*, 19:1 (March 1985), p. 3. Other groups included: Physiotherapists – 260; Remedial Gymnasts – 55; Chiropodists – 87; Other clinical professions – 35; PE and sports sciences – 266; and Administrators – 28.

92   'Honorary Treasurer's Report for the year 1987', *BJSM*, nd.

93   M. Cullen and M. Batt, 'Sport and exercise medicine in the United Kingdom comes of age', *BJSM*, 39: (2005), pp. 250–1.

94   BASM Executive Minutes, 1 December 1999.

95   Zweiniger-Bargielowska, *Managing the Body*, pp. 51–61.

96   *Guardian*, 26 August 2006, p. 6.

97   Tony Blair's speech on healthy living, http://politics.guardian.co.uk/print/0,,329538655-1070979,00.html [Accessed 26 July 2006].

98   *Guardian* (Sport), 25 October 2004, p. 25; *Observer*, 30 July 2006.

99   The establishment of the IABSEM brought the Scottish royal colleges exam and the Apothecaries' diploma under its wing and so there was only a single diploma.

100   *Witness Seminar*, p. xxvi n.13.

101   By contrast, the ACPSM had 1,200, almost exclusively physiotherapists and the osteopaths' group, OSCA had 250 members. 'The Future of BASEM: Opinion Poll of BASEM Members', BASEM Archives, in possession of author.

102   *Witness Seminar*, pp. 78–9, 136.

103   Paul McCrory, 'Evidence-based sports medicine', *BJSM*, 35 (2001), pp. 79–80.

104   These included IOC member, Kevin O'Flannagan, an Irish rugby international who also played for Arsenal in the 1940s. *Guardian*, 22 June 2006. James Marshall played for Glasgow Rangers between 1925 and 1935 when he moved to West Ham. He also won three England caps.

105 Anne Digby, *Making a medical living: Doctors and patients in the English market for medicine* (Cambridge: Cambridge University Pres, 1994), p. 170; Irvine Loudon, *Medical Care and the General Practitioner, 1750–1850* (Oxford: Oxford University Press, 1986), pp. 282–301. In the 1840s there had been an unsuccessful attempt to establish a College of General Practitioners.

106 Loudon, *Medical Care*, p. 205.

107 R. Woods, 'Physician, Heal Thyself: the Health and Mortality of Victorian Doctors', *Social History of Medicine*, 9:1 (1996), pp. 1–30.

108 Interview with Neil Phillips, 21 June 2005.

109 Interview with Ian Adams.

110 Simon Inglis, *League Football and the Men Who Made It: The Official Centenary History of the Football League* (London: Collins Willow, 1988), p. 391; *FA News*, November 1970, p. 4.

111 Royal Society, Harold W. Thompson papers (HWT), E149, Coaching scheme reports, Report: Re-structuring of the Football Association Coaching Scheme, Charles Hughes, 1976, p. 6.

112 Barrie Smith, *Doc: Jottings of a Football Club Doctor* (Birmingham: Self-published, 2003), p. 7; Interview with Stuart Carne, 13 August 2008.

113 West Bromwich Albion FC Minutes, 1895–1920.

114 Questionnaire survey of football club doctors.

115 Stuart Carne, 'General practitioner to a football club', *BMJ*, 283 (19 September 1981), pp. 765–6.

116 Interview with Ian Adams.

117 Smith, *Doc*, p. 16.

118 Ellen Welch and Sara Kelly, 'Premier league doctor', *Student BMJ*, 12 (2004), p. 265.

119 Carne, 'General practitioner', p. 766.

120 Interview with John Rowlands, 17 February 2005.

121 It was renamed the Centre of Medicine and Exercise Science in 2000.

122 Interview with Alan Hodson, 31 August 2005.

123 *Ibid*.

124 Welch and Kelly, 'Premier league doctor', p. 265.

125 One example was Sheffield Wednesday. Waddington *et al*, *Managing Injuries*, pp. 56–7.

126 In 2006 the average salary for a general practitioner was £100,000. *Guardian*, (London), 5 May 2006.

127 John Pickstone, 'Production, Community and Consumption: The Political Economy of Twentieth Century Medicine' in Cooter and Pickstone (eds), p. 16.

128 Porter, *Greatest Benefit*, pp. 717–18.

Chapter 4   Science and the Making of the Athletic Body

1 Huntington-Whiteley (ed.), *British Sporting Heroes*, p. 214.

2 Porter, *Greatest Benefit*, p. 39.

3 The terms 'coach' and 'trainer' used here are interchangeable.

4 For example, see Dave Day, 'London Swimming Professors: Victorian Craftsmen and Aquatic Entrepreneurs', *Sport in History*, 30:1 (March 2010), pp. 32–54. See also Neil Carter (ed.), *Coaching Cultures* (London: Routledge, 2011).

5 McNab *et al*, *Athletics*, pp. xxxv–i. David Day, 'From Barclay to Brickett: Coaching Practices and Coaching Lives in Nineteenth and Early Twentieth Century England', (Unpublished PhD: De Montfort University, Leicester 2008),

pp. 91–2; Wray Vamplew, 'Training', in Tony Collins, John Martin and Wray Vamplew (eds), *Encyclopedia of Traditional British Rural Sports* (London: Routledge, 2005), pp. 270–1.

6 Thomas Schlich, 'The Emergence of Modern Surgery' in Brunton (ed.), p. 68.

7 Vamplew, 'Training', pp. 270–1.

8 Day, 'From Barclay to Brickett', p. 92.

9 *Ibid.*, pp. 91–2; Vamplew, 'Training', pp. 270–1.

10 Peter Radford, 'The good, the bad and the ugly', *Sociology of Sport Online*, vol. 1 (1), 1998.

11 Tony Collins, 'Captain Robert Barclay' in Collins *et al* (eds), p. 40; John Bryant, *3:59.4: The Quest to Break the 4 Minute Mile* (London: Arrow, 2004), pp. 20–1.

12 McNab *et al*, *Athletics*, p. xxxvi.

13 Roberta J. Park, 'Athletes and their training in Britain and America, 1800–1914' in Berryman and Park (eds), p. 70.

14 See Deborah Brunton, 'The Rise of Laboratory Medicine' in Brunton (ed.), pp. 92–118.

15 Brunton, 'Introduction', pp. 4–5; Day, 'From Barclay to Brickett', pp. 82–3.

16 Brunton, 'Laboratory Medicine', pp. 100–1.

17 Bergdolt, *Wellbeing*, p. 202; Porter, *Greatest Benefit*, pp. 218, 337–41; Bivins, *Alternative Medicine?*, p. 33.

18 Holt, 'Amateur Body', p. 360; Porter, *Greatest Benefit*, pp. 337–41.

19 Cronin, 'Not Taking the Medicine', p. 27.

20 Hoberman, *Mortal Engines*, pp. 80–3.

21 Anon., 'History of sports medicine in the Netherlands', *BJSM*, 23:4 (1989), p. 219.

22 Hoberman, *Mortal Engines*, p. 78.

23 See Whorton, "Athlete's Heart", pp. 30–52.

24 *The Times*, 10 October 1867, p. 9.

25 Vanessa Heggie, 'A Century of Cardiomythology: Exercise and the Heart c. 1880s–1980', *Social History of Medicine*, 23:2 (August 2010), p. 293.

26 Day, 'From Barclay to Brickett', p. 131; Patricia Vertinsky, 'Embodying Normalcy: Anthropometry and the Long Arm of William H. Sheldon's Somatotyping Project', *Journal of Sport History*, 29:1 (Spring 2002), p. 96.

27 Park, 'Physiologists, Physicians', pp. 44–5; Vertinsky, 'Embodying Normalcy', pp. 103–4.

28 Zweiniger-Bargielowska, *Managing the Body*, pp. 36–50.

29 Park, 'Athletes', p. 90.

30 Holt, 'Amateur Body', p. 361.

31 Day, 'From Barclay to Brickett', p. 108.

32 Whorton, "Athlete's Heart", pp. 38–9.

33 Day, 'From Barclay to Brickett', pp. 102, 108.

34 Park, 'Athletes', pp. 76–8. McNab *et al*, *Athletics*, p. xxxvi.

35 Day, 'From Barclay to Brickett', pp. 98–9.

36 *Ibid.*, p. 134.

37 James Irvine Lupton and James Money Kyrle Lupton, *The Pedestrian's Record: To which is added a description of the external human form* (London: WH Allen, 1890), p. 4.

38 *Ibid.*, p. 24.

39 Day, 'From Barclay to Brickett', p. 132.

40 This exercise was still used by Steve Ovett's coach, Harry Wilson, a century later.

41 Bryant, *3:59.4*, p. 35.
42 Bryant, *3:59.4*, pp. 40–5; Ian Buchanan, 'Jackson, Arnold Nugent Strode Strode- (1891–1972)', *Oxford Dictionary of National Biography* [accessed 10 Feb 2006].
43 Harry Andrews, *Training for Athletics and General Health* (London: Bloomsbury, 2005), p. 18, 70. First published in 1911.
44 Sam Mussabini, *The Complete Athletic Trainer* (London: Methuen, 1913), p. 10; David Terry, 'An Athletic Coach Ahead of his Time', *British Society of Sports History Newsletter*, 11 (Spring 2000), pp. 34–8.
45 Mussabini, *Athletic Trainer*, p. 143.
46 *Ibid.*, p. 141; Andrews, *Training*, chapter 2.
47 Andrews, *Training*, pp. 87–8.
48 *The Times*, 6 May 1906, quoted in British Olympic Council (BOC), *Aims and Objects of the Olympic Games Fund* (London: British Olympic Association, 1913), p. 5.
49 *Ibid.*, pp. 5–6.
50 Stockholm Organising Committee, *The Olympic Games of Stockholm 1912* (Stockholm: Swedish Olympic Committee, 1912) pp. 286–92. In 1912 Sweden 'won' the Olympics with 24 gold medals, 24 silvers and 17 bronzes. Britain was third overall behind America with 10, 15 and 16. The Swedes also had employed coaches in other sports such as tug of war, football and lawn tennis.
51 Carter, 'From Knox to Dyson', pp. 55–81.
52 *Athletic News*, 6 July 1914.
53 Bourne, 'Fast Science', pp. 133–45.
54 Oriard, *Reading Football*, pp. 35–56.
55 J. Kenneth Doherty, *Modern Training for Running* (Englewood Cliffs, NJ: Prentice-Hall, 1964), pp. 13–14.
56 Quoted from Alex Natan (ed.), *Sport and Society* (London: Bowes and Bowes, 1958), p. 87 in Doherty, *Modern Training*, p. 14.
57 Park, 'Athletes', pp. 93–4; F.A.M. Webster, *Coaching and Care of Athletes* (London: George G. Harrap, 1938), pp. 26–9; Bourne, 'Fast Science', p. 120.
58 Bourne, 'Fast Science', pp. 145–53.
59 Rob Beamish and Ian Ritchie, 'From Fixed Capacities to Performance-Enhancement: The Paradigm Shift in the Science of "Training" and the Use of Performance-Enhancing Substances', *Sport in History*, 25:3 (December 2005), pp. 417–20.
60 Cronin, 'Not taking the Medicine'.
61 Arnd Kruger, 'Training Theory and Why Roger Bannister was the First Four-Minute Miler', *Sport in History*, 26:2 (August 2006), p. 312.
62 For an early history of German sports science, see John Hoberman, 'The Early Development of Sports Medicine in Germany' in Berryman and Park (eds), pp. 233–82 and Beamish and Ritchie, *Fastest, Highest, Strongest*.
63 Wrynn, 'Athlete in the Making', p. 127.
64 Beamish and Ritchie, 'From Fixed Capacities', pp. 418–19.
65 Ernst Jokl, 'Pioneers: 90th Birthday of Professor A.V. Hill', *Journal of Sports Medicine*, 16 (1976), p. 349.
66 See also National Archives, FD 1/1948, File on A.V. Hill's work during 1920s.
67 Quoted in Berryman, *Out of Many*, p. 10.

68   David R. Bassett, 'Scientific contributions of A.V. Hill: exercise physiology pioneer', *Journal of Applied Physiology*, 93 (2002), pp. 1567–82.

69   *Ibid.*, pp. 1573–8.

70   Bryant, *3:59.4*, pp. 64–5.

71   Bourne, 'Fast Science', p. 158.

72   Kruger, 'Training Theory', pp. 306–12.

73   *Ibid.*; Doherty, *Modern Training*, p. 20.

74   Bourne, 'Fast Science', pp.175–6.

75   The ideas of Achilles members gradually replaced those of the old trainer-coaches, although clubs and universities continued to employ 'trainer-type coaches' until the late 1950s. McNab *et al*, *Athletics*, pp. xv-xlv.

76   Adolphe Abrahams and Harold Abrahams, *Training for Athletes* (London: G. Bell and Son, 1928), p. 14.

77   *Ibid.*, p. 7.

78   *Ibid.*, p. 31.

79   Douglas G.A. Lowe and Arthur E. Porritt, *Athletics* (London: Longmans, 1929), p. 84.

80   Christopher Lawrence and Anna-K. Mayer, 'Regenerating England: An Introduction' in Christopher Lawrence and Anna-K. Mayer (eds), *Regeneration England: Science, Medicine and Culture in Inter-War Britain* (Amsterdam: Rodopi, 2000), p. 2.

81   Arthur Porritt, 'General Health' in H.A. Meyer (ed.), *Athletics: By members of the Achilles Club* (London: J.M. Dent and Sons, 1955), pp. 342–3.

82   Abrahams and Abrahams, *Training*, p. 57.

83   Douglas G. A. Lowe, *Track and Field Athletics* (London: Sir Issac Pitman and Sons, 1936), p. 20.

84   Lowe and Porritt, *Athletics*, p. 103.

85   *Ibid.*

86   F.A.M. Webster and J.A. Heys, *Athletic Training for Men and Boys* (London: John F. Shaw, 1933), p. 13.

87   *Ibid.*, p. 11.

88   R.M.N. Tisdall and F. Sherie, *The Young Athlete* (London: Blackie, 1933), p. 21.

89   Carter, 'From Knox to Dyson', pp. 70–4.

90   A.J. Newton, *Boxing* (London: Bloomsbury, 2005), p. 71. First published in 1910.

91   Andrews, *Training*, p. 86.

92   Lowe and Porritt, *Athletics*, pp. 90–1.

93   Graham Vaughan and Bernard Guerin, 'A Neglected Innovator in Sports Psychology: Norman Triplett and the Early History of Competitive Performance', *IJHS*, 14:2 (August 1997), pp. 84–5.

94   Diane L. Gill, 'Sport and Exercise Psychology' in Massengale and Swanson (eds), pp. 297–9.

95   Hoberman, 'Sports Medicine in Germany', pp. 254–61.

96   Neil Carter, *The Football Manager: A History* (London: Routledge, 2006), pp. 74–5.

97   Mathew Thomson, 'The Psychological Body' in Cooter and Pickstone (eds), pp. 302–4.

98   *The Football Association Coaching Manual* (London: Evans, 1938), pp. 11–12.

99   Peter Beck, 'Britain and the Cold War's "Cultural Olympics": Responding to the Political Drive of Soviet Sport, 1945–58', *Contemporary British History*, 19:2 (June 2005), p. 170.

100 Interestingly, the likes of Nurmi, Hagg and Zátopek served in the army and military life enabled them to spend more time training than they would have been able to in civilian life.

101 Bourne, 'Fast Science', p. 279.

102 *Ibid.*, pp. 277–80.

103 *World Sports*, April 1953, pp. 9–10; September 1953, pp. 5–6.

104 Bryant, *3:59.4*, pp. 284–5. It was perhaps the effects of the sun as much as over-training that were the cause. Ironically, Peters' ordeal took place just 20 minutes after Bannister had defeated Landy in the so-called 'Mile of the Century'.

105 For a critical view on Bannister's achievement see a collection of essays in *Sport in History, Special Issue, The Sporting Barrier: Historical and Cultural Interpretations of the Four-Minute Mile*, 26:2 (August 2006).

106 John Bale, 'How Much of a Hero? The Fractured Image of Roger Bannister', *Sport in History*, 26:2 (August 2006), pp. 237–40.

107 Kruger, 'Training Theory'.

108 Beamish and Ian Ritchie, 'From Fixed Capacities', p. 425.

109 *World Sports*, November 1953, p. 12.

110 Bourne, 'Fast Science', pp. 315–25.

111 Cronin, 'Not Taking the Medicine', p. 27.

112 Beamish and Ritchie, 'From Fixed Capacities', p. 427.

113 Patrick Mignon, 'The Tour de France and the Doping Issue', *IJHS*, 20:2 (June 2003), p. 233.

114 Bourne, 'Fast Science', pp. 301–8.

115 *Ibid.*, pp. 309–10.

116 *Ibid.*, pp. 352–4; Geoff Dyson, *The Mechanics of Athletics: seventh edition* (London: Hodder and Stoughton, 1977).

117 McNab *et al*, pp. xlii–iii.

118 Interview between Geoff Dyson and Tom McNab.

119 Heggie, "Only the British", pp. 213–35.

120 Hopman is one of the few coaches to have a trophy named after him: the Hopman Cup. The most famous example is the Vince Lombardi Trophy in American football.

121 Murray Phillips, *From Sidelines to Centre Field: A History of Sports Coaching in Australia* (Sydney: University of NSW Press, 2000), pp. 52–3.

122 Forbes Carlile, *Forbes Carlile on Swimming* (London: Sphere, 1963), p. 15.

123 *Ibid.*, pp. 87–98; Bourne, 'Fast Science', p. 311.

124 Carlile, *Forbes Carlile*, p. 9.

125 Phillips, *From Sidelines*, pp. 73–81.

126 Percy Wells Cerruty, *Middle-Distance Running* (London: Pelham Books, 1964); Doherty, *Modern Training*, pp. 17–19, 82–4; Phillips, *From Sidelines*, pp. 73–81.

127 Nicholas Bourne, Jan Todd and Terry Todd, 'The Cold War's Impact on the Evolution of Training Theory in Boxing', *Iron Game History*, 2:2&3 (July 2002), p. 27.

128 *Ibid.*, pp. 26–30.

129 Beamish and Ritchie, *Fastest, Highest, Strongest*, pp. 52–65.

130 Riordan, 'Sports Medicine', pp. 19–26.

131 Bourne, 'Fast Science', pp. 375–401.

132 *Ibid.*, pp. 360–1.

133 *Ibid.*, p. 360.

134 *Ibid.*, pp. 344–5.

135   Mick Green, 'Olympic Glory or Grassroots Development?: Sport Policy Priorities in Australia, Canada and the United Kingdom, 1960–2006', *IJHS*, 24:7 (July 2007), p. 922.

136   *The Coaching Task Force – Final Report* (London: Department for Culture, Media and Sport, 2002), p. 31 n9.

137   Green, 'Olympic Glory', p. 940.

138   B. Bloom, *Developing Talent in Young People* (New York: Ballantines, 1985).

139   Dave Day, 'Craft Coaching and the "Discerning Eye" of the Coach', *International Journal of Sports Science and Coaching*, 6:1 (2011), pp. 179–95.

140   *Ibid.*, p. 181.

141   *Ibid.*

142   Steve Cram, Distinguished Lecture Series, De Montfort University, 2 December 2010.

143   C. Hencken and C. White, 'Anthropometric Assessment of Premiership Soccer Players in Relation to Playing Position', *European Journal of Sport Science*, 6:4 (2006), pp. 205–11.

144   Day, 'Craft Coaching', p. 189.

145   David Simons, 'The Evolution of the Endurance Athlete: Training, Diet and Performance, c.1750–1914', (Unpublished MA Dissertation: De Montfort University, Leicester, 2008), pp. 81–2; Paula Radcliffe, *Paula: My Story So Far* (London: Simon and Schuster, 2004); *Observer* (Sport), 6 January 2008.

Chapter 5   Testing Times: Drugs, Anti-Doping and Ethics

1   For this particular 'battle' see William Fotheringham, *Put Me Back On My Bike: In Search of Tom Simpson* (London: Yellow Jersey Press, 2002), pp. 1–20.

2   *Cycling Weekly*, 22–29 December 2001, pp. 72–3.

3   The term 'anti-doping' refers to attitudes against the use of what have been deemed performance-enhancing drugs in sport. Doping though can mean either to impair or enhance performance. 'Dope' usually refers to a substance that impairs performance.

4   For example, Waddington, *Sport, Health*.

5   Dimeo, *Drug Use in Sport*.

6   Hoberman, *Mortal Engines*.

7   For example, Steven Ungerleider, *Faust's Gold: Inside the East German Doping Machine* (New York: St. Martin's Press, 2001). Although strictly not an academic book, it is based on interviews with former athletes.

8   Philip Ball, *Unnatural: The heretical idea of making people* (London: Bodley Head, 2011).

9   Mike McNamee, 'Whose Prometheus? Transhumanism, biotechnology and the moral typography of sports medicine', *Sport, Ethics and Philosophy*, 1:2 (2007), p. 178.

10   Alex Mold, '"Consuming Habits"': Histories of Drugs in Modern Societies', *Cultural and Social History*, 2:2 (2007), p. 261–70.

11   Dimeo, *Drug Use*, pp. 3–16.

12   Domhanll MacAuley, 'Fortnightly Review: Drugs in sport', *BMJ* 313, (27 July 1996), pp. 211–15.

13   Charles E. Yesalis and Michael S. Bahrke, 'Anabolic Steroid and Stimulant Use in North American Sport between 1850 and 1980', *Sport in History*, 25:3 (December 2005), p. 441.

14   Day, 'From Barclay to Brickett', p. 126.

15 Wray Vamplew, 'Alcohol and the Sportsperson: An Anomalous Alliance', *Sport in History*, 25:3 (December 2005), p. 391.
16 Lucas, *1904 Olympic Report*, p. 51.
17 James Nicholls, *The Politics of Alcohol: A history of the drink question in England* (Manchester: Manchester University Press, 2009), chapters 10–12.
18 Porter, *Greatest Benefit*, pp. 663–5.
19 Day, 'From Barclay to Brickett', p. 129.
20 Porter, *Greatest Benefit*, pp. 663–5.
21 Dimeo, *Drug Use*, p. 31.
22 For a more in-depth analysis of horses and sports science, see Hoberman, *Mortal Engines*, Chapter 8.
23 Mike Huggins, *Flat Racing and British Society 1790–1914: A Social and Economic History* (London: Frank Cass, 2000), pp. 193–4; Erkki Vettenniemi, 'Runners, Rumors, and Reams of Representations: An Inquiry into Drug Use by Athletes in the 1920s', *Journal of Sport History*, 37:3 (Fall 2010), p. 419.
24 Andrews, *Training*, p. 83.
25 Dimeo, *Drug Use*, p. 33.
26 *Ibid.*, p. 39.
27 Lowe and Porritt, *Athletics*, pp. 108–9.
28 Abrahams and Abrahams, *Training*, pp. 34–5. The practice in Germany was later brought to the attention of the British athletics administrator, Jack Crump. See Jack Crump, *Running Round the World* (London: Hale, 1966), p. 54.
29 Quoted in Vettenniemi, 'Runners, Rumors', p. 419.
30 Martin Pugh, *We Danced All Night: A Social History of Britain Between the Wars* (London: Vintage, 2009), p. 223.
31 Virginia Berridge, 'The Origins of the English Drug "Scene"', *Medical History*, 32 (1988), pp. 51–64.
32 Vettenniemi, 'Runners, Rumors', p. 421.
33 *Ibid.*
34 See Bernard Joy, *Forward Arsenal: A History of the Arsenal Football Club* (London: Phoenix House, 1952), pp. 32–3.
35 See also Heggie, *British Sports Medicine*, pp. 81–2.
36 Brunton, 'Laboratory Medicine', pp. 101–2.
37 David Hamilton, *The Monkey Gland Affair* (London: Chatto & Windus, 1986), pp. 102, 114–19.
38 *News of the World*, 3 April 1938, p. 19; *Express and Star* (Wolverhampton), 29 March 1939, p. 12.
39 *Daily Mirror*, 15 March 1938, p. 12.
40 Bob Ferrier, *Soccer Partnership: Billy Wright and Walter Winterbottom* (London: Heinemann, 1960), pp. 88–9.
41 *Daily Mirror*, 31 May 1938, p. 27.
42 *Express and Star*, 29 March 1939, p. 12.
43 Dimeo, *Drug Use*, p. 45.
44 Hardy, *Health and Medicine*, pp. 152–7; Jordan Goodman, 'Pharmaceutical Industry' in Cooter and Pickstone (eds), pp. 146–50.
45 Hunt, *Drug Games*, p. 21.
46 John Hoberman, 'Amphetamine and the Four-Minute Mile', *Sport in History*, 26:2 (August 2006), pp. 289–304.
47 Paul Dimeo, 'Introduction', *Sport in History*, 25:3 (December 2005), p. 352.
48 Dimeo, *Drug Use*, p. 58.

49 Ruy Castro, *Garrincha: The triumph and tragedy of Brazil's forgotten footballing hero* (London: Yellow Jersey Press, 2004), p. 86.

50 Roger Bannister, *The First Four Minutes* (Stroud: Sutton, 2004), pp. 89–101.

51 Anon., 'Is the oxygenation of athletes a form of "doping"?', *Olympic Bulletin*, 1954, no. 45, pp. 24–5.

52 *Ibid.*

53 Thompson, *Tour de France*, p. 224.

54 Paul Kimmage, *Rough Ride: Behind the Wheel with a Pro Cyclist, second edition* (London: Yellow Jersey Press, 2001), pp. 93–4.

55 Thompson, *Tour de France*, pp. 225–6.

56 Mignon, 'Tour de France', p. 230.

57 Thompson argues this about the Tour de France. Thompson, *Tour de France*, pp. 249–53.

58 Fotheringham, *Tom Simpson*, pp. 137–53.

59 *Ibid.*, p. 143.

60 *Ibid.*, p. 146.

61 See Dimeo, *Drug Use*, pp. 87–95.

62 A.J. Ryan, 'Use of Amphetamines in Athletics', *Journal of American Medical Association*, 170:5 (30 May 1959), p. 562.

63 Dimeo, *Drug Use*, pp. 90–1.

64 Les Woodland (ed.), *The Yellow Jersey Companion to the Tour de France* (London: Yellow Jersey Press, 2003), pp. 38, 94. Coppi died of malaria in 1960.

65 Dimeo, *Drug Use*, p. 57.

66 Alison Wrynn, 'The Human Factor: Science, Medicine and the International Olympic Committee, 1900–70', *Sport in Society*, 7:2 (2004), pp. 211–31.

67 Adolphe Abrahams, *The Human Machine* (London: Penguin, 1956), p. 125.

68 Williams, 'The Athlete's Life', pp. 402–3.

69 For an in-depth examination of the reasons and myths surrounding his death, see Vernon Moller, 'Knud Enemark Jensen's Death During the 1960 Rome Olympics: A Search for Truth?', *Sport in History*, 25:3 (December 2005), pp. 452–71.

70 Hunt, *Drug Games*, p. 11.

71 Mike Saks, 'Medicine and the Counter Culture' in Cooter and Pickstone (eds), pp. 113–23.

72 John Davis, 'The London Drug Scene and the Making of Drug Policy, 1965–73', *Twentieth Century British History* (Advanced Access, 11 January 2006), pp. 1–24.

73 Dimeo, *Drug Use*, p. 14.

74 *Ibid.*, p. 128.

75 BASM Committee Minutes, 5 October 1966.

76 Quoted in Hunt, *Drug Games*, pp. 22–3.

77 *Ibid.*, p. 14.

78 Krasnoff, 'French Sports Policy'.

79 Thompson, *Tour de France*, pp. 228–41.

80 Hunt, *Drug Games*, p. 14.

81 Dimeo, *Drug Use*, pp. 105–6; Waddington, *Sport, Health*, p. 154.

82 Thompson, *Tour de France*, p. 237.

83 Vanessa Heggie, 'Testing sex and gender in sports: reinventing, reimagining and reconstructing histories', *Endeavour*, 34:4 (December 2010), pp. 157–63.

84 See Heggie, "Only the British".

85 Yesalis and Bahrke, 'Anabolic Steroid', p. 438.
86 Hunt, *Drug Games*, p. 45.
87 See Ungerleider, *Faust's Gold*.
88 Cole, 'East German Sports System'; Paul Dimeo, Thomas M. Hunt and Richard Horbury, 'The Individual and the State: A Social Historical Analysis of the East German "Doping System"', *Sport in History*, 31:2 (June 2011), pp. 218–37; Paul Dimeo and Thomas Hunt, 'The doping of athletes in the former East Germany: A critical assessment of comparisons with Nazi medical experiments', *International Review for the Sociology of Sport* (Published on-line 11 April 2011), pp. 1–13.
89 Hunt, *Drug Games*, p. 53.
90 *Ibid*.
91 Yesalis and Bahrke, 'Anabolic Steroid', p. 440.
92 Hunt, *Drug Games*, pp. 49–60.
93 *Ibid*., pp. 68–79.
94 *The Times*, 27 May 1987.
95 *The Times*, 21 November 1986.
96 *The Times*, 19 September 1987.
97 Ivan Waddington, 'Changing Patterns of Drug Use in British Sport from the 1960', *Sport in History*, 25:3 (December 2005), p. 480.
98 *Ibid*., pp. 481–92.
99 Hunt, *Drug Games*, p. 78.
100 *The Times*, 20 April 1987.
101 *The Times*, 5 October 1985.
102 *Sunday Times*, 27 October 1985.
103 *The Times*, 24 April 1987.
104 *Sunday Times*, 20 October 1985.
105 *The Times*, 19 April 1988.
106 Elsewhere, Clive Everton has claimed that the tremor was the result of a car accident. *Guardian* (Sport), 19 April 1997, p. 9.
107 He later claimed this as an overhead for the purposes of income tax.
108 *Independent* (Sport), 20 April 2002, p. 6; *The Times* (Features), 23 January 2003, p. 34; *The Times*, 1 April 1989.
109 *The Times*, 5 October 1988.
110 *The Times* 10 April 1985, p. 1. That this story made page one of *The Times*, indicates the popularity of the game at this time.
111 *The Times*, 20 April 1987.
112 *The Times*, 25 April 1987.
113 *The Times*, 2 September 1988.
114 *The Times*, 4 October 1988.
115 Hunt, *Drug Games*, p. 69.
116 *Ibid*., see Chapter 6.
117 *Ibid*., pp. 100–2.
118 See Hunt, *Drug Games*, Chapter 6.
119 Ruud Stokvis, 'Moral Entrepreneurship and Doping Cultures in Sport' (Amsterdam School for Social Science Research, Working Papers 03/04, November 2003), pp. 19–20; Barrie Houlihan, 'Building an international regime to combat doping in sport' in Roger Levermore and Adrian Budd (eds), *Sport and International Relations: An Emerging Relationship* (London: Routledge, 2004), pp. 72–3.
120 Hunt, *Drug Games*, pp. 110–11, 132.

121 Waddington, *Sport, Health*, p. 168.

122 Hunt, *Drug Games*, pp. 88–9, Chapter 9.

123 Stokvis, 'Moral Entrepreneurship', pp. 19–20: Hunt, *Drug Games*, p. 130. Cycling still retains some independent control over drug testing as the case of Alberto Contador has recently demonstrated, even if his initial acquittal was overthrown by the Court of Arbitration for Sport following an appeal from WADA.

124 http://www.telegraph.co.uk/sport/othersports/drugsinsport [accessed 21 March 2011].

125 Hunt, *Drug Games*, pp. 136–7.

126 David Runciman, 'Is the rise of the super-athlete ruining sport? *Observer*, 10 January 2010.

Chapter 6 Repairing the Athletic Body: Treatments, Practices and Ethics

1 *Athletics Weekly*, 10 December 2009, p. 38. A cortisone injection is classified as a therapeutic drug rather than one that enhances performance.

2 Quoted in Herman Weiskopf, 'The Good Hands Man', *Sports Illustrated*, 16 July 1979.

3 Saks, *Orthodox and Alternative Medicine*, p. 3.

4 William C. Cockerham, *Medical Sociology, Sixth Edition* (Englewood Cliffs, NJ: Prentice Hall, 1995), Chapter 7.

5 Saks, *Orthodox and Alternative Medicine*.

6 Park, 'Training'; Day 'From Barclay to Brickett', Chapters 2–4.

7 Day From Barclay to Brickett', pp. 136–8; Andrews, *Training*, p. 45.

8 *Boxing News*, 2 August 1950, p. 5; *The Times*, 23 November 1963, p. 4.

9 J.W. Graham, *Eight, Nine, Out! Fifty Years as a Boxer's Doctor* (Manchester: Protel, 1975), p. 61; *The Times*, 23 November 1963, p. 4.

10 *Ibid.*, p. 70.

11 Savage *et al*, *American College Athletics*, p. 146.

12 Correspondence with Robin Harland, Belfast, UK, 17 February 2006 and Gerry McFadam, December 2006.

13 Correspondence with Tom Hunt, 23 November 2007. O'Neill was the owner of the famous racehorse, Danoli.

14 Sean Boylan, *The Will To Win* (Dublin: O'Brien Press, 2006), p. 190.

15 In Williams (ed.), *Sports Medicine*, the book's first plate is that of a football trainer running on to the pitch.

16 Carter, *Football Manager*, Introduction.

17 Ian Nannestad, 'No ball practice! Training Methods in the Period to 1914', *Soccer History*, 13 (2005–6), pp. 3–6.

18 In 1920, the organization was awarded a royal charter and re-named the Chartered Society of Massage and Medical Gymnastics (CSMMG).

19 Heggie, *British Sports Medicine*, pp. 43–51.

20 Barclay, *In Good Hands*, pp. 8–9, 28. In 1921 its membership was 2,655, 191 of whom were men. *Ibid.*, p. 74.

21 P. Vaughan, '"Secret Remedies" in the Late Nineteenth and Early Twentieth Centuries' in Mike Saks (ed.), *Alternative Medicine in Britain* (Oxford: Clarendon Press, 1992), p. 101.

22 Mason, *Association Football*, p. 98.

23 G. Larkin, *Occupational Monopoly and Modern Medicine* (London: Tavistock, 1983), p. 94.

24 *Birmingham Mail*, 3 October 1936, p. 3.

25 Barclay, *In Good Hands*, pp. 50–69; Roger Cooter, *Surgery and Society in Peace and War: Orthopaedics and the Organization of Modern Medicine, 1880–1948* (Basingstoke: Macmillan, 1993), pp. 134–6. For a more detailed analysis of the rehabilitation of disabled soldiers after both world wars, see Julie Anderson, *War, Disability and Rehabilitation in Britain: 'Soul of a Nation'* (Manchester: Manchester University Press, 2011).

26 Larkin, *Occupational Monopoly*, pp. 100–18.

27 Charles Heald, *Injuries and Sport: A General Guide for the Practitioner* (Oxford: Oxford University Press, 1931).

28 W. E. Tucker, 'Athletic Injuries' in H. Rolleston (ed.), *The British Encyclopaedia of Medical Practice, volume 2* (London: Butterworth, 1936).

29 It was probably written by a former rugby union international, Dr Ronald Cove-Smith, who himself had written a training manual on Rugby Football in 1925.

30 *Albion News*, 26 August 1922, p. 2.

31 *Sports Budget*, 15 January, p. 14; 5 February, p. 15; 30 April, p. 14; 17 September 1938, p. 22. These 'qualifications' may have been gained through correspondence courses. One such organization was the Swedish Massage Institute. See *Athletic News*, 17 October 1921.

32 For Jones's role in the development of orthopaedics, see Cooter, *Surgery and Society*, pp. 30–4; Barclay *In Good Hands*, pp. 17, 66; Roy Peskett (ed.), *Tom Whittaker's Arsenal Story* (London: The Sportsmans Book Club, 1958), pp. 44, 194–200; George Allison, *Allison Calling* (London: Staples Press, 1948), pp. 234–7. Whittaker was later the manager of Arsenal from 1947 until 1956 when he died in office.

33 Taylor, *The Leaguers*, pp. 147–60.

34 *Aston Villa News and Record*, 8 August 1914, pp. 661–9.

35 *Sports Budget*, 15 January, p. 14; 5 February, p. 15; 30 April, p. 14; 17 September 1938, p. 22.

36 Barclay, *In Good Hands*, p. 113. Electrotherapy was part of the growing consumption of electricity during the inter-war period.

37 Questionnaire survey of professional footballers.

38 J.W. Mowles, 'Injuries at Sport', *Journal of the Chartered Society of Massage and Medical Gymnastics* (September 1937), pp. 75–6.

39 Barclay, *In Good Hands*, p. 164.

40 FA Minutes, Report on the Regional Conferences of Club Doctors, May 1962. In 1999, it was found from a survey of 53 physiotherapists, that 27 were chartered. Most of them worked in the Premier League. Waddington, 'Jobs', p. 60.

41 Matthew Taylor, *The Association Game: A History of British Football* (Harlow: Pearson, 2007), chapter 5.

42 Barclay, *In Good Hands*, pp. 141–3; *FA News*, August 1956, p. 6.

43 John Colson and William Armour, *Sports Injuries and their Treatment* (London: Stanley Paul, 1968).

44 Barclay, *In Good Hands*, p. 142. The Society of Remedial Gymnasts merged with the CSP in 1985. The former head of the FA's Medical and Exercise Science Department, Alan Hodson, also trained as a remedial gymnast at Pinderfields.

45 This form of treatment would lead to the establishment of the Stoke Mandeville Games and eventually the Paralympics. See Anderson, *War, Disability*.

46 Wrynn, "'Under the Showers'", p. 46.

47 Barclay, *In Good Hands*, pp. 141–4; Interview with Alan Hodson, 31 August 2005.

48 Cooter, *Surgery and Society*, p. 239.

49   Interview with Norman Pilgrim, 5 January 2007.
50   *Practitioner*, July 1981, p. 1047.
51   Barclay, *In Good Hands*, pp. 125–51; Anderson, *War, Disability*; Larkin, *Occupational Monopoly*, pp. 118–24; Saks, *Orthodox and Alternative Medicine*, pp. 97–8.
52   Porter, *Greatest Benefit*, pp. 686–9; Saks, *Orthodox and Alternative Medicine*, Chapter 4; Hardy, *Health and Medicine*, p. 140.
53   Mike Saks, 'Alternative Medicine and the Health Care Division of Labour: Present Trends and Future Prospects', *Current Sociology*, 49 (2001), p. 124.
54   Initially, the courses were aimed at the coaching of schoolboys but contained treatment of injury lectures. FA Minutes, Instructional Classes for Boys in Association Football, Report of Committee, 1935–6.
55   FA Minutes, Report on the Regional Conferences of Club Doctors, May 1962.
56   FA Minutes, Coaching Report 1957–8.
57   *Ibid*.
58   See Carter, *Football Manager*, Chapter 5.
59   Barclay, *In Good Hands*, pp. 163–4, 245, 294. In 1994 the CSP had 26,000 members.
60   Interview with Alan Hodson.
61   *Doctor*, 2 December 1982, p. 72.
62   *Football News*, March 1976, p. 10.
63   *Four Four Two*, May 2001, p. 9.
64   Waddington, 'Jobs', p. 59.
65   By 2000 89 per cent of chartered physiotherapists were women.
66   Personal correspondence with Amanda Johnson, March 2008. She claimed that Wimbledon was the first to employ a female physiotherapist in the mid-1980s. Female physiotherapists had also begun working at professional rugby league clubs from the late 1980s. Viv Gleave at Widnes was the first.
67   Amanda Johnson, 'Society of Sports Therapists – A Response', *BJSM*, 24 (1990), p. 78.
68   Interview with Laurie Brown, 7 June 2005.
69   Interview with Alan Hodson.
70   R. Verdonk, "Alternative Treatments of Meniscal Injuries", *Journal of Bone and Joint Surgery*, 79:B (1997), p. 866.
71   Peskett, *Tom Whittaker's*, pp. 37–41.
72   *Athletic News*, 16 September 1912.
73   *Albion News*, 11 December 1937, p. 139.
74   William B. Mead, 'The surgeon general of baseball', *National Pastime*, Annual 2002, p. 95.
75   M. Randal Roberts, 'A Footballers' Hospital', *Windsor Magazine*, March 1899, pp. 511–16.
76   Hardy, *Health and Medicine*, 16.
77   *Athletic News*, 18 August 1913.
78   Harding, *Living to Play*, pp. 108–10; Ian Nannestad, 'John Allison and His Football Hospital', *Soccer History* 9 (2004), pp. 42–3.
79   Charlton Athletic Football Co. Ltd Minutes, 18 November 1943.
80   Peskett (ed.), *Tom Whittaker*, pp. 44, 194–200; Allison, *Allison Calling*, pp. 234–7.
81   BASM Executive Committee Minutes, 1 December 1955.

82   Obituaries: *BJSM*, 25:4 (1991), p. 241; *BJSM*, 25:3 (1991), p. 170; *BMJ*, 19 October 1991, pp. 988–9; *Independent*, 8 August 1991, p. 25; *The Times*, 16 August 1991. His father was also called William Eldon Tucker, was also a surgeon and also played rugby for England. 'Obituary', *BMJ*, 7 November 1953, p. 1051.

83   John Oaksey, *Mince Pie for Starters* (London: Headline, 2003), p. 264.

84   Stephen Chalke, *Tom Cartwright: The Flame Still Burns* (Bath: Fairfields, 2007), pp. 150, 155.

85   Porter, *Greatest Benefit*, pp. 383–4; G. Larkin, 'Orthodox and Osteopathic Medicine in the Inter-War Years' in Mike Saks (ed.), *Alternative Medicine in Britain* (Oxford: Clarendon Press, 1992), pp. 112–23; Norman Gevitz, 'Unorthodox Medical Theories' in Bynum and Porter (eds), pp. 620–6; Cooter, *Surgery and Society*, pp. 1–10; 'The Meaning of Fractures: Orthopaedics and the Reform of British Hospitals in the Inter-War Period', *Medical History*, 31 (1987), pp. 306–32.

86   BASM Executive Committee Minutes, 1 March 1963.

87   Denis Law, *The King: My Autobiography* (London: Bantam, 2003), pp. 216–18.

88   See Martin Roderick, *The Work of Professional Football: A labour of love?* (London: Routledge, 2006).

89   Cockerham, *Medical Sociology*, pp. 134–6. In 1987 a federal court ruled that the AMA had conspired to undermine chiropractic and was ordered to cease its campaign.

90   Herman Weiskopf, 'The Good Hands Man', *Sports Illustrated*, 16 July 1979.

91   Kevin Keegan, *Kevin Keegan: My Autobiography* (London: Little, Brown, 1997), pp. 188–93.

92   Glenn Hoddle, *Glenn Hoddle: My 1998 World Cup Story* (London: Andre Deutsch, 1998), pp. 49–55, 232; Tony Adams, *Addicted* (London: Collins Willow, 1998), pp. 159–60; David Davies, *FA Confidential: Sex, Drugs and Penalties: The Inside Story of English Football* (London: Simon & Schuster, 2008), pp. 115–16. Davies, the FA's spokesman at the time, also visited Drewery about a long-standing back injury.

93   *The Times* (The Game), 11 April 2005, p. 21.

94   Simon Compton, 'The most feared man in football', *The Times*, 3 June 2006; Steven Downes, 'Mystery of marathon proportions over Ethiopian runner's death', *Scotsman*, 9 January 2005; Simon Turnbull, 'Healing Hans' adds needle to 'burn-up in Berlin', *Independent*, 14 August 2009; Radcliffe, *Paula Radcliffe*, pp. 85–6, 277–8.

95   *Independent*, 19 November 2009, pp. 56–7.

96   *Times* (London), 16 December 2002, p. 4; *Guardian* (London) 20 August 2002; *Guardian* (Sport) (London), 13 October 2005, p. 8.

97   Quoted from Ivan Waddington, 'Ethical problems in the medical management of sports injuries: A case study of English professional football' in Loland *et al* (eds), *Pain and Injury in Sport*, p. 182.

98   Brunton, 'Medical Profession', pp. 133–4.

99   Mike Saks, 'Bringing together the orthodox and alternative in health care', *Complementary Therapies in Medicine*, 11 (2003), pp. 142–5.

100   Waddington, 'Ethical problems', p. 182.

101   Hence the title of his book, Rob Huizenga, *"You're Okay, It's Just a Bruise": A Doctor's Sideline Secrets About Pro Football's Most Outrageous Team* (New York: St. Martin's Griffin, 1994), pp. 124, 259.

102   William Nack, 'Playing Hurt – the Doctors' Dilemma', *Sports Illustrated*, 11 June 1979.

103 Huizenga, *"You're Okay"*, pp. 74–5.
104 Lester Munson, 'Fast Operators', *Sports Illustrated*, 6 November 1995.
105 Carter, *Football Manager*.
106 Questionnaire survey of football club doctors.
107 Ted Farmer, *The Heartbreak Game* (Wolverhampton, U.K.: Hillburgh, 1987), 53–4.
108 Roderick, *Professional Football*, p. x, Chapter 2.
109 Interview with Ian Adams. By the time Adams had worked off his notice, relations had thawed and he resumed his position.
110 Interview with Ian Adams.
111 For a post-1992 analysis of this issue, see Waddington *et al*, *Managing Injuries*.
112 Interview with Norman Pilgrim.
113 Questionnaire survey of football club physiotherapists.
114 Interview with Laurie Brown.
115 European Rugby Cup, Decision of Appeal Committee in Appeal by Tom Williams, held at the Radisson SAS Hotle, 301 Argyle Street, Glasgow, 17 August 2009; *Guardian*, 26 August 2009.
116 European Rugby Cup, Decision of Appeal Committee in Appeal by Tom Williams.
117 http://www.telegraph.co.uk/sport/rugbyunion/club/8002256/Harlequins-Bloodgate-physio-Steph-Brennan-struck-off-by-Health-Professions-Council.html; http://www.guardian.co.uk/sport/2010/sep/14/steph-brennan-harlequins-bloodgate; *Frontline*, 19 May 2011. *Guardian*, 22 January 2011.
118 *The Times*, 21 August 2009.
119 Radcliffe, *Paula Radcliffe*, pp. 161–2, 248.
120 The Football League did not permit substitutions until 1965.
121 Law, *The King*, pp. 216–18.
122 Ian St. John, *The Saint: My Autobiography* (London: Hodder, 2005), pp. 66–9.
123 Roderick, *Professional Football*, pp. 60–1.
124 Smith, *Doc*, 36.
125 Huizenga, *"You're Okay"*, pp. 72–8.
126 *The Times*, 9 November 1971, p. 2.
127 Interview with Ian Adams. Hartford's condition did not have a detrimental effect on his career, however. He played in a total of 731 Football League games between 1967 and 1990 for nine clubs. In 1997 this put him nineteenth on the all-time list for league appearances.
128 *Guardian* (Sport) (London), 29 April 2000. Van Nistelrooy broke down in training a few days later but following a successful knee operation was signed by United in 2001.
129 Roderick, *Professional Football*, p. 37.
130 Queen's Bench Division, 2 April 1998.
131 Joseph Nocera, 'Bitter Medicine', *Sports Illustrated*, 6 November 1995.
132 William Oscar Johnson, 'This Strange and Perilous Joint', *Sports Illustrated*, 24 October 1977; http://query.nytimes.com/gst/fullpage.html?res=990DEFDE173BF93BA1574C0A9649C8B63&sec=health&spon=&pagewanted=3 [accessed 24 June 2011].
133 William Nack, 'Playing Hurt – the Doctors' Dilemma', *Sports Illustrated*, 11 June 1979. Pappas had been team physician since 1977.
134 Joseph Nocera, 'Bitter Medicine', *Sports Illustrated*, 6 November 1995.
135 *Daily Telegraph* (Sport), 3 January 2003, p. 4.
136 *BASEM Today*, Issue 12, Autumn 2008, p. 8.
137 Roderick, *Professional Football*, pp. 62–5.

Chapter 7 Medicine, Sport and the Female Body

1 *Daily Telegraph* (Sport), 6 September 2007, p. S18.
2 Heggie, 'Testing sex', pp. 157–63.
3 Jennifer Hargreaves, *Sporting Females: Critical issues in the history and sociology of women's sports* (London: Routledge, 1994), p. 8.
4 Carol A. Osborne and Fiona Skillen, 'Introduction. The State of Play: Women in British Sport History', *Sport in History*, 30:2 (June 2010), p. 190.
5 Claire Langhamer, *Women's leisure in England 1920–60* (Manchester: Manchester University Press, 2000), pp. 16–18.
6 See for example, Judy Lee, 'Media Portrayals of Male and Female Olympic Athletes: Analyses of Newspaper Accounts of the 1984 and the 1988 Summer Games', *International Review for the Sociology of Sport*, 27:3 (1992), pp. 197–219.
7 Zweiniger-Bargielowska, *Managing the Body*, p. 335.
8 Mason and Riedi, *Sport and the Military*, p. 249.
9 Mary Louise Adams, 'From Mixed-Sex Sport to Sport for Girls: The Feminization of Figure Skating', *Sport in History*, 30:2 (June 2010), p. 237. This also included boys playing so-called 'girl's' sports.
10 Allen Guttmann, *Women's Sports: A History* (New York: Columbia University Press, 1991), pp. 48–9.
11 *Times Higher Education*, 15 October 2009, p. 47.
12 See Catriona Parratt, 'Little Means or Time: Working-Class Women and Leisure in Late Victorian and Edwardian England', *IJHS*, 15:2 (August 1998), pp. 22–53.
13 Neil Tranter, *Sport, Economy and Society in Britain, 1750–1914* (Cambridge: Cambridge University Press, 1998), p. 89.
14 Gertrud Pfister, 'Women and the Olympic Games: 1900–97' in B.L. Drinkwater (ed.), *Women in Sport, Volume 8 of the Encyclopedia of Sports Medicine* (Oxford: Blackwell Science, 2000), p. 10.
15 Gertrud Pfister, 'The Medical Discourse on Female Physical Culture in Germany in the 19th and Early 20th Centuries', *Journal of Sport History*, 17:2 (Summer, 1990), p. 183.
16 Vertinsky, 'Exercise, Physical Capability', pp. 183–6.
17 *Practitioner*, 1 July to 31 December 1904, p. 719.
18 Jennifer Hargreaves, '"Playing Like Gentlemen While Behaving Like Ladies": Contradictory Features of the Formative Years of Women's Sport', *British Journal of Sports History*, 2:1 (May 1985), p. 43.
19 Quoted in Nicky Fossey, 'Gender' in Richard Cox, Grant Jarvie and Wray Vamplew (eds), *Encyclopedia of British Sport* (Oxford: ABC-Clio, 2000), p. 149–51.
20 Gregory P. Moon, 'A New Dawn Rising: An Empirical and Social Study concerning the emergence and development of English Women's athletics until 1960' (Unpublished PhD: Roehampton Institute, 1997), p. 246.
21 Zweiniger-Bargielowska, *Managing the Body*, p. 12.
22 *Ibid.*, p. 117.
23 *Ibid.*, pp. 105–48; Tranter, *Sport, Economy*, pp. 85–6.
24 *Practitioner*, 1 July to 31 December 1904, p. 719.
25 Guttmann, *Women's Sports*, p. 95.
26 Quoted in Jean Williams, *A Game for Rough Girls? A history of women's football in Britain* (London: Routledge, 2003), p. 35.
27 Catherine Horwood, '"Girls who arouse dangerous passions"': women and bathing, 1900–39', *Women's History Review*, 9:4 (2000), pp. 653–73.
28 Guttmann, *Women's Sports*, pp. 87–9.

29 Abrahams and Abrahams, *Training*, p. 15.
30 Abrahams, *Human Machine*, pp. 68–9.
31 These were the 4 sports that prospective teachers taking the examination to enter the Ling Association had to learn the rules of. *Journal of Scientific Physical Training* 6:16 (Autumn 1913), p. 36.
32 Shelia Fletcher, 'The Making and Breaking of a Female Tradition: Women's Physical Education in England 1880–1980', *British Journal of Sports History*, 2:1 (May 1985), pp. 29–31.
33 Nicky Fossey, 'Netball' in Cox *et al* (eds), p. 279.
34 Quoted in Ali Melling, 'Women and Football' in Cox *et al* (eds), p. 325.
35 Tranter, *Sport, Economy*, p. 85. See Chapter 6 for a comprehensive survey of women's sport during this period.
36 In 1904 there were 8 women; in 1908, 36; and in 1912, 57.
37 Tipton, 'Sports Medicine', pp. 878s–85s.
38 Jennifer Hargreaves, 'Women's sports between the wars: Continuities and Discontinuities', *Warwick Centre for the Study of Sport in Society, Working Papers* (1994), p. 119.
39 Jeremy Crump, 'Athletics' in Tony Mason (ed.), *Sport in Britain: A Social History* (Cambridge: Cambridge University Press, 1989), p. 60.
40 Hargreaves, 'Women's sports', pp. 122–6.
41 Shelia Rowbotham, *A Century of Women: The History of Women in Britain and the United States* (London: Viking, 1997), p. 162.
42 Guttmann, *Women's Sports*, pp. 144–6.
43 *Ibid.*, pp. 157–9.
44 Football Association, Consultative Committee Minutes, 5 December 1921. The FA was also unhappy with the distribution of the receipts from these charity games. For a fuller discussion on the FA ban see Williams, *A Game*, pp. 32–7.
45 See Zweiniger-Bargielowska, *Managing the Body*, pp. 236–78.
46 Moon, 'Women's athletics', p. 86.
47 Ina Zweiniger-Bargielowska, 'Building a British Superman: Physical Culture in Interwar Britain', *Journal of Contemporary History*, 41:4 (2006), p. 595.
48 Jill Matthews, 'They had Such a Lot of Fun: The Women's League of Health and Beauty Between the Wars', *History Workshop Journal*, 30 (Autumn 1990), pp. 22–54.
49 *Recreation and Physical Fitness for Girls and Women* (London: Board of Education, Physical Training Series, no. 16, 1938).
50 Moon, 'Women's athletics', pp. 251–2.
51 Langhamer, *Women's Leisure*, p. 49.
52 Lynne Robinson, '"Tripping Daintily into the Arena": A Social History of English Women's Athletics 1921–1960' (Unpublished PhD: University of Warwick, 1996), p. 289.
53 *Ibid.*, p. 287. The perception of the home-bound woman in order to bring up her children was given greater legitimacy in the post-war period through the influence of psychologists such as Benjamin Spock and John Bowlby. Mathew Thomson, 'The Psychological Body' in Cooter and Pickstone (eds), p. 302.
54 Heald, *Injuries and Sport*, p. 119.
55 Berlin Olympic Committee, *The Official Report of the XIth Olympiad, Berlin* (Berlin: Olympic Committee of the Berlin Olympic Games, 1936), vol. 1, p. 225.
56 Moon, 'Women's athletics', p. 249. In addition, it was said that they were restricted in their training and sporting efforts because of their glandular structure and were liable to organic upsets.
57 *Ibid.*, p. 88.

58   Robinson, 'Women's athletics', p. 17. Tug-of-war was attached to the AAA.
      Peter Lovesey, *The Official History of the Amateur Athletic Association*
      (London: Guinness Superlatives, 1979), p. 116.
59   Robinson, 'Women's athletics', p. 17.
60   *Ibid.*, p. 21.
61   See Heggie, 'Testing Sex'.
62   Moon, 'Women's athletics', pp. 261–2; Robinson, 'Women's athletics', pp. 17–18.
63   Kevin B. Wamsley, 'Womanizing Olympic Athletes: Policy and Practice during
      the Avery Brundage Era' in Gerald P. Schaus and Stephen R. Wenn (eds),
      Onwards to the Olympics: Historical Perspectives on the Olympic Games
      (Waterloo, Ontario: Wilfred Laurier University Press, 2007), p. 274.
64   James Riordan, 'The Social Emancipation of Women Through Sport', *British
      Journal of Sports History*, 2:1 (May 1985), p. 57; Tipton, 'Sports Medicine',
      pp. 878s–85s.
65   Wamsley, 'Womanizing Olympic Athletes', pp. 276–8.
66   Shelia Mitchell, 'Women's Participation in the Olympic Games 1900–1926',
      Journal of Sport History, 4:2 (1977), pp. 208–19.
67   Guttmann, *Women's Sports*, pp. 166–8.
68   *Ibid.*, pp. 163–71; Wamsley, 'Womanizing Olympic Athletes', p. 265. Florence
      Carpentier and Jean-Pierre Lefevre, 'The Modern Olympic Movement, Women's
      Sport and the Social Order During the Inter-War Period', *IJHS*, 23:7 (November
      2006), pp. 1112–27.
69   Moon, 'Women's athletics', p. 263.
70   *Ibid.*, p. 264; Hargreaves, *Sporting Females*, p. 44.
71   In 1933 the WAAA abolished their distance limit but this did not result in any
      new distances in practice.
72   Robinson, 'Women's athletics', pp. 18–22; Moon, 'Women's athletics', pp. 264–5.
73   Guttmann, *Women's Sports*, pp. 163–71; Wamsley, 'Womanizing Olympic
      Athletes', p. 265.
74   Elidh Macrae, '"Scotland for Fitness": The National Fitness Campaign and
      Scottish Women', *Women's History Magazine*, 62 (2010), pp. 26–36.
75   For other accounts of this episode see, Heggie, *British Sports Medicine*, pp.
      87–8; Zweiniger-Bargielowska, *Managing the Body*, pp. 255–6.
76   National Archives (TNA), ED 113/49, National Fitness Council (hereafter NFC),
      Sports and Games Committee, 2 February 1938.
77   TNA, ED 113/49, NFC Sports and Games Committee, 29 April 1938.
78   TNA, ED 113/49, NFC, Medical Sub-committee on the Desirability of Athletics
      for Women and Girls, 8 March 1939.
79   The four were: Miss K. Doman – Team Games – Games lecturer at Dartford PT
      College, Games Mistress Roedean School, former Captain of All England hockey
      team, member of the All England Lacrosse team, international selector of hockey,
      lacrosse and cricket teams; Miss Verrall Newman – Swimming and water
      polo – President of the Southern Counties Amateur Swimming Association,
      Olympic Diver; Mrs L.A. Godfree – Tennis – Wightman Cup player; Dr Violet
      Cyriax – Rowing – All England rower.
80   TNA, ED 113/49, NFC, Sub-Committee, 3 July 1939.
81   Miss M. Fountain – Physical Training – Headmistress, Chelsea PE College;
      Dr Garrow – Physical Training – MO at Chelsea College of PE; Miss R. Foster –
      Physical Training – PT Organiser to Willesden LEA, international hockey player
      and captain for Lancashire and the North.
82   TNA, ED 113/49, NFC, Medical Sub-committee, 26 April 1939.

83 Lara Freidenfelds, *The Modern Period: Menstruation in Twentieth-Century America* (Baltimore: Johns Hopkins University Press, 2009), pp. 1–4.
84 TNA, ED 113/49, NFC, Medical Committee, 15 June 1939.
85 *Ibid.*
86 *The Times*, 28 December 1959, p. 8.
87 TNA, ED 113/49, NFC, Sub-Committee, 3 July 1939.
88 Pfister, 'Medical Discourse', p. 193.
89 Stephan Westmann, *Sport, Physical Training and Womanhood* (London, 1939), p. ix.
90 *Ibid.*, p. 77.
91 *Ibid.*, p. ix.
92 *Lancet*, 18 November 1939, p. 1091.
93 *Lancet*, 4 November 1939, p. 988.
94 Joyce Kay, 'A Window of Opportunity? Preliminary Thoughts on Women's Sport in Post-war Britain', *Sport in History*, 30:2 (June 2010), pp. 196–217.
95 Abrahams, *Human Machine*, p. 69.
96 Ernst Jokl, 'The Athletic Status of Women: An Analysis of a Social Phenomenon', *British Journal of Physical Medicine* (November 1957).
97 Moon, 'Women's athletics', p. 249.
98 Sophie Eliott Lynn, *Athletics for Women and Girls* (London: Robert Scott, 1925), p. xiv.
99 Lynne Duval, 'The Development of Women's Track and Field in England: The Role of the Athletic Club, 1920s–1950s', *The Sports Historian*, 21:1 (May 2001), pp. 15–16.
100 Kay, 'Window of Opportunity', p. 211.
101 Wamsley, 'Womanizing Olympic Athletes', p. 276.
102 FR M Messerli, 'Women's participation to the Modern Olympic Games', *Olympic Bulletin*, no. 33, 1952, p. 31.
103 *Ibid.*, p. 26. He had been a judge in this event.
104 *Ibid.*, p. 30.
105 *Ibid.*, p. 30.
106 It has also been referred to at various times as femininity controls, sex control and gender verification.
107 Heggie, 'Testing sex', pp. 157–63.
108 *Ibid.*
109 Stefan Wiederkehr, '"We shall never know the exact number of men who have competed in the Olympics posing as women": Sport, Gender Verification and the Cold War', *IJHS*, 26:4 (2009), p. 559.
110 Tamara won gold in the shot putt and silver in the discus in 1960, and gold in both events in 1964. Irina won gold in the 80 metres hurdles in 1960 and gold in the Pentathlon in 1964.
111 Wrynn, 'Human Factor', p. 221.
112 *Guardian* (Olympics 2004 Souvenir), p. 82.
113 M.A. Ferguson-Smith and Elizabeth Ferris, 'Gender verification in sport: the need for change?', *BJSM*, 25:1 (1991), pp. 17–20.
114 *Ibid.*
115 *The Times*, 7 June 1971, p. 9.
116 *The Times*, 29 October 1976, p. 13; *Guardian* (Sport), 22 May 2004, p. 19.
117 Ferguson-Smith and Ferris, 'Gender verification', pp. 17–20; Anon., 'Editor's Note', *BJSM*, 25:2 (1991), p. 104; Heggie, 'Testing sex', pp. 157–63.
118 Guttmann, *Sports*, p. 308.

119 'American College of Sports Medicine Opinion Statement on: The Participation of the Female Athlete in Long-Distance Running, November 1979', FIMS, 1967–1981 et Executif 1981.

120 Annemarie Jutel, '"Thou Dost Run as in Flotation": Femininity, Reassurance and the Emergence of the Women's Marathon', *IJHS* 20:) (September 2003), pp. 27–30.

121 *Ibid.*, p. 17.

122 *The Times*, 2 February, p. 4; 14 April, p. 2; 15 June, p. 4; 16 June, p. 2; 3 July, p. 8; 29 July 1978.

123 House of Commons Culture, Media and Sport Committee, *Women's Football: Fourth Report of Session 2005–06* (London: Houses of Commons, 2006), p. 7; Evidence 38, 2.9.

124 Amanda N. Schweinbenz, 'Selling Femininity: The Introduction of Women's Rowing at the 1976 Olympic Games', *IJHS*, 26:5 (2009), p. 660.

125 Adams, 'From Mixed-Sex', pp. 218–41.

126 Ann Chisholm, 'Acrobats, Contortionists, and Cute Children: The Promise and Perversity of U.S. Women's Gymnastics', *Signs*, 27:2 (Winter, 2002), pp. 415–50.

127 Natalie Barker-Ruchti, 'Ballerinas and Pixies: a Genealogy of the Changing Female Gymnastics Body', *IJHS*, 26:1 (January 2009), p. 47.

128 *Ibid.*, pp. 52–5.

129 Joan Ryan, *Little Girls in Pretty Boxes: The Making and Breaking of Elite Gymnasts and Figure Skaters* (New York: Warner, 1995), p. 65.

130 *Ibid.*, pp. 47–53.

131 See Chisolm, 'Acrobats', pp. 444–5.

132 Karen Stabiner, *Courting Fame: The hazardous road to women's tennis stardom* (London: Kingswood Press, 1986).

133 Ryan, *Little Girls*, p. 11.

134 *Guardian* (Sport), 14 November 1997, p. 11; *The Times*, 4 March 1999.

135 *Observer* (Sport), 8 October 1995.

136 Wendy Varney, 'Legitimation and Limitations: How the Opie Report on Women's Gymnastics Missed its Mark', *Sporting Traditions*, 15:2 (May 1999), pp. 73–90. The Australian government actually set up an enquiry, although its outcome was criticised due to the narrowness of its parameters. *Ibid.*

137 *Guardian* (Education), 6 October 1998, p. 9.

138 Varney, 'Legitimation', p. 83.

139 Women had been boxing as far back as the early eighteenth century and an exhibition of women's boxing was included in the 1904 Games.

140 Osborne and Skillen, 'Introduction', p. 191.

141 *Ibid.*

142 Dave Russell, 'Mum's the Word: The Cycling Career of Beryl Burton, 1956–1986', *Women's History Review*, 17:5 (2008), pp. 787–806.

143 Adams, 'From Mixed-Sex', p. 238.

144 Kay, 'Window of Opportunity', pp. 197–8.

Chapter 8 Boxing: A Medical History

1 Although it would have shed greater light on the subject, I was unable to gain access to the records of the British Boxing Board of Control.

2 Timothy Chandler, Mike Cronin and Wray Vamplew, *Sport and Physical Education: The Key Concepts* (London: Routledge, 2002), 'Boxing Debate'.

3   While head injuries have aroused the most controversy, other common boxing injuries include the 'boxer's nose' in which there is a flattening of the nasal bones from previous fractures with dislocation of the nasal septum. Eye injuries, like detached retinas, are treated very seriously and have led to the mandatory retirement of fighters like Sugar Ray Leonard and Frank Bruno.

4   Mandler, *English National Character*, pp. 24–40.

5   Ken Sheard, 'Boxing in the western civilizing process' in Eric Dunning *et al* (eds), *Sport Histories: Figurational Studies of the Development of Modern Sports* (London: Routledge, 2004), pp. 15–30.

6   Sheard, '"Brutal and degrading"', pp. 74–102; Welshman, 'Only Connect', pp. 1–21.

7   The last significant prizefight was in 1860 between Tom Sayers of Brighton and the American, John Heenan.

8   For an early history of boxing see Dennis Brailsford, *Bareknuckles: A Social History of Prize-Fighting* (Cambridge: Lutterworth Press, 1988) and Kasia Boddy, *Boxing: A Cultural History* (London: Reaktion, 2008) Chapters 1–4.

9   Stonehenge 'Forrest' [aka Rev JG Wood], *The Handbook of Manly Exercises: Comprising Boxing, Walking, Running, Leaping, Vaulting, etc. with chapters on Training for Pedestrianism and other purposes* (London: Routledge, Warne and Routledge, 1864), pp. 7–18.

10   *BMJ*, 8 January 1955, p. 102.

11   *BMJ*, 2 July 1960, Supplement, p. 15.

12   *Lancet*, 11 May 1901, p. 1366.

13   J.L. Blonstein, *Boxing Doctor* (London: Stanley Paul, 1965), pp. 17, 22–4.

14   Graham, *Eight, Nine, Out!*, p. 21.

15   Peter Koehler, 'The evolution of British neurology in comparison with other countries' in F. Clifford Rose (ed.), *A Short History of Neurology: The British Contribution 1660–1910* (Oxford: Butterworth-Heinemann, 1999), pp. 58–74.

16   Porter, *Greatest Benefit*, pp. 534–51, 612–13.

17   *Lancet*, 11 May 1901, p. 1336.

18   Byles and Osborn, 'First Aid'.

19   Brailsford, *Bareknuckles*, p. 158.

20   Originally comprising 12 clubs, the ABA held its first championship a year later where four weight classes (Feather, Light, Middle, Heavy) were contested. In prize-fighting there were generally no weight classes.

21   Michael Gunn and David Ormerod, 'The legality of boxing', *Legal Studies*, 15:2 (July 1995), pp. 190–1.

22   *Ibid.*, p. 183.

23   In 1919 a British Board of Boxing Control was formed but was essentially ran by the NSC. An initial meeting had taken place in February 1914 between 10 members of the NSC together with representatives from the Army and Navy Boxing Association, the ABA and various boxing promoters. Sheard, 'Boxing', p. 302.

24   Sheard, 'Boxing', pp. 295–6. Arthur Conan Doyle was a regular and in his novel, *Rodney Stone*, he used a prize-fighter as one of the characters.

25   In 1898, following the death of Thomas Turner, six men including his opponent, Nathaniel Smith, the club's owners and its manager, Arthur Bettinson, were charged with manslaughter. They were found not guilty. *The Times*, 11 November 1898, p. 13; 18 November 1898, p. 14. Following the death of Michael Riley on its premises in 1900 a similar verdict was reached. *The Times*, 13 March 1900, p. 14.

26   *The Times*, 2 May 1901, p. 7.

27   *The Times*, 16 May 1901, p. 14.

28   *The Times*, 29 June 1901, p. 19.
29   *The Times*, 14 November 1911, p. 7.
30   *The Times*, 15 March 1912, p. 13.
31   K.B. Wamsley and D. Whitson, 'Celebrating Violent Masculinities: The Boxing Death of Luther McGrory', *Journal of Sport History*, 25:3 (Fall 1998), pp. 419–31.
32   http://www.boxrec.com/media/index.php/USA:_New_York_Laws; http://www.boxrec.com/media/index.php/Walker_Law.
33   *The Times*, 21 March 1911, p. 4.
34   *The Times*, 30 April 1901, p. 10.
35   Norman Clark, *The Boxing Referee* (London: Methuen, 1926), p. 59.
36   Sheard, 'Boxing', p. 289.
37   *Boxing*, 29 May 1929, p. 1.
38   Lewis Carroll had been a champion at Rugby school.
39   George Saintsbury and Jeff James, *Boys Will Be Boxers* (London: Lonsdale, 1997), pp. 13–23; Mason and Riedi, *Sport and the Military*, p. 18.
40   Stan Shipley, 'Boxing', in Mason (ed.), p. 93.
41   Matthew Taylor, 'Round the London Ring: Boxing, Class and Community in Interwar London', *The London Journal*, 34:2 (July 2009), pp. 139–62.
42   James Morton, *Fighters: The Lives and Sad Deaths of Freddie Mills and Randolph Turpin* (London: Time Warner, 2004), p. 73.
43   Matthew Taylor, 'Boxers United: Trade Unionism in British Boxing in the 1930s', *Sport in History*, 29:3 (September 2009), pp. 462–70.
44   Jack Birtley, *The Tragedy of Randolph Turpin* (London: New English Library, 1975), pp. 24–5.
45   Graham, *Eight, Nine, Out!*, p. 11.
46   Morton, *Fighters*, p. 7.
47   *Ibid.*, pp. 10–11. It was unusual for a boxer who had been knocked out to be required to box a second time on the same bill.
48   Holt, *Sport and the British*, p. 302.
49   Morton, *Fighters*, p. 55.
50   *Ibid.*, pp. 87–8.
51   *Ibid.*, p. 8.
52   *Ibid.*, p. 96.
53   In a fictional story about baseball in the *Washington Times*, 17, 18 November 1913, p. 9, titled 'The Girl and the Pennant', the phrase is used in connection with drink. Thereafter, other references are in connection with boxing, e.g. *Washington Herald*, 13 January 1914, p. 10.
54   I am grateful to Kasia Boddy for this reference.
55   *The Times*, 6 July 1953, p. 5.
56   Harrison Martland, 'Punch Drunk', *Journal of the American Medical Association*, 91:15 (13 October 1928), pp. 1103–7.
57   C.E. Winterstein, 'Head Injuries Attributable to Boxing' *Lancet*, 18 September 1937, pp. 719–20. Winterstein, a German by birth, had been an amateur boxer from 1923–29. He had carried out his research at Guy's Hospital in 1934. *The Times*, 20 January 1939, p. 4.
58   Jokl, *Boxing*, pp. 154–5.
59   *Boxing*, 3 October 1933, p. 8.
60   *Ibid.*, p. 2.
61   *The Times*, 6 October 1939, p. 15.
62   *Daily Mirror*, 4 February 1938, p. 31.

63   Although unnamed in the article, the paper was successfully sued by Henry Wiseman and his son, Cyril (his fighting name was Charlie Wise).

64   *The Times*, 18 January 1939, p. 4. In court, it was said that Wise, due to a low score in intelligence tests, had been sent to a 'special school for mental deficients'.

65   *The Times*, 17 January 1939, pp. 5, 18, pp. 4, 19, pp. 4, 20, p. 4.

66   Peter Leese, *Shell Shock: Traumatic Neurosis and the British Soldiers of the First World War* (Basingstoke: Palgrave Macmillan, 2002), p. 3.

67   *Boxing*, 3 October 1933, p. 8.

68   By the 1920s the definition of mental deficiency had been extended to include later-onset cerebral trauma. Sharon Morris, "Human dregs at the bottom of our national vats': The interwar debate on sterilization of the mentally deficient' in David M. Turner and Kevin Staggs (eds), *Social Histories of Disability and Deformity* (London: Routledge, 2006), p. 143.

69   Mark Mazower, *Dark Continent: Europe's Twentieth Century* (London: Penguin, 1998), p. 97.

70   See Ross McKibbin, *Classes and Cultures: England 1918–1951* (Oxford: Oxford University Press, 1998).

71   Ronnie Johnston and Arthur McIvor, 'Marginalising the Body at Work? Employers' Occupational Health Strategies and Occupational Medicine in Scotland c.1930–1974, *Social History of Medicine*, 21:3 (April 2008), p. 131.

72   *Empire News*, 30 September 1951, p. 7.

73   *Empire News*, 7 October, p. 7; 14 October, p. 7; 16 December 1951, p. 7.

74   Graham, *Eight, Nine, Out!*, pp. 57–8.

75   *International Olympic Committee Bulletin*, no. 29, September 1951, pp. 16–17.

76   International Olympic Committee, 45th Session Minutes, Paris, 1955. In 1952, no bronze medals were awarded, only golds and silvers.

77   International Olympic Committee, 52nd Session Minutes, Sofia, 1957.

78   *Boxing News*, 11 January 1950, p. 6.

79   *Boxing News*, 22 March 1950, p. 6.

80   *Boxing News*, 14 June 1950, p. 15.

81   Blonstein, *Boxing Doctor*, pp. 67–8; J.L. Blonstein and Edwin Clarke, 'The Medical Aspects of Amateur Boxing', *BMJ*, 25 December 1954, pp. 1523–5.

82   Graham, *Eight, Nine, Out!*, pp. 66–9.

83   Blonstein, *Boxing Doctor*, pp. 126–7.

84   In conversation with Teddy Carter, 1 December 2004.

85   Henry Cooper, *Henry Cooper: An Autobiography* (London: Coronet Books, 1972), p. 54.

86   J.W. Graham, 'Professional Boxing and the Doctor, *BMJ*, 22 January 1955, pp. 219–21.

87   *The Times*, 5 June 1959, p. 9.

88   *BMJ*, 2 July 1960, Supplement, p. 15.

89   Anon., 'Brain Injury in Boxing', *BMJ*, 25 December 1954, p. 1535.

90   Blonstein and Clarke, 'Medical Aspects', pp. 1523–5; Graham, 'Professional Boxing', pp. 219–21.

91   *BMJ*, 16 February 1957, p. 392.

92   MacDonald Critchley, 'Medical aspects of boxing, particularly from a neurological standpoint', *BMJ*, 16 February 1957, pp. 358–9.

93   J.L. Blonstein and Edwin Clarke, 'Further observations on the medical aspects of amateur boxing', *BMJ*, 16 February 1957, pp. 362–4.

94   *BMJ*, 16 February 1957, pp. 392–3.

95   *The Times*, 1 March 1982, p. 6.

96   *Lancet*, 7 February 1953, pp. 282–3; *BMJ*, 25 December 1954, pp. 1525, 1535.

97   *BMJ*, 16 February 1957, pp. 392–3.

98   Fielding *et al*, 'England Arise!', Chapter 6.

99   Penny Summerfield, '"Our Amazonian Colleague": Edith Summerskill's problematic reputation' in R. Toye and J. Gottlieg (eds), *Making Reputations: Power, Persuasion and the Individual in Modern British Politics* (London: I.B. Tauris, 2005), pp. 135–50.

100   *The Times*, 27 November 1950, p. 3; 21 May 1953, p. 8.

101   Edith Summerskill, *The Ignoble Art* (London: William Heinemann, 1956), p. 47.

102   *Ibid.*, pp. 43–4.

103   *The Times*, 12 December 1953, p. 6.

104   Sheard, '"Brutal and Degrading"', pp. 93–4.

105   Macdonald Critchely, 'Summary' in A.L. Bass, J.L. Blonstein, R.D. James and J.G.P. Williams (eds), *Medical Aspects of Boxing: Proceedings of a Conference held at the Goldsmiths' College London, November 1963* (London: Pergamon Press, 1965), p. 66.

106   *The Times*, 25 November 1963, p. 3.

107   Geoffrey Nicholson, *The Professionals* (London: Andre Deutsch, 1964), p. 22; *The Times*, 11 January 1964, p. 8; Blonstein, *Boxing Doctor*, p. 126.

108   This is not to argue that the impact of debates over boxing's safety was the sole reason for the sport's decline. Factors such as changes in the economy, the increase in leisure opportunities and an increase in living standards would also need to be taken into consideration.

109   Cunningham, *Invention of Childhood*, pp. 211–45.

110   Freddie Mills had received a pair of boxing gloves on his birthday. Morton, *Fighters*, p. 9.

111   BASM Executive Committee Minutes, 11 October 1954.

112   National Archives, FD 23/1894, Letter 21 January 1960 Mr Casson to Medical Research Council. He was directed to articles in the *Lancet*, 6 June 1959. p. 1185 and correspondence plus London ABA's booklet, 'Medical Aspects of Amateur Boxing'. Letter MRC, PJ Chapman M.B., 28 January 1960.

113   *Evening Standard*, 24 November 1966, p. 13; *The Times*, 25 November 1966, p. 10. Only 41 out of 700 schools offered boxing either on its curriculum or as an evening club activity.

114   *The Times*, 17 September 1984, p. 11.

115   Anthony Quick, *Charterhouse: A History of the School* (London: James and James, 1990), p. 126.

116   *Lancet*, 22 November 1969, p. 1114. An interim report in 1964 had reached the conclusion that the existing evidence concerning the medical dangers of boxing was insufficient.

117   The report came out a year later in the form of a book. A.H. Roberts, *Brain Damage in Boxers: A Study of the Prevalence of Traumatic Encephalopathy Among Ex-Professional Boxers* (London: Pitman Medical and Scientific Publishing, 1969), pp. 56–69.

118   *Ibid*, p. 50.

119   Virginia Berridge, 'Medicine and the Public: The 1962 Report of the Royal College of Physicians and the New Public Health, *Bulletin of the History of Medicine*, 81 (2007), pp. 286–311; 'Medicine, public health and the media in Britain from the nineteen-fifties to the nineteen-seventies', *Historical Research*, 82:2 (May 2009), pp. 360–73.

120 Roberts, *Brain Damage*, p. 56.

121 *The Times*, 4 November 1969, p. 1.

122 *The Times*, 28 October 1970, p. 7.

123 For a more detailed discussion of how this decision was reached see Sheard, '"Brutal and Degrading"', p. 98.

124 *The Times*, 1 March 1982, p. 6; *Practitioner*, July 1981, p. 1054.

125 *The Times*, 8 March 1980, p. 12.

126 Sheard, 'Boxing', p. 341.

127 Barry J. Hugman (ed.), *British Boxing Yearbook 1985* (London: Hamlyn, 1984), p. 522.

128 *The Times*, 24 July 1978, p. 6; 20 March 1985, p. 26.

129 *The Times*, 15 December, p. 1; 20 December 1979, p. 15.

130 *The Times*, 17 November 1982, p. 22.

131 *The Times*, 23 September 1980, p. 18.

132 *The Times*, 15 January 1983, p. 19.

133 *Doctor*, 29 July 1982, p. 16.

134 *The Times*, 2 December 1980, p. 11; Hugman (ed.), *British Boxing Yearbook 1985*, p. 523.

135 *The Times*, 27 November 1981, p. 12.

136 J. Corsellis, C. Burton and D. Freeman-Browne, 'The aftermath of boxing', *Psychological Medicine*, 3 (1973), pp. 270–303; *The Times*, 1 March 1982, p. 6; *BMJ*, 24 November 1973, pp. 439–40.

137 *BJSM*, April 1972, vol. 6 (2), p. 85.

138 *BJSM*, June 1983, vol. 17 (2), p. 75.

139 *BJSM*, September 1986, vol. 20 (3), p. 98.

140 Porter, *Health, Civilization*, pp. 236–7.

141 Professional boxing had been banned in Iceland in 1957.

142 *BMJ*, 17 March 1984, p. 874.

143 *The Times*, 8 July 1982, p. 19.

144 *The Times*, 15 January 1983, p. 19.

145 Council on Scientific Affairs, 'Brain Injury in Boxing', *Journal of American Medical Association*, 14 January 1983, p. 256.

146 *The Times*, 9 March 1984, p. 3; *BMJ*, 17 March 1984, p. 876.

147 *The Times*, 4 July 1984, p. 1.

148 *The Times*, 9 March 1984, p. 13.

149 *BMJ*, 4 August 1984, p. 324.

150 *The Times*, 23 January 1985, p. 22.

151 *BMJ*, 31 March 1984, p. 1007; Hugman (ed.), *British Boxing Yearbook 1985*, p. 522; *The Times*, 3 May 1984, p. 28.

152 *The Times*, 3 May 1984, p. 28.

153 Porter, *Greatest Benefit*, p. 610; Sheard, '"Brutal and Degrading"', p. 95.

154 *The Times*, 4 April 1984, p. 23.

155 COMMI-MEDIC-SCOMM, 1982–84 (203621), Minutes of the Meeting Concerning Problems of Boxing, Brussels, 11 May 1983; COMMI-MEDIC-SCOMM, 1977–84 (2036843), Meeting of the IOC Medical Sub-commission 'sports medicine and orthopaedics', Cologne, 28 September 1983, IOC Historical Archives, Lausanne; 85th IOC Session, Sarajevo 1984, re: Medical Report – Annex 22; 94th IOC Session, Tokyo 1990, re: Medical Report – Annex 9.

156 LM Adams and PJ Wren, 'The doctor at the boxing ring: amateur boxing' in Simon DW Payne (ed.), *Medicine, Sport and the Law* (London: Blackwell Scientific Publications, 1990), pp. 230–76.

157   *The Times*, 13 January 1983, p. 18. The European Boxing Union had made the
      reduction in 1978 after the death of Jacopucci. Following the death of Duk Koo
      Kim in 1983, the World Boxing Council followed.
158   One honorary area medical officer recalled how after a few years of not doing
      the job, he rang up the area secretary anonymously to ask for the details on
      the area MO, who then repeated the doctor's own name and address. Sheard,
      'Boxing', p. 326.
159   A.L. Whiteson, 'The doctor at the boxing ring: professional boxing' in Payne (ed.),
      Medicine, pp. 278–81.
160   *Daily Telegraph*, 10 July 1999.
161   *Guardian*, 31 October 1996, p. 13.
162   *Guardian*, 16 June 1994, p. 5; 16 October 1995, p. 3.
163   *Guardian*, 31 October 1996, p. 13.
164   *Guardian*, 27 February 1995, p. 19.
165   *Guardian*, 16 November 1994, p. 26.
166   *Guardian*, 16 October 1995, p. 3.
167   *Guardian*, 15 March 1996, p. 26.
168   *Guardian*, 24 October 1995, p. 24.
169   *Guardian*, 4 May 1994, p. 17.
170   *Guardian*, 28 February 1995, p. 6.
171   *Daily Telegraph*, 10 July 1999.
172   *Guardian* (Sport), 11 January 1994, p. 15; (Education) 16 March 1994, p. 10.
173   *Guardian*, 5 May 1994, p. 23.
174   British Medical Association, *The Boxing Debate* (London: BMA Scientific
      Department, 1993), pp. 70–1; *Guardian*, 10 June 1993, p. 6.
175   *Guardian*, 31 October 1996, p. 13.
176   *Guardian*, 23 September 1991.
177   *Guardian* (Education), 14 March 1994, p. 11.
178   Middleweight boxers used 10-ounce gloves and were permitted 18 feet of
      bandages, held in place by 9 to 11 feet of zinc-oxide tape for each hand.
      Economist, 4 March 1995.
179   *Guardian*, 25 September 1999, p. 2.
180   *Guardian*, 15 November 1991.
181   *Guardian*, 27 February 1995, p. 19.
182   *Guardian*, 26 October 1995, p. 27.
183   *Guardian*, 27 March 1997, p. 27.
184   *Independent*, 18 December 2000.
185   *Guardian*, 16 February 2001, p. 35.
186   *Independent*, 19 December 2000.
187   *Guardian*, 16 February 2001, p. 35.
188   Hugh Brayne, Lincoln Sargeant, Carol Brayne, 'Could boxing be banned?
      A legal and epidemiological perspective' *BMJ*, 316 (13 June 1998),
      pp. 1813–15.
189   *Guardian*, 16 July 1984.
190   *Guardian*, 28 February 2000, p. 8; http://sport.independent.co.uk/general/
      article2214804.ece.
191   *Observer*, 2 October 2005.
192   Contests only went ahead under stringent medical conditions. This included: 6
      two minute rounds, boxers had to be over 20 and had to wear 10 oz. gloves, and
      the doctor had the right to stop the fight when he, and not the referee, wanted.
      Boxing News, 8 December 2006, p. 9.

Conclusion

1 Susan Barton, Neil Carter, Richard Holt and John Williams, *Learning Disability, Sport and Legacy: A Report by the Legacy Research Group on the Special Olympics GB National Summer Games Leicester 2009* (Leicester: De Montfort University, 2011).
2 See Anderson, *War, Disability*, Chapter 5.
3 David Howe, 'The Paralympic Movement: Identity and (Dis)ability' in John Harris and Andrew Parker (eds), *Sport and Social Identities* (Basingstoke: Palgrave, 2009), pp. 32–5.
4 *Guardian*, 10 July 2007.
5 *Guardian*, 14 January 2008, 28 April 2008. Medical debate and evidence has continued over the merits of both sides of the argument e.g. *Guardian*, 4 November 2009.
6 Porter, *Health, Civilization*, p. 314.
7 Runciman, 'Super-athlete?'.
8 *Ibid.*
9 Andy Miah, 'The engineered athlete: Human rights in the genetic revolution', *Sport in Society*, 3:3 (2000), pp. 25–40. Miah actually advocates the removal of barriers to sporting performance.
10 Runciman, 'Super-athlete?'.

Bibliography

Archives

British Association of Sport and Exercise Medicine
(Photocopies of records in possession of author. Archives subsequently deposited in Wellcome Trust Library, London, reference: SA/BSM: Collection, British Association of Sport and Exercise)

British Olympic Association, London
British Olympic Council (BOC), *Aims and Objects of the Olympic Games Fund* (London: British Olympic Association, 1913)

Charlton Athletic Football Co. Ltd, London
Minutes of Directors Meetings, 1930–55

Football Association, London
Minutes of Football Association, 1900–90

International Olympic Committee, Records, 1894–1990, International Olympic Museum, Lausanne, Switzerland
IOC Medical Commission:
COMMI-MEDIC-SCOMM, 1982–84 (203621)
COMMI-MEDIC-SCOMM, 1977–84 (2036843)
Medical Reports
Fédération Internationale de Médecine Sportive Executive Records, 1967–1981

Middlesbrough Football Club, Middlesbrough
Minutes of Directors Meetings, 1898–1939

National Archives (TNA), Kew, London
TNA, ED 113/49, National Fitness Council (NFC), Sports and Games Committee, 1938–39
TNA, ED 113/49, NFC, Medical Committee
TNA, ED 113/49, NFC, Medical Sub-committee on the Desirability of Athletics for Women and Girls, 8 March 1939.
TNA, ED 113/49, NFC, Medical Sub-committee, 26 April 1939.
TNA, ED 113/49, NFC, Sub-Committee, 3 July 1939.
TNA, FD 1/1948, File on A.V. Hill's work during 1920s.
TNA, FD 23/1894, Medical Research Council

Royal Society, Harold W. Thompson papers (HWT)

Sport England, London
Wolfenden Committee on Sport, Draft Report and Proceedings

West Bromwich Albion FC, West Bromwich
Minutes of Directors Meetings, 1895–1920

Wolverhampton Wanderers FC, Wolverhampton
Minutes of Directors Meetings, 1924–39

Interviews

Interview between Geoff Dyson (former AAA head coach) and Tom McNab (former athletics coach), c. 1968.

Interview with Alan Hodson, Head of FA Medical and Exercise Science Department (1990–2008), 31 August 2005.

Interview with Ian Adams, club doctor Leeds United (1961–75), 22 August 2005.

Interview with John Rowlands, general practitioner, 17 February 2005.

Interview with Laurie Brown, physiotherapist Manchester United (1970–82), 7 June 2005.

Interview with Neil Phillips, club doctor and director Middlesbrough (1962–74), 21 June 2005.

Interview with Norman Pilgrim, physiotherapist Coventry City (1964–76), 5 January 2007.

Interview with Stuart Carne, club doctor Queen's Park Rangers and past President of Royal College of General Practitioners, 13 August 2008.

These interviews, except Geoff Dyson were a product of survey, undertaken by the author between 2004 and 2006, which also included questionnaires:

Football club doctors – current and former – 14 in total survey

Football physiotherapists – current and former – 8

Professional footballers – retired – 20

Unattributed statements in the book are the result of the survey. An assurance of confidentiality was a condition of their participation. Results are in the possession of the author.

Newspapers and Periodicals

Albion News
Aston Villa News and Record
Athletic News
Athletics Weekly
BASEM Today
BASM Bulletin
Birmingham Mail
Boxing News
British Medical Journal (BMJ)
Cycling Weekly
Daily Mirror
Daily Record
Daily Telegraph
Doctor
Economist
Empire News
Evening News (Glasgow)
Evening Standard
Express and Star (Wolverhampton)
FA Bulletin
FA News
Four Four Two
Frontline

Guardian
Independent
International Olympic Committee Bulletin
Lancet
New York Times
News of the World
Observer
Sports Budget
Practitioner
Sports Illustrated
Sunday Times
Sunderland Echo
The Times
Times Higher Education
Washington Herald
Washington Times
World Sports

Secondary Sources

Abrahams, Adolphe and Abrahams, Harold, *Training for Athletes* (London: G. Bell and Son, 1928).

Abrahams, Adolphe, 'Athletics' in Humphrey Rolleston (ed.) *The British Encyclopaedia of Medical Practice: Volume 2* (London: Butterworth, 1936).

Abrahams, Adolphe, *The Human Machine* (London: Penguin, 1956).

Adams, Mary Louise, 'From Mixed-Sex Sport to Sport for Girls: The Feminization of Figure Skating', *Sport in History*, 30:2 (June 2010).

Adams, Tony, *Addicted* (London: Collins Willow, 1998).

Adams. L.M. and Wren, P.J., 'The doctor at the boxing ring: amateur boxing' in Simon D.W. Payne (ed.), *Medicine, Sport and the Law* (London: Blackwell Scientific Publications, 1990).

Allison, George, *Allison Calling* (London: Staples Press, 1948).

Anderson, Julie, '"Turned into Taxpayers": Paraplegia, Rehabilitation and Sport at Stoke Mandeville, 1944–56', *Journal of Contemporary History*, 38: (2003).

Anderson, Julie, *War, Disability and Rehabilitation in Britain: 'Soul of a Nation'* (Manchester: Manchester University Press, 2011).

Andrews, Harry, *Training for Athletics and General Health* (London: Bloomsbury, 2005). First published in 1911.

Anon., 'Brain Injury in Boxing', *BMJ*, 25 December 1954, p. 1535.

Anon., 'History of sports medicine in the Netherlands', *BJSM*, 23:4 (1989), p. 219.

Anon., 'Inauguration of sports medicine at the University of Giessen 1920', *International Journal of Sports Medicine*, 23 (2002).

Anon., 'Is the oxygenation of athletes a form of "doping"?', *Olympic Bulletin*, 45 (1954).

Anon., *BASM Bulletin* (1968) pp. 96–104.

Arlott, John, *Fred: Portrait of a Fast Bowler* (London: Coronet, 1971).

Armstrong, J.R. and Tucker, W.E. (eds), *Injury in Sport: The Physiology, Prevention and Treatment of Injuries associated with Sport* (London: Staples Press, 1964).

August, Andrew, 'A culture of consolation? Rethinking politics in working-class London, 1870–1914', *Historical Research*, 74:183 (August 2001).

Bailey, Peter, *Leisure and Class in Victorian England: Rational recreation and the contest for control, 1830–1885* (London: Methuen, 1987).

Baker, N., 'The Amateur Ideal in a Society of Equality: Change and Continuity in post-Second World War British Sport, 1945–48', *IJHS*, 12:1 (April 1995).

Bale, John and Howe, P. David (eds), *Sport in History, Special Issue, The Sporting Barrier: Historical and Cultural Interpretations of the Four-Minute Mile*, 26:2 (August 2006).

Bale, John, 'How Much of a Hero? The Fractured Image of Roger Bannister', *Sport in History*, 26:2 (August 2006).

Bale, John, 'Lassitutde and Latitude: Observations on Sport and Environmental Determinism', *International Review for the Sociology of Sport*, 37 (2002).

Bale, John, 'The Mysterious Professor Jokl' in John Bale, Mette K. Christensen and Gertrud Pfister (eds), *Writing Lives in Sport: Biographies, Life-histories and Methods* (Aarhus: Aarhus University Press, 2004).

Ball, Philip, *Unnatural: The heretical idea of making people* (London: Bodley Head, 2011).

Bannister, Roger, 'Sport, Physical Recreation, and the National Health', *BMJ* (23 December 1972).

Bannister, Roger, *The First Four Minutes* (Stroud: Sutton, 2004).

Barclay, Jean, *In Good Hands: The History of the Chartered Society of Physiotherapy 1894–1994* (Oxford: Butterworth Heinemann, 1994).

Barker-Ruchti, Natalie, 'Ballerinas and Pixies: a Genealogy of the Changing Female Gymnastics Body', *IJHS*, 26:1 (January 2009).

Bascomb, Neal, *The Perfect Mile: Three Athletes. One Goal. And less than Four Minutes to achieve it* (London: Harper Collins, 2004.

Bassett, David R., 'Scientific contributions of A.V. Hill: exercise physiology pioneer', *Journal of Applied Physiology*, 93: (2002).

Beamish, Rob and Ritchie, Ian, 'From Fixed Capacities to Performance-Enhancement: The Paradigm Shift in the Science of "Training" and the Use of Performance-Enhancing Substances', *Sport in History*, 25:3 (December 2005).

Beamish, Rob and Ritchie, Ian, *Fastest, Highest, Strongest: A Critique of High-Performance Sport* (London: Routledge, 2006).

Beaven, Brad, *Leisure, citizenship and working-class men in Britain, 1850–1945* (Manchester: Manchester University Press, 2005).

Beck, Peter, 'Britain and the Cold War's "Cultural Olympics": Responding to the Political Drive of Soviet Sport, 1945–58', *Contemporary British History*, 19:2 (June 2005).

Behringer, Wolfgang, 'Arena and Pall Mall: Sport in the Early Modern Period', *German History*, 27:3 (2009).

Bergoldt, Klaus, *Wellbeing: A Cultural History of Healthy Living* (translated by Jane Dewhurst) (Cambridge: Polity, 2008).

Berridge, Virginia, 'Medicine and the Public: The 1962 Report of the Royal College of Physicians and the New Public Health', *Bulletin of the History of Medicine*, 81 (2007).

Berridge, Virginia, 'Medicine, public health and the media in Britain from the nineteen-fifties to the nineteen-seventies', *Historical Research*, 82:2 (May 2009).

Berridge, Virginia, 'The Origins of the English Drug "Scene"', *Medical History*, 32 (1988).

Berridge, Virginia, *Health and Society in Britain since 1939* (Cambridge: Cambridge University Press, 1999).

Berryman, Jack W. and Park, Roberta J. (eds), *Sport and Exercise Science: Essays in the History of Sports Medicine* (Urbana: University of Illinois Press, 1992).

Berryman, Jack W., 'Exercise and the Medical Tradition from Hippocrates through Antebellum America: A Review Essay' in Jack W. Berryman and Roberta J. Park (eds), *Sport and Exercise Science: Essays in the History of Sports Medicine* (Urbana: University of Illinois Press, 1992).

Berryman, Jack, *Out of Many, One: A History of the American College of Sports Medicine* (Champaign, Ill: Human Kinetics, 1995).

Biasca, N., Wirth, S. and Tegner, Y., 'The avoidability of head and neck injuries in ice hockey: an historical review', *BJSM*, 36:6 (2002).

Birtley, Jack, *The Tragedy of Randolph Turpin* (London: New English Library, 1975).

Bivins, Roberta, *Alternative Medicine? A History* (Oxford: Oxford University Press, 2007).

Blonstein, J.L. and Clarke, Edwin, 'Further observations on the medical aspects of amateur boxing', *BMJ* (16 February 1957).

Blonstein, J.L. and Clarke, Edwin, 'The Medical Aspects of Amateur Boxing', *BMJ* (25 December 1954).

Blonstein, J.L., *Boxing Doctor* (London: Stanley Paul, 1965).

Bloom, B., *Developing Talent in Young People* (New York: Ballantines, 1985).

Boddy, Kasia, *Boxing: A Cultural History* (London: Reaktion, 2008).

Bonde, Hans, 'I.P. Muller: Danish Apostle of Health', *IJHS*, 8:1 (December 1991).

Bourke, Joanna, 'Wartime' in Roger Cooter and John Pickstone (eds), *Medicine in the Twentieth Century* (Amsterdam: Harwood, 2000).

Bourne, Nicholas, Todd, Jan and Todd, Terry, 'The Cold War's Impact on the Evolution of Training Theory in Boxing', *Iron Game History*, 2:2&3 (July 2002).

Boylan, Sean, *The Will To Win* (Dublin: O'Brien Press, 2006).

Brailsford, Dennis, *Bareknuckles: A Social History of Prize-Fighting* (Cambridge: Lutterworth Press, 1988).

Braun, Jutta, 'The People's Sport? Popular Sport and Fans in the Later Years of the German Democratic Republic', *German History*, 27:3 (2009).

Brayne, Hugh, Sargeant, Lincoln and Brayne, Carol , 'Could boxing be banned? A legal and epidemiological perspective' *BMJ*, 316 (13 June 1998).

Brittain, Ian, *The Paralympic Games Explained* (London: Routledge, 2010).

Brooks, John and Fuller, Colin, *England Rugby Injury and Training Audit* (London: Professional Rugby Players' Association, 2005).

Brunton, Deborah, 'Dealing with Disease in Populations: Public Health, 1830–1880' in Deborah Brunton (ed.), *Medicine Transformed: Health, Disease and Society in Europe 1800–1930* (Manchester: Manchester University Press, 2004).

Brunton, Deborah, 'Introduction' in Deborah Brunton' (ed.) *Medicine Transformed: Health, Disease and Society in Europe, 1800–1930* (Manchester: Manchester University Press, 2004).

Brunton, Deborah, 'The Emergence of a Modern Profession?' in Deborah Brunton (ed.), *Medicine Transformed: Health, Disease and Society in Europe 1800–1930* (Manchester: Manchester University Press, 2004).

Brunton, Deborah, 'The Rise of Laboratory Medicine' in Deborah Brunton (ed.), *Medicine Transformed: Health, Disease and Society in Europe 1800–1930* (Manchester: Manchester University Press, 2004).

Bryant, John, *3:59.4: The Quest to Break the 4 Minute Mile* (London: Arrow, 2004).

Bryant, John, *The London Marathon: The History of the Greatest Race on Earth* (London: Arrow, 2005).

Buchan, Charles, *A Lifetime in Football* (London: Sportsmans Book Club, 1956).

Buchanan, Ian, 'Jackson, Arnold Nugent Strode Strode- (1891–1972)', *Oxford Dictionary of National Biography* [accessed 10 Feb 2006].

Buskirk, Elsworth R. and Tipton, Charles M., 'Exercise Physiology' in John D. Massengale and Richard A. Swanson (eds), *The History of Exercise and Sport Science* (New York: Human Kinetics, 1997).

Byles, J.B. and Osborn, Samuel, 'First Aid' in *Encyclopedia of Sport* (London: G.R. Putnam, 1912).

Carlile, Forbes, *Forbes Carlile on Swimming* (London: Sphere, 1963).

Carne, Stuart, 'General practitioner to a football club', *BMJ*, 283: (19 September 1981).

Carpentier, Florence and Lefevre, Jean-Pierre, 'The Modern Olympic Movement, Women's Sport and the Social Order During the Inter-War Period', *IJHS*, 23:7 (November 2006).

Carrington, Ben and McDonald, Ian (eds), *'Race', Sport and British Society* (London: Routledge, 2001).

Carter, Neil (ed.) *Coaching Cultures* (London: Routledge, 2011).

Carter, Neil, 'From Knox to Dyson: Coaching, Amateurism and British Athletics, 1912–1947', *Sport in History*, 30:1 (March 2010).

Carter, Neil, 'Metatarsals and Magic Sponges: English Football and the Development of Sports Medicine', *Journal of Sport History*, 34:1 (Spring 2007).

Carter, Neil, 'Mixing Business with Leisure? The Football Club Doctor, Sports Medicine and the Voluntary Tradition', *Sport in History*, 29:1 (March 2009).

Carter, Neil, 'The Rise and Fall of the Magic Sponge: Medicine and the Transformation of the Football Trainer', *Social History of Medicine*, 23:2 (August 2010).

Carter, Neil, *The Football Manager: A History* (London: Routledge, 2006).

Castro, Ruy, *Garrincha: The triumph and tragedy of Brazil's forgotten footballing hero* (London: Yellow Jersey Press, 2004).

Cerruty, Percy Wells, *Middle-Distance Running* (London: Pelham Books, 1964).

Chalke, Stephen, *Tom Cartwright: The Flame Still Burns* (Bath: Fairfields, 2007).

Chandler, Timothy, Cronin, Mike and Vamplew, Wray, *Sport and Physical Education: The Key Concepts* (London: Routledge, 2002).

Chisholm, Ann, 'Acrobats, Contortionists, and Cute Children: The Promise and Perversity of U.S. Women's Gymnastics', *Signs*, 27:2 (Winter, 2002).

Clark, Norman, *The Boxing Referee* (London: Methuen, 1926).

Cockerham, William C., *Medical Sociology, Sixth Edition* (Englewood Cliffs, NJ: Prentice Hall, 1995).

Collings, Timothy and Sykes, Stuart, *Jackie Stewart: A Restless Life* (London: Virgin, 2003).

Collins, Tony, 'Captain Robert Barclay' in Tony Collins, John Martin and Wray Vamplew (eds), *Encyclopedia of Traditional British Rural Sports* (London: Routledge, 2005).

Collins, Tony, 'History, Theory and the "Civilizing Process"', *Sport in History*, 25:2 (August 2005).

Collins, Tony, *A Social History of English Rugby Union* (London: Routledge, 2009).

Collins, Tony, *Rugby League in Twentieth Century Britain* (London: Routledge, 2006).

Collins, Tony, *Rugby's Great Split: Class, Culture and the Origins of Rugby League Football* (London: Frank Cass, 1998).

Colson, John and Armour, William, *Sports Injuries and their Treatment* (London: Stanley Paul, 1968).

Cooper, Henry, *Henry Cooper: An Autobiography* (London: Coronet Books, 1972).

Cooter, Roger and Pickstone, John, 'Introduction' in Roger Cooter and John Pickstone (eds), *Medicine in the Twentieth Century* (Amsterdam: Harwood, 2000).

Cooter, Roger, 'The meaning of fractures: orthopaedics and the reform of British hospitals in the inter-war period', *Medical History*, 31: (1987).

Cooter, Roger, 'The Moment of the Accident: Culture, Militarism and Modernity in Late-Victorian Britain', in Roger Cooter and Brian Luckin (eds), *Accidents in History: Injuries, Fatalities and Social Relations* (Amsterdam: Rodopi, 1997).

Cooter, Roger, *Surgery and Society in Peace and War: Orthopaedics and the Organization of Modern Medicine, 1880–1948* (Basingstoke: Macmillan, 1993).

Corsellis, J., Burton, C. and Freeman-Browne, D., 'The aftermath of boxing', *Psychological Medicine*, 3 (1973).

Council on Scientific Affairs, 'Brain Injury in Boxing', *Journal of American Medical Association*, 14 January 1983.

Cram, Steve, Distinguished Lecture Series, De Montfort University, 2 December 2010.

Crawford, Robert, 'Healthism and the Medicalization of Everyday Life', *International Journal of Health Services*, 10:3 (1980).

Critchely, Macdonald, 'Summary' in A.L. Bass, J.L. Blonstein, R.D. James and J.G.P. Williams (eds), *Medical Aspects of Boxing: Proceedings of a Conference held at the Goldsmiths' College London, November 1963* (London: Pergamon Press, 1965).

Critchley, MacDonald, 'Medical aspects of boxing, particularly from a neurological standpoint', *BMJ* (16 February 1957).

Crump, Jack, *Running Round the World* (London: Hale, 1966).

Crump, Jeremy, 'Athletics' in Tony Mason (ed.), *Sport in Britain: A Social History* (Cambridge: Cambridge University Press, 1989).

Cullen, M. and Batt, M., 'Sport and exercise medicine in the United Kingdom comes of age', *BJSM*, 39 (2005).

Cunningham, Hugh, 'Leisure and Culture' in FML Thompson (ed.) *The Cambridge Social History of Britain, 1750–1950* (Cambridge: Cambridge University Press, 1990).

Cunningham, Hugh, *The Invention of Childhood* (London: BBC Books 2006).

Davies, David, *FA Confidential: Sex, Drugs and Penalties: The Inside Story of English Football* (London: Simon & Schuster, 2008).

Davies, Elsa, "National Playing Fields Association," in Richard Cox, Grant Jarvie and Wrav Vamplew (eds) *Encyclopedia of British Sport* (Oxford: ABC-Clio, 2000).

Davis, John, 'The London Drug Scene and the Making of Drug Policy, 1965–73', *Twentieth Century British History* (Advanced Access, 11 January 2006).

Day, Dave, 'Craft Coaching and the "Discerning Eye" of the Coach', *International Journal of Sports Science and Coaching*, 6:1 (2011).

Day, Dave, 'London Swimming Professors: Victorian Craftsmen and Aquatic Entrepreneurs', *Sport in History*, 30:1 (March 2010).

Dear, Peter, *Revolutionizing the Sciences: European Knowledge and its Ambitions, 1500–1700, Second Edition*, (Basingstoke: Palgrave Macmillan, 2009).

Devitt, Patrick F., *May the Best Man Win: Sport, Masculinity, and Nationalism in Great Britain and the Empire 1880–1935* (Basingstoke: Palgrave, 2004).

Digby, Anne, *Making a medical living: Doctors and patients in the English market for medicine* (Cambridge: Cambridge University Press, 1994).

Dimeo, Paul and Hunt, Thomas, 'The doping of athletes in the former East Germany: A critical assessment of comparisons with Nazi medical experiments', *International Review for the Sociology of Sport* (Published on-line 11 April 2011).

Dimeo, Paul, 'Introduction', *Sport in History*, 25:3 (December 2005).

Dimeo, Paul, *A History of Drug Use in Sport 1876–1976: Beyond Good and Evil* (London: Routledge, 2007).

Dimeo, Paul, Hunt, Thomas M. and Horbury, Richard, 'The Individual and the State: A Social Historical Analysis of the East German "Doping System"', *Sport in History*, 31:2 (June 2011).

Dine, Phil, 'Sport and the State in contemporary France: from la Charte des Sports to decentralisation', *Modern and Contemporary France*, 6:3 (1998).

Doherty, J. Kenneth, *Modern Training for Running* (Englewood Cliffs, NJ: Prentice-Hall, 1964).

Drawer, S. and Fuller, C.W., 'Propensity for osteoarthritis and lower limb joint pain in retired professional soccer players', *BJSM*, 35 (2001).

Duval, Lynne, 'The Development of Women's Track and Field in England: The Role of the Athletic Club, 1920s–1950s', *The Sports Historian*, 21:1 (May 2001).

Dyreson, Mark, 'Johnny Weissmuller and the Old Global Capitalism: The Origins of the Federal Blueprint for Selling American Culture to the World', *IJHS*, 25:2 (2008).

Dyson, Geoff, *The Mechanics of Athletics: seventh edition* (London: Hodder and Stoughton, 1977).

Eaton, K.K., 'Motor Racing', *Journal of the Royal College of General Practitioners*, 20 (1970).

Edwards, A. Clement, *The Compensation Act 1906* (London: Chatto and Windus, 1907).

Eisenberg, Christiane, 'Charismatic Nationalist Leader: Turnvater Jahn', *IJHS*, 13:1 (March 1996).

Eliott Lynn, Sophie, *Athletics for Women and Girls* (London: Robert Scott, 1925).

Erdozain, Dominic, *The Problem of Pleasure: Sport, Recreation and the Crisis of Victorian Religion* (Woodbridge: Boydell Press, 2010).

Ergen, E. *et al*, 'Sports medicine: a European perspective. Historical roots, definitions and scope', *Journal of Sports Medicine and Physical Fitness*, 46: 2 (June 2006).

Evans, H. Justin, *Service to Sport: The Story of the CCPR – 1935–1972* (London: Pelham, 1974).

Farmer, Ted, *The Heartbreak Game* (Wolverhampton, U.K.: Hillburgh, 1987).

Ferguson-Smith, M.A. and Ferris, Elizabeth, 'Gender verification in sport: the need for change?', *BJSM*, 25:1 (1991).

Ferrier, Bob, *Soccer Partnership: Billy Wright and Walter Winterbottom* (London: Heinemann, 1960).

Fielding, Steven, Thompson, Peter and Tiratsoo, Nick, *'England Arise!' The Labour Party and Popular Politics in 1940s Britain* (Manchester: Manchester University Press, 1995).

Fletcher, Shelia, 'The Making and Breaking of a Female Tradition: Women's Physical Education in England 1880–1980', *British Journal of Sports History*, 2:1 (May 1985).

Football Association Coaching Manual (London: Evans, 1938).

Fossey, Nicky, 'Gender' in Richard Cox, Grant Jarvie and Wray Vamplew (eds), *Encyclopedia of British Sport* (Oxford: ABC-Clio, 2000).

Fossey, Nicky, 'Netball' in Richard Cox, Grant Jarvie and Wray Vamplew (eds), *Encyclopedia of British Sport* (Oxford: ABC-Clio, 2000).

Foster, Ken, 'Developments in Sports Law' in Lincoln Allison (ed.), *The Changing Politics of Sport* (Manchester: Manchester University Press, 1993).

Fotheringham, William, *Put Me Back On My Bike: In Search of Tom Simpson* (London: Yellow Jersey Press, 2002).

Francis, Dick, *Lester: The Official Biography* (London: Michael Joseph, 1986).

Freidenfelds, Lara, *The Modern Period: Menstruation in Twentieth-Century America* (Baltimore: Johns Hopkins University Press, 2009).

Frew, Matthew and McGillivray, David, 'Health Clubs and Body Politics: Aesthetics and the Quest for Physical Capital', *Leisure Studies*, 24:2, (2005).

Fuller, Colin, 'Implications of health and safety legislation for the professional sportsperson', *BJSM*, 29:1 (1995).

Gelfand, Toby, 'The history of the medical profession' in W. F. Bynum and R. Porter (eds.), *Companion Encyclopaedia of the History of Medicine, Volume 2* (London: Routledge, 1993).

Gevitz, Norman, 'Unorthodox Medical Theories' in W. F. Bynum and R. Porter (eds.), *Companion Encyclopaedia of the History of Medicine, Volume 1* (London: Routledge, 1993).

Gill, Diane L., 'Sport and Exercise Psychology' in John D. Massengale and Richard A. Swanson (eds), *The History of Exercise and Sport Science* (Champaign, IL: Human Kinetics, 1997).

Goodman, Jordan, 'Pharmaceutical Industry' in Roger Cooter and John Pickstone (eds), *Medicine in the Twentieth Century* (Amsterdam: Harwood, 2000).

Gori, Gigliola, *Italian Fascism and the Female Body: Sport, Submissive Women and Strong Mothers* (London: Routledge, 2004).

Graham, J.W., 'Professional Boxing and the Doctor', *BMJ* (22 January 1955).

Graham, J.W., *Eight, Nine, Out! Fifty Years as a Boxer's Doctor* (Manchester: Protel, 1975).

Green, Harvey, *Fit For America: Health, Fitness, Sport and American Society* (London: Johns Hopkins University Press, 1986).

Green, Mick, 'Olympic Glory or Grassroots Development?: Sport Policy Priorities in Australia, Canada and the United Kingdom, 1960–2000', *IJHS*, 24:7 (July 2007).

Gunn, Michael and Ormerod, David, 'The legality of boxing', *Legal Studies*, 15:2 (July 1995).

Guttmann, Allen, *Women's Sports: A History* (New York: Columbia University Press, 1991).

Haley, Bruce, *The Healthy Body and Victorian Culture* (London: Harvard University Press, 1978).

Hamilton, David, *The Monkey Gland Affair* (London: Chatto & Windus, 1986).

Harding, John, *Living to Play: From Soccer Slaves to Socceratti – A Social History of the Professionals* (London: Robson, 2003).

Hardy, Anne, *Health and Medicine in Britain since 1860* (Basingstoke: Palgrave, 2001).

Hargreaves, Jennifer, 'Women's sports between the wars: Continuities and Discontinuities', *Warwick Centre for the Study of Sport in Society, Working Papers* (1994).

Hargreaves, Jennifer, "Playing Like Gentlemen While Behaving Like Ladies': Contradictory Features of the Formative Years of Women's Sport', *British Journal of Sports History*, 2:1 (May 1985), p. 43.

Hargreaves, Jennifer, *Sporting Females: Critical issues in the history and sociology of women's sports* (London: Routledge, 1994).

Harris, Bernard, *The Origins of the British Welfare State: Social Welfare in England and Wales, 1800–1945* (Basingstoke: Palgrave, 2004).

Harris, Jose, *Private Lives, Public Spirit: Britain 1870–1914* (London: Penguin, 1993).

Hawkins, R.D. *et al*, 'The association football medical research programme: an audit of injuries in professional football', *BJSM*, 35 (2001).

Hawkins, Richard D. and Fuller, Colin W., 'A prospective epidemiological study of injuries in four English professional football clubs', *BJSM*, 33 (1999).

Heald, Charles, *Injuries and Sport: A General Guide for the Practitioner* (Oxford: Oxford University Press, 1931).

Heggie, Vanessa, '"Only the British Appear to be Making a Fuss": The Science of Success and the Myth of Amateurism at the Mexico Olympiad, 1968', *Sport in History*, 28:2 (June 2008).

Heggie, Vanessa, 'A Century of Cardiomythology: Exercise and the Heart c. 1880s–1980', *Social History of Medicine*, 23:2 (August 2010).

Heggie, Vanessa, 'Only the British Appear to be Making a Fuss': The Science of Success and the Myth of Amateurism at the Mexico Olympiad, 1968', *Sport in History*, 28:2 (June 2008).

Heggie, Vanessa, 'Specialization without the Hospital: The Case of British Sports Medicine, *Medical History*, 54: (2010).

Heggie, Vanessa, *A History of British Sports Medicine* (Manchester: Manchester University Press, 2011).

Hencken, C. and White, C., 'Anthropometric Assessment of Premiership Soccer Players in Relation to Playing Position', *European Journal of Sport Science*, 6:4 (2006).

Hill, Jeffrey, 'British Sports History: A Post-Modern Future?', *Journal of Sport History*, 23:1 (Spring 1996).

Hill, Jeffrey, *Sport, Leisure and Culture in Twentieth Century Britain* (Basingstoke: Palgrave, 2002).

Hoberman, John, 'Amphetamine and the Four-Minute Mile', *Sport in History*, 26:2 (August 2006).

Hoberman, John, 'The Early Development of Sports Medicine in Germany' in Jack W. Berryman and Roberta J. Park (eds), *Sport and Exercise Science: Essays in the History of Sports Medicine* (Urbana: University of Illinois Press, 1992).

Hoberman, John, *Darwin's Athletes: How Sport has Damaged Black America and Preserved the Myth of Race* (Boston: Houghton Mifflin, 1997).

Hoberman, John, *Mortal Engines: The Science of Performance and the Dehumanization of Sport* (London: Macmillan, 1992).

Hoddle, Glenn, *Glenn Hoddle: My 1998 World Cup Story* (London: Andre Deutsch, 1998).

Holgate, Virginia, *Ginny: An Autobiography* (London: Stanley Paul, 1986).

Hollmann, W., 'Sports medicine in the Federal Republic of Germany', *BJSM*, 23:3 (1989).

Holt, Richard and Mason, Tony, *Sport in Britain 1945–2000* (Oxford: Blackwell, 2000).

Holt, Richard, 'Sport, the French, and the Third Republic', *Modern and Contemporary France*, 6:3 (1998).

Holt, Richard, 'The Amateur Body and the Middle-Class Man: Work, Health and Style in Victorian Britain', *Sport in History*, 26:3 (December 2006).

Holt, Richard, *Sport and the British: A Modern History* (Oxford: Oxford University Press, 1989).

Horwood Catherine, '"Girls who arouse dangerous passions": women and bathing, 1900–39', *Women's History Review*, 9:4 (2000).

Houlihan, Barrie, 'Building an international regime to combat doping in sport' in Roger Levermore and Adrian Budd (eds), *Sport and International Relations: An Emerging Relationship* (London: Routledge, 2004).

Houlihan, Barrie, *The Government and Politics of Sport* (London: Routledge, 1991).

Howe, David, 'The Paralympic Movement: Identity and (Dis)ability' in John Harris and Andrew Parker (eds), *Sport and Social Identities* (Basingstoke: Palgrave, 2009).

Howe, P. David, 'The tail is wagging the dog: Body culture, classification and the Paralympic movement', *Ethnography*, 9: (2008).

Huggins, Mike, *Flat Racing and British Society 1790–1914: A Social and Economic History* (London: Frank Cass, 2000).

Hugman, Barry J. (ed.), *British Boxing Yearbook 1985* (London: Hamlyn, 1984).

Huizenga, Rob, *"You're Okay, It's Just a Bruise": A Doctor's Sideline Secrets About Pro Football's Most Outrageous Team* (New York: St. Martin's Griffin, 1994).

Hunt, Thomas M., 'Countering the Soviet Threat in the Olympic Medals Race: The Amateur Sports Act of 1978 and American Athletics Policy Reform, *IJHS*, 24:6 (June 2007).

Hunt, Thomas, *Drug Games: The International Olympic Committee and the Politics of Doping, 1960–2008* (Austin: University of Texas Press, 2011).

Huntington-Whiteley, James (ed.), *The Book of British Sporting Heroes* (London: National Portrait Gallery, 1998).

Hurt, J., 'Drill, discipline and the elementary school ethos' in W.P. McCann (ed.) *Popular Education and Socialization in the Nineteenth Century* (London: Methuen, 1977).

Inglis, Simon, *League Football and the Men Who Made It: The Official Centenary History of the Football League* (London: Collins Willow, 1988).

Jensen, Erik, *Body By Weimar: Athletes, Gender and German Modernity* (Oxford: Oxford University Press, 2010).

Johnes, Martin, '"Heads in the Sand": Football, Politics and Crowd Disasters in Twentieth-Century Britain', *Soccer in Society*, 5:2 (Summer 2004).

Johnson, Amanda, 'Society of Sports Therapists – A Response', *BJSM*, 24 (1990).

Johnson, William Oscar, 'This Strange and Perilous Joint', *Sports Illustrated*, 24 October 1977.

Johnston, Ronnie and McIvor, Arthur, 'Marginalising the Body at Work? Employers' Occupational Health Strategies and Occupational Medicine in Scotland c.1930–1974', *Social History of Medicine*, 21:3 (April 2008).

Jokl, Ernst, 'Pioneers: 90th Birthday of Professor A.V. Hill', *Journal of Sports Medicine*, 16 (1976).

Jokl, Ernst, 'The Athletic Status of Women: An Analysis of a Social Phenomenon', *British Journal of Physical Medicine* (November 1957).

Jokl, Ernst, *The Medical Aspect of Boxing* (Pretoria: J.L. Van Schaik, 1941).

Jones, Kathleen, *The Making of Social Policy in Britain 1830–1990* (London: Athlone, 1994).

Jones, Stephen G., 'State Intervention in Sport and Leisure in Britain between the Wars', *Journal of Contemporary History*, 22 (1987).

Joy, Bernard, *Forward Arsenal: A History of the Arsenal Football Club* (London: Phoenix House, 1952).

Jutel, Annemarie, '"Thou Dost Run as in Flotation": Femininity, Reassurance and the Emergence of the Women's Marathon', *IJHS*, 20 (September 2003).

Katzer, Nikolaus, 'Soviet physical culture and sport: A European legacy?' in Alan Tomlinson, Christopher Young and Richard Holt (eds), *Sport and the Transformation of Modern Europe: States, media and markets 1950–2010* (London: Routledge, 2011).

Kay, Joyce, 'A Window of Opportunity? Preliminary Thoughts on Women's Sport in Post-war Britain', *Sport in History*, 30:2 (June 2010).

Keegan, Kevin, *Kevin Keegan: My Autobiography* (London: Little, Brown, 1997).

Kerrigan, Colm, 'London Schoolboys and Professional Football, 1899–1915', *IJHS*, 11:2 (August 1994), pp. 287–97.

Keys, Barbara, *Globalizing Sport: National Rivalry and International Community in the 1930s* (Harvard: Harvard University Press, 2006).

Kimmage, Paul, *Rough Ride: Behind the Wheel with a Pro Cyclist, second edition* (London: Yellow Jersey Press, 2001).

Koehler, Peter, 'The evolution of British neurology in comparison with other countries' in F. Clifford Rose (ed.), *A Short History of Neurology: The British Contribution 1660–1910* Oxford: Butterworth-Heinemann, 1999).

Krasnoff, Lindsay Sarah, 'Resurrecting the nation: The evolution of French sports policy from de Gaulle to Mitterand' in Alan Tomlinson, Christopher Young and Richard Holt (eds), *Sport and the Transformation of Modern Europe: States, media and markets 1950–2010* (London: Routledge, 2011).

Kruger, Arnd, 'The role of sport in German international politics, 1918–1945' in P. Arnaud and J. Riordan, (eds), *Sport and international politics* (London: E. & F.N. Spon, 1998).

Kruger, Arnd, 'Training Theory and Why Roger Bannister was the First Four-Minute Miler', *Sport in History*, 26:2 (August 2006).

La Cava, Guiseppe , 'The International Federation for Sports Medicine', *Journal of the American Medical Association*, 162: (17 November 1956).

La Cava, Guiseppe, 'Sports medicine in modern times: A short historical survey', *Journal of Sports Medicine and Physical Fitness*, 13:3 (July–September 1973).

Langhamer, Claire, *Women's leisure in England 1920–60* (Manchester: Manchester University Press, 2000).

Larkin, G., 'Orthodox and Osteopathic Medicine in the Inter-War Years' in Mike Saks (ed.), *Alternative Medicine in Britain* (Oxford: Clarendon Press, 1992).

Larkin, G., *Occupational Monopoly and Modern Medicine* (London: Tavistock, 1983).

Law, Denis, *The King: My Autobiography* (London: Bantam, 2003).

Lawrence, Christopher and Mayer, Anna-K., 'Regenerating England: An Introduction' in Christopher Lawrence and Anna-K. Mayer (eds), *Regeneration England: Science, Medicine and Culture in Inter-War Britain* (Amsterdam: Rodopi, 2000).

Lee, Judy, 'Media Portrayals of Male and Female Olympic Athletes: Analyses of Newspaper Accounts of the 1984 and the 1988 Summer Games', *International Review for the Sociology of Sport*, 27:3 (1992).

Leese, Peter, *Shell Shock: Traumatic Neurosis and the British Soldiers of the First World War* (Basingstoke: Palgrave Macmillan, 2002).

Loland, Sigmund, Skirstad, Berit and Waddington, Ivan, (eds), *Pain and Injury in Sport: Social and Ethical Analysis* (London: Routledge, 2006).

Loudon, Irvine, *Medical Care and the General Practitioner, 1750–1850* (Oxford: Oxford University Press, 1986).

Lovell, Richard, 'Choosing People: An Aspect of the Life of Lord Moran (1882–1977)', *Medical History*, 36 (1992).

Lovesey, Peter, *The Official History of the Amateur Athletic Association* (London: Guinness Superlatives, 1979).

Lowe, Douglas G. A., *Track and Field Athletics* (London: Sir Issac Pitman and Sons, 1936).

Lowe, Douglas G.A. and Porritt, Arthur E., *Athletics* (London: Longmans, 1929).

Lupton, James Irvine and Lupton, James Money Kyrle, *The Pedestrian's Record: To which is added a description of the external human form* (London: WH Allen, 1890).

MacAuley, Domhanll, 'Fortnightly Review: Drugs in sport', *BMJ* 313, (27 July 1996).

Macdonald, Charlotte, *Strong, Beautiful, and Modern: National Fitness in Britain, New Zealand, Australia and Canada, 1935–1960* (Wellington, NZ: Bridget Williams Books, 2011).

MacMillan, Margaret, *Peacemakers: The Paris Conference of 1919 and Its Attempt to End War* (London: Hodder, 2001).

Macrae, Elidh, '"Scotland for Fitness": The National Fitness Campaign and Scottish Women', *Women's History Magazine* 62 (2010).

Malcolm, Dominic and Sheard, Ken, '"Pain in the Assets": The Effects of Commercialization and Professionalization on the Management of Injury in English Rugby Union.' *Sociology of Sport Journal* 19: (2002).

Malcolm, Dominic, 'Sports medicine: A very peculiar practice? Doctors and physiotherapists in elite English rugby union' in Sigmund Loland, Berit Skirstad and Ivan Waddington (eds), *Pain and Injury in Sport: Social and ethical analysis* (London: Routledge, 2006).

Malcolm, Dominic, 'Unprofessional Practice? The Status and Power of Sport Physicians', *Sociology of Sport Journal*, 23: (2006).

Malcolm, Dominic, Sheard, Ken and Smith, Stuart, 'Protected Research: Sports Medicine and Rugby Injuries', *Sport in Society*, 7:1 (2004).

Mandler, Peter, *The English National Character: The History of an Idea from Edmund Burke to Tony Blair* (New Haven: Yale University Press, 2006).

Martin, Simon, *Sport Italia: The Italian Love Affair with Sport* (London: I.B. Tauris, 2011).

Martland, Harrison, 'Punch Drunk', *Journal of the American Medical Association*, 91:15 (13 October 1928).

Mason, Fred, 'R. Tait McKenzie's Medical Work and Early Exercise Therapies for People with Disabilities', *Sport History Review*, 39:1 (2008).

Mason, Tony and Riedi, Eliza, *Sport and the Military: The British Armed Forces 1880–1960* (Cambridge: Cambridge University Press, 2010).

Mason, Tony, *Association Football and English Society 1863–1915* (Brighton; Harvester Press, 1980).

Mason, Tony, *Sport in Britain* (London: Faber and Faber, 1988).

Massengale, John D. and Swanson, Richard A. (eds), *The History of Exercise and Sport Science* (New York: Human Kinetics, 1997).

Matthews, Jill, 'They had Such a Lot of Fun: The Women's League of Health and Beauty Between the Wars', *History Workshop Journal*, 30 (Autumn 1990).

Mazower, Mark, *Dark Continent: Europe's Twentieth Century* (London: Penguin, 1998).

McCrory, Paul, 'Evidence-based sports medicine', *BJSM*, 35 (2001).

McCrory, Paul, 'What is sports and exercise medicine?' *BJSM*, 40 (2006).

McCrory, Peter, 'Warm Up', *BJSM*, 35 (2001).

McCullough, Carol Porter, *The Alexander Technique and the String Pedagogy of Paul Rolland* (Phoenix: Arizona State University Press, 1996).

McIntosh, Peter, 'Archibald Maclaren', *Dictionary of National Biography*, 2004 [accessed 18 Nov 2004: http://www.oxforddnb.com/view/article/50298].

McKibbin, Ross, *Classes and Cultures: England 1918–1951* (Oxford: Oxford University Press, 1998).

McNab, Tom, Lovesey, Peter and Huxtable, Andrew, *An Athletics Compendium: An annotated guide to the UK Literature of track and field* (Boston Spa: British Library, 2001).

McNamee, Mike, 'Whose Prometheus? Transhumanism, biotechnology and the moral typography of sports medicine', *Sport, Ethics and Philosophy*, 1:2 (2007).

Mead, William B., 'The surgeon general of baseball', *National Pastime*, Annual 2002.

Melling, Ali, 'Women and Football' in Richard Cox, Grant Jarvie and Wrav Vamplew (eds) *Encyclopedia of British Sport* (Oxford: ABC-Clio, 2000).

Messerli, F.R.M, 'Women's participation to the Modern Olympic Games', *Olympic Bulletin*, 33 (1952).

Miah, Andy, 'The engineered athlete: Human rights in the genetic revolution', *Sport in Society*, 3:3 (2000).

Mignon, Patrick, 'The Tour de France and the Doping Issue', *IJHS*, 20:2 (June 2003), p. 233.

Miles, J.R., 'The racecourse medical officer', *Journal of the Royal College of General Practitioners*, 19 (1970).

Mitchell, Shelia, 'Women's Participation in the Olympic Games 1900–1926', *Journal of Sport History*, 4:2 (1977).

Mold, Alex, '"Consuming Habits": Histories of Drugs in Modern Societies', *Cultural and Social History*, 2:2 (2007).

Moller, Vernon, 'Knud Enemark Jensen's Death During the 1960 Rome Olympics: A Search for Truth?', *Sport in History*, 25:3 (December 2005).

Moore, James, 'The Fortunes of Eugenics' in Deborah Brunton (ed.), *Medicine Transformed: Health, Disease and Society in Europe 1800–1930* (Manchester: Manchester University Press, 2004).

Morris, Sharon, '"Human dregs at the bottom of our national vats': The interwar debate on sterilization of the mentally deficient' in David M. Turner and Kevin Staggs (eds), *Social Histories of Disability and Deformity* (London: Routledge, 2006).

Morton, James, *Fighters: The Lives and Sad Deaths of Freddie Mills and Randolph Turpin* (London: Time Warner, 2004).

Mowles, J.W., 'Injuries at Sport', *Journal of the Chartered Society of Massage and Medical Gymnastics* (September 1937).

Muller, I.P., *My System: 15 Minutes' Exercise a Day for Health's Sake* (London: Link House, 1904).

Munson, Lester, 'Fast Operators', *Sports Illustrated*, 6 November 1995.

Munting, Roger, 'The Games Ethic and Industrial Capitalism before 1914: The Provision of Company Sports', *Sport in History*, 23:1 (Summer 2003).

Murphy, Patrick, *'Tiger' Smith of Warwickshire and England* (Guildford: Lutterworth Press, 1981).

Mussabini, Sam, *The Complete Athletic Trainer* (London: Methuen, 1913).

Nack, William, 'Playing Hurt – the Doctors' Dilemma', *Sports Illustrated*, 11 June 1979.

Nannestad, Ian, 'John Allison and His Football Hospital', *Soccer History* 9 (2004).

Nannestad, Ian, 'No ball practice! Training Methods in the Period to 1914', *Soccer History*, 13 (2005–6).

Newton, A.J., *Boxing* (London: Bloomsbury, 2005). First published in 1910.

Nicholls, James, *The Politics of Alcohol: A history of the drink question in England* (Manchester: Manchester University Press, 2009).

Nicholson, Geoffrey, *The Professionals* (London: Andre Deutsch, 1964).

Noakes, Timothy and Jakoet, Ismail, 'Spinal cord injuries in rugby union players', *BMJ*, 310 (27 May 1995).

Nocera, Joseph, 'Bitter Medicine', *Sports Illustrated*, 6 November 1995.

Nutton, Vivian, 'Humoralism', in W. F. Bynum and R. Porter (eds.), *Companion Encyclopaedia of the History of Medicine, Volume 1* (London: Routledge, 1993).

Oaksey, John, *Mince Pie for Starters* (London: Headline, 2003).

Oriard, Michael, *King Football: Sport and Spectacle in the Golden Age of Radio and Newsreels, Movies and Magazines, the Weekly and the Daily Press* (Chapel Hill: North Carolina Press, 2001).

Oriard, Michael, *Reading Football: How the Popular Press Created an American Spectacle* (London: University of North Carolina Press, 1993).

Osborne, Carol A. and Skillen, Fiona, 'Introduction. The State of Play: Women in British Sport History', *Sport in History*, 30:2 (June 2010).

Park, Roberta J, 'Setting the Scene – Bridging the Gap between Knowledge and Practice: When Americans Really Built Programmes to Foster Healthy Lifestyles, 1918–1940', *IJHS*, 25:11 (2008).

Park, Roberta J., 'Sharing, arguing, and seeking recognition: International congresses, meetings, and physical education, 1867–1915', *IJHS*, 25:5 (2008).

Park, Roberta J., '"Cells or Soaring?": Historical reflections on "visions" of body, athletics, and Modern Olympism', *IJHS*, 24:12 (2007).

Park, Roberta J., 'Physiologists, physicians, and physical educators: Nineteenth century biology and exercise, hygienic and educative', *IJHS*, 24:12 (2007).

Park, Roberta J., '"Cells or Soaring?": Historical reflections of 'visions' of the body, athletics and Modern Olympism', *Olympika: the international journal of Olympic Studies*, 9 (2000).

Park, Roberta J., 'Boys' Clubs Are Better Than Policemen's Clubs': Endeavours by Philanthropists, Social Reformers, and Others to Prevent Juvenile Crime, the Late 1800s to 1917, *IJHS*, 24:6 (June 2007).

Park, Roberta J., 'Physicians, Scientists, Exercise and Athletics in Britain and America from the 1867 Boat Race to the Four-Minute Mile', *Sport in History*, 31:1 (March 2011), pp. 1–31.

Park, Roberta J., 'Physiologists, Physicians, and Physical Educators: Nineteenth-Century Biology and Exercise, Hygienic and Educative' in Jack W. Berryman and Roberta J. Park (eds), *Sport and Exercise Science: Essays in the History of Sports Medicine* (Urbana: University of Illinois Press, 1992).

Park, Roberta J., 'Physiologists, Physicians, and Physical Educators: Nineteenth Century Biology and Exercise', *Journal of Sport History*, 14:1 (Spring 1987).

Park, Roberta J., 'Physiology and Anatomy are Destiny!?: Brains, Bodies and Exercise in Nineteenth Century American Thought', *Journal of Sport History*, 18:1 (Spring 1991).

Park, Roberta J., 'Setting the Scene – Bridging the Gap between Knowledge and Practice: When Americans Really Built Programmes to Foster Healthy Lifestyles, 1918–1940', *IJHS*, 25:11 (September 2008).

Park, Roberta J., 'Sharing, arguing and seeking recognition: International congresses, meetings, and physical education, 1867–1915', *IJHS*, 25:5 (2008).

Park, Roberta J., '"Mended or Ended?": Football Injuries and the British and American Medical Press, 1870–1910', *IJHS*, 18:2 (June 2001).

Park, Roberta, 'Athletes and their training in Britain and America, 1800–1914' in Jack W. Berryman and Roberta J. Park (eds), *Sport and Exercise Science: Essays in the History of Sports Medicine* (Urbana: University of Illinois Press, 1992).

Parker, Claire, 'The Rise of Competitive Swimming 1840 to 1878', *The Sports Historian*, 21:2 (November 2001).

Parratt Catriona, 'Little Means or Time: Working-Class Women and Leisure in Late Victorian and Edwardian England', *IJHS*, 15:2 (August 1998).

Perkin, Harold, *The Rise of Professional Society: England Since 1880* (London: Routledge, 1989).

Perkin, Harold, *The Third Revolution: Professional Elites in the Modern World* (London: Routledge, 1996).

Peskett, Roy (ed.), *Tom Whittaker's Arsenal Story* (London: The Sportsmans Book Club, 1958).

Pfister, Gertrud, 'The Medical Discourse on Female Physical Culture in Germany in the 19th and Early 20th Centuries', *Journal of Sport History*, 17:2 (Summer, 1990).

Pfister, Gertrud, 'The Role of German Turners in American Physical Education', *IJHS*, 26:13 (2009).

Pfister, Gertrud, 'Women and the Olympic Games: 1900–97' in B.L. Drinkwater (ed.), *Women in Sport, Volume 8 of the Encyclopedia of Sports Medicine* (Oxford: Blackwell Science, 2000).

Phelan, Nancy and Volin, Michael, *Yoga for Women* (London: Arrow, 1963).

Phillips, Murray, *From Sidelines to Centre Field: A History of Sports Coaching in Australia* (Sydney: University of NSW Press, 2000).

Pickstone, John, 'Production, Community and Consumption: The Political Economy of Twentieth Century Medicine' in Roger Cooter and John Pickstone (eds), *Medicine in the Twentieth Century* (Amsterdam: Harwood, 2000).

Pipkin, James, *Sporting Lives: Metaphor and Myth in American Sports Autobiographies* (London: University of Missouri Press, 2008).

Polley, Martin, *Moving the Goalposts: A history of sport and society since 1945* (London: Routledge, 1998).

Porritt, Arthur, 'General Health' in H.A. Meyer (ed.), *Athletics: By members of the Achilles Club* (London: J.M. Dent and Sons, 1955.

Porter Dorothy, 'The Healthy Body' in Roger Cooter and John Pickstone (eds), *Medicine in the Twentieth Century* (Amsterdam: Harwood, 2000).

Porter, Dorothy, *Health, Civilization and the State: A history of public health from ancient to modern times* (London: Routledge, 1999).

Porter, Roy, *The Greatest Benefit to Mankind: A Medical History of Humanity* (New York: W.W. Norton, 1997).

Proctor, Tammy, '(Uni)Forming Youth: Girl Guides and Boy Scouts in Britain, 1908–39', *History Workshop Journal*, 45: (1998).

Pugh, Martin, *We Danced All Night: A Social History of Britain Between the Wars* (London: Vintage, 2009).

Quick, Anthony, *Charterhouse: A History of the School* (London: James and James, 1990).

Radcliffe, Paula, *Paula: My Story So Far* (London: Simon & Schuster, 2004).

Radford, Peter, 'The good, the bad and the ugly', *Sociology of Sport Online*, 1:1 (1998).

Radford, Peter, *The Celebrated Captain Barclay: Sport, Money and Fame in Regency Britain* (London: Headline, 2001).

Ramsey, Matthew, 'Public Health in France' in Dorothy Porter (ed.), *The History of Public Health and the Modern State* (Amsterdam: Rodopi, 1994).

Reynolds, L.A. and Tansey, E.M., *The Development of Sports Medicine in Twentieth Century Britain* (Transcript of a Witness Seminar) (London: Wellcome Trust, 2009).

Riedi, Eliza and Mason, Tony, '"Leather" and the Fighting Spirit: Sport in the British Army in World War I', *Canadian Journal of History*, 41: (2006).

Riess, Steven A., *Sport in Industrial America 1850–1920* (Wheeling, Il: Harlan Davidson, 1995).

Riordan, James, 'The Social Emancipation of Women Through Sport', *British Journal of Sports History*, 2:1 (May 1985).

Riordan, Jim, 'Sports Medicine in the Soviet Union and German Democratic Republic', *Social Science and Medicine*, 25:1 (1987).

Roberts, A.H., *Brain Damage in Boxers: A Study of the Prevalence of Traumatic Encephalopathy Among Ex-Professional Boxers* (London: Pitman Medical and Scientific Publishing, 1969).

Roberts, M. Randal, 'A Footballers' Hospital', *Windsor Magazine*, March 1899.

Robson, Henry, 'Editorial', *BJSM*, 19:1 (March 1985).

Robson, Henry, 'Honorary Treasurer's Report for the year 1987', *BJSM*, nd.

Robson, Henry, 'Obituary: William Eldon Tucker', *BJSM*, 25:4 (1991).

Roderick, Martin, 'The sociology of pain and injury in sport' in Sigmund Loland, Berit Skirstad and Ivan Waddington (eds), *Pain and Injury in Sport: Social and ethical analysis* (London: Routledge, 2006).

Roderick, Martin, *The Work of Professional Footbal: A labour of love?* (London: Routledge, 2006).

Roderick, Martin, Waddington, Ivan and Parker, Graham, 'Playing Hurt: Managing Injuries in English Professional Football, *International Review for the Sociology of Sport*, 35:2 (2000).

Roemer, Milton I., 'Internationalism in Medicine and Public Health' in W. F. Bynum and R. Porter (eds.), *Companion Encyclopaedia of the History of Medicine, Volume 2* (London: Routledge, 1993).

Rowbotham, Shelia, *A Century of Women: The History of Women in Britain and the United States* (London: Viking, 1997).

Runciman, David, 'Is the rise of the super-athlete ruining sport?', *Observer*, 10 January 2010.

Russell, Dave, 'Mum's the Word: The Cycling Career of Beryl Burton, 1956–1986', *Women's History Review*, 17:5 (2008).

Russell, Dave, *Popular Music in England, 1840–1914: A social history, Second edition* (Manchester: Manchester University Press, 1997).

Ryan, A.J., 'History of sports medicine' in A.J. Ryan and F. Allman (eds), *Sports Medicine* (London: Academic Press, 1974).

Ryan, A.J., 'Use of Amphetamines in Athletics', *Journal of American Medical Association*, 170:5 (30 May 1959).

Ryan, Allan J., 'Sportsmedicine History', *Physician and Sportsmedicine* (October 1978).

Ryan, Allan J., 'Sports Medicine in the World Today' in Allan J. Ryan and Fred L. Allman Jr. (eds), *Sports Medicine 2nd Edition* (London: Academic Press, 1989).

Ryan, Joan, *Little Girls in Pretty Boxes: The Making and Breaking of Elite Gymnasts and Figure Skaters* (New York: Warner, 1995).

Safai, Parissa, 'A critical analysis of the development of sport medicine in Canada', *International Review for the Sociology of Sport*, 42: (2007).

Saintsbury, George and James, Jeff, *Boys Will Be Boxers* (London: Lonsdale, 1997).

Saks, Mike, 'Alternative Medicine and the Health Care Division of Labour: Present Trends and Future Prospects', *Current Sociology*, 49 (2001).

Saks, Mike, 'Bringing together the orthodox and alternative in health care', *Complementary Therapies in Medicine*, 11 (2003).

Saks, Mike, 'Introduction' in Mike Saks (ed.), *Alternative Medicine in Britain* (Oxford: Clarendon Press, 1992).

Saks, Mike, 'Medicine and the Counter Culture' in Roger Cooter and John Pickstone (eds), *Medicine in the Twentieth Century* (Amsterdam: Harwood, 2000).

Saks, Mike, *Orthodox and Alternative Medicine: Politics, Professionalization and Health Care* (London: Continuum, 2003).

Sandow, Eugen, *Life is Movement: The Physical Reconstruction and Regeneration of the People* (London: National Health Press, 1919).

Sassatelli, Roberta, 'The Commercialization of Discipline: Keep-Fit Culture and Its Values', *Journal of Modern Italian Studies*, 5:3 (2000).

Saure, Felix, 'Beautiful Bodies, Exercising Warriors and Original Peoples: Sports, Greek Antiquity and National Identity from Winckelmann to "Turnvater Jahn"', *German History*, 27:3 (2009).

Savage, Mike and Miles, Andrew, *The Remaking of the British Working Class 1840–1940* (London: Routledge, 1994).

Schiller, Kay and Young, Christopher, 'The History and Historiography of Sport in Germany: Social, Cultural and Political Perspectives', *German History*, 27:3 (2009).

Schlich, Thomas, 'The Emergence of Modern Surgery' in Deborah Brunton (ed.), *Medicine Transformed: Health, Disease and Society in Europe 1800–1930* (Manchester: Manchester University Press, 2004).

Schweinbenz, Amanda N., 'Selling Femininity: The Introduction of Women's Rowing at the 1976 Olympic Games', *IJHS*, 26:5 (2009), p. 660.

Searle, Geoffrey, *The Quest for National Efficiency: A study of British politics and British political thought 1899-1914* (Oxford: Blackwell, 1971).

Sheard, K.G., '"Brutal and degrading": the medical profession and boxing, 1838–1984', *IJHS*, 15:3, (1998).

Sheard, Ken, 'Boxing in the western civilizing process' in Eric Dunning *et al* (eds), *Sport Histories: Figurational Studies of the Development of Modern Sports* (London: Routledge, 2004).

Shipley, Stan, 'Boxing' in Tony Mason (ed.), *Sport in Britain: A Social History* (Cambridge: Cambridge University Press, 1989).

Shipley, Stan, 'Tom Causer of Bermondsey: A Boxer Hero of the 1890s', *History Workshop Journal*, 15 (1983).

Silver, J.R., 'The impact of the 21st century on rugby injuries', *Spinal Cord*, 40 (2002).

Skelton, Nick, *Only Falls and Horses* (London: Greenwater, 2001).

Smith Maguire, J., 'Leisure and the Obligations of Self-Work: An Examination of the Fitness Field', *Leisure Studies*, 27:1 (2008).

Smith, Barrie, *Doc: Jottings of a Football Club Doctor* (Birmingham: Self-published, 2003).

Sperryn, Peter, 'A personal letter from the retiring honorary secretary', *BJSM*, 17:3 (September 1983).

Sperryn, Peter, 'Secretary's Column', *BJSM*, 11:2 (June 1977).

Springhall, John, *Youth, Empire and Society; British Youth Movements, 1883–1940* (London: Croom Helm, 1977).

St. John, Ian, *The Saint: My Autobiography* (London: Hodder, 2005).

Stabiner, Karen, *Courting Fame: The hazardous road to women's tennis stardom* (London: Kingswood Press, 1986).

Stokvis, Ruud, 'Moral Entrepreneurship and Doping Cultures in Sport' (Amsterdam School for Social Science Research, Working Papers 03/04, November 2003).

Stonehenge 'Forrest' [aka Rev JG Wood], *The Handbook of Manly Exercises: Comprising Boxing, Walking, Running, Leaping, Vaulting, etc. with chapters on Training for Pedestrianism and other purposes* (London: Routledge, Warne and Routledge, 1864).

Sturdy, Steve, 'The Industrial Body' in Roger Cooter and John Pickstone (eds), *Medicine in the Twentieth Century* (Amsterdam: Harwood, 2000).

Summerfield, Penny, '"Our Amazonian Colleague": Edith Summerskill's problematic reputation' in R. Toye and J. Gottlieg (eds), *Making Reputations: Power, Persuasion and the Individual in Modern British Politics* (London: I.B. Tauris, 2005).

Summerskill, Edith, *The Ignoble Art* (London: William Heinemann, 1956).

Taylor, Matthew, 'Boxers United: Trade Unionism in British Boxing in the 1930s', *Sport in History*, 29:3 (September 2009).

Taylor, Matthew, 'Round the London Ring: Boxing, Class and Community in Interwar London', *The London Journal*, 34:2 (July 2009).

Taylor, Matthew, *The Association Game: A History of British Football* (Harlow: Pearson, 2007).

Taylor, Matthew, *The Leaguers: The Making of Professional Football in England, 1900–1939* (Liverpool: Liverpool University Press, 2005).

Teja, Angela, 'Italian sport and international relations under fascism' in P. Arnaud and J. Riordan, (eds), *Sport and international politics* (London: E. & F.N. Spon, 1998).

Terry, David, 'An Athletic Coach Ahead of his Time', *British Society of Sports History Newsletter*, 11 (Spring 2000).

Thompson, B. *et al*, 'Defining the Sports Medicine Specialist in the United Kingdom: A Delphi Study', *BJSM*, 38 (2004).

Thompson, Christopher S., *The Tour de France: A Cultural History* (Los Angeles: University of California Press, 2008).

Thomson, Mathew, 'The Psychological Body' in Roger Cooter and John Pickstone (eds), *Medicine in the Twentieth Century* (Amsterdam: Harwood, 2000).

Tinkler, Penny, 'Cause for Concern: young women and leisure, 1930–50', *Women's History Review*, 12:2 (2003).

Tipton, Charles M., 'Sports Medicine: A Century of Progress', *Journal of Nutrition*, 127:5 (May 1996).

Tisdall, R.M.N and Sherie, F., *The Young Athlete* (London: Blackie, 1933).

Tittel, K. and Knuttgen, H.G., 'The development, objectives and activities of the International Federation of Sports Medicine (FIMS)' in A. Drix, H.G. Knuttgen and K. Tittel (eds), *The Olympic Book of Sports Medicine, Volume 1 of the Encyclopedia of Sports Medicine* (Oxford: International Olympic Committee, 1988).

Todd, Jan, 'Bernarr Macfadden: Reformer of Feminine Form' in Jack W. Berryman and Roberta J. Park (eds), *Sport and Exercise Science: Essays in the History of Sports Medicine* (Urbana: University of Illinois Press, 1992).

Todd, Jan, 'The Classical Ideal and its Impact on the Search for Suitable Exercise: 1774–1830', *Iron Game History*, 2:4 (1992).

Tolich, Martin and Bell, Martha, 'The Commodification of Jockeys' Working Bodies: Anorexia or Work Discipline' in Chris McConville (ed.), *A Global Racecourse: Work, Culture and Horse Sports* (Melbourne: Australian Society for Sports History, 2008).

Tranter, Neil, *Sport, Economy and Society in Britain, 1750–1914* (Cambridge: Cambridge University Press, 1998).

Trescothick, Marcus, *Coming back to me: The Autobiography* (London: Harper, 2008).

Tucker, W. E., 'Athletic Injuries' in H. Rolleston (ed.), *The British Encyclopaedia of Medical Practice, volume 2* (London: Butterworth, 1936).

Tunstall-Pedoe, Dan, 'Obituary: Dr John G.P. Williams', *BJSM*, 29:4 (1995).

Underwood, John, 'An Unfolding Tragedy', *Sports Illustrated*, 14 August 1978.

Ungerleider, Steven, *Faust's Gold: Inside the East German Doping Machine* (New York: Thomas Dunne, 2001).

Vamplew, Wray, 'Alcohol and the Sportsperson: An Anomalous Alliance', *Sport in History*, 25:3 (December 2005).

Vamplew, Wray, 'Playing with the rules: Influences on the development of regulation in sport', *IJHS*, 24:7 (2007).

Vamplew, Wray, 'Still Crazy after All Those Years: Continuity in a Changing Labour Market for Professional Jockeys' in Adrian Smith and Dilwyn Porter (eds), *Amateurs and Professionals in Post-War British Sport* (London: Frank Cass, 2000).

Vamplew, Wray, 'Training', in Tony Collins, John Martin and Wray Vamplew, (eds), *Encyclopedia of Traditional British Rural Sports* (London: Routledge, 2005).

Van Der Merwe, Floris, 'Ernst Franz Jokl as the Father of Physical Education in South Africa', NASSH Proceedings 1990.

Varney, Wendy, 'Legitimation and Limitations: How the Opie Report on Women's Gymnastics Missed its Mark', *Sporting Traditions*, 15:2 (May 1999).

Vaughan, Graham and Guerin, Bernard, 'A Neglected Innovator in Sports Psychology: Norman Triplett and the Early History of Competitive Performance', *IJHS*, 14:2 (August 1997).

Vaughan, P., '"Secret Remedies" in the Late Nineteenth and Early Twentieth Centuries' in Mike Saks (ed.) *Alternative Medicine in Britain* (Oxford: Clarendon Press, 1992).

Verdonk, R., "Alternative Treatments of Meniscal Injuries", *Journal of Bone and Joint Surgery*, 79:B (1997).

Vertinsky, Patricia, 'Body Shapes: The Role of the Medical Establishment in Informing Female Exercise and Physical Education in Nineteenth-Century North America' in J.A. Mangan and Roberta Park (eds) *From 'Fair Sex' to Feminism: Sport and Socialization of Women in the Industrial and Post-industrial Era* (London: Frank Cass, 1987).

Vertinsky, Patricia, 'Embodying Normalcy: Anthropometry and the Long Arm of William H. Sheldon's Somatotyping Project', *Journal of Sport History*, 29:1 (Spring 2002).

Vertinsky, Patricia, 'Exercise, Physical Capability, and the Eternally Wounded Woman in Late Nineteenth-Century North America' in Jack W. Berryman and Roberta J. Park (eds), *Sport and Exercise Science: Essays in the History of Sports Medicine* (Urbana: University of Illinois Press, 1992).

Vertinsky, Patricia, 'Making and marking gender: Bodybuilding and the medicalization of the body from one century's end to another', *Sport in Society*, 2:1 (1999).

Vertinsky, Patricia, 'What is Sports Medicine?' *Journal of Sport History*, 34:1 (Spring 2007).

Vettenniemi, Erkki, 'Runners, Rumors, and Reams of Representations: An Inquiry into Drug Use by Athletes in the 1920s', *Journal of Sport History*, 37:3 (Fall 2010).

Waddington, I., Roderick, M. and Naik, R., 'Methods of Appointment and Qualifications of Club Doctors and Physiotherapists in English Professional Football: Some Problems and Issues', *BJSM*, 35: (2001).

Waddington, Ivan, 'Changing Patterns of Drug Use in British Sport from the 1960', *Sport in History*, 25:3 (December 2005).

Waddington, Ivan, 'Ethical problems in the medical management of sports injuries: A case study of English professional football' Sigmund Loland, Berit Skirstad and Ivan Waddington (eds), *Pain and Injury in Sport: Social and ethical analysis* (London: Routledge, 2006).

Waddington, Ivan, 'Jobs for the Boys: A Study of the Employment of Club Doctors and Physiotherapists in English Professional Football', *Soccer and Society*, 3 (2002).

Waddington, Ivan, Roderick, Martin and Parker, Graham, *Managing Injuries in Professional Football: A Study of the Roles of the Club Doctor and Physiotherapist* (Leicester: Leicester University Press, 1999).

Waddington, Ivan, *Sport, Health and Drugs: A Critical Sociological Perspective* (London: E and F.N. Spon, 2000).

Wamsley, K.B. and Whitson, D., 'Celebrating Violent Masculinities: The Boxing Death of Luther McGrory', *Journal of Sport History*, 25:3 (Fall 1998).

Wamsley, Kevin B., 'Womanizing Olympic Athletes: Policy and Practice during the Avery Brundage Era' in Gerald P. Schaus and Stephen R. Wenn (eds), *Onwards to the Olympics: Historical Perspectives on the Olympic Games* (Waterloo, Ontario: Wilfred Laurier University Press, 2007).

Watkins, Sid, *Beyond the Limit* (Basingstoke: Macmillan, 2001).

Watkins, Sid, *Life at the Limit: Triumph and Tragedy in Formula One* (London: Pan, 1996).

Watt, Carey, Book Review of John J. MacAloon (ed.), *Muscular Christianity in Colonial and Post-Colonial Worlds* (London: Routledge, 2008), *IJHS*, 26:15 (2009).

Weber, Eugen, 'Gymnastics and Sports in *Fin-de-Siècle* France', *American Historical Review*, 76:1 (February 1971).

Webster, Charles, 'The Health of the School Child During the Depression' in N. Parry and D. McNair (eds) *The Fitness of the Nation-Physical and Health Education in the Nineteenth and Twentieth Centuries: Proceedings of the 1982 Annual Conference of the History of Education Society of Great Britain* (History of Education Society, 1983).

Webster, F.A.M. and Heys, J.A., *Athletic Training for Men and Boys* (London: John F. Shaw, 1933).

Webster, F.A.M., *Care of Athletes* (London: George G. Harrap, 1938).

Weightman, Doris and Browne, R.C., 'Injuries in Rugby and Association Football', *BJSM*, 8:4 (December 1974).

Weindling, Paul, 'From Germ Theory to Social Medicine: Public Health, 1880–1930' in Deborah Brunton (ed.), *Medicine Transformed: Health, Disease and Society in Europe 1800–1930* (Manchester: Manchester University Press, 2004).

Weiskopf, Herman, 'The Good Hands Man', *Sports Illustrated*, 16 July 1979.

Welch, Ellen and Kelly, Sara, 'Premier league doctor', *Student BMJ*, 12 (2004).

Welshman, John, 'Boxing and the historians', *IJHS*, 14:1 (1997), pp. 195–203.

Welshman, John, 'Only Connect: The History of Sport, Medicine and Society', *IJHS*, 15:2 (August 1998).

Welshman, John, 'Physical Culture and Sport in Schools in England and Wales, 1900–40', *IJHS*, 15:1 (April 1998).

Welshman, John, 'Physical Education and the School Medical Service in England and Wales, 1907–1939', *Social History of Medicine*, 9:1 (1996).

Westmann, Stephan, Sport, Physical Training and Womanhood (London, 1939).

Whitelocke, R.H. Anglin, *Football Injuries* (London: Medical Officers of Schools Association, 1904).

Whiteson, A.L., 'The doctor at the boxing ring: professional boxing' in Simon D.W. Payne (ed.), *Medicine, Sport and the Law* (London: Blackwell Scientific Publications, 1990).

Whorton, James, '"Athlete's Heart"': The Medical Debate Over Athleticism, 1870–1920', *Journal of Sport History*, 9:1 (Spring 1982).

Wiederkehr, Stefan, '"We shall never know the exact number of men who have competed in the Olympics posing as women": Sport, Gender Verification and the Cold War', *IJHS*, 26:4 (2009).

Wiggins, David, *Glory Bound: Black Athletes in a White America* (Syracuse: Syracuse University Press, 1997).

Williams, J.G.P. (ed.), *Sports Medicine* (London: Edward Arnold, 1962).

Williams, J.P.R., *JPR: Given the Breaks: My Life in Rugby* (London: Hodder, 2006).

Williams, Jean, *A Game for Rough Girls? A history of women's football in Britain* (London: Routledge, 2003).

Williams, John A., 'Winter Sports' in J.R. Armstrong and W.E. Tucker (eds), *Injury in Sport: The Physiology, Prevention and Treatment of Injuries associated with Sport* (London: Staples Press, 1964).

Williams, John G.P., *Medical Aspects of Sport and Physical Fitness* (London: Pergamon Press, 1965).

Williams, John, *Red Men* (Edinburgh: Mainstream, 2011).

Winterstein, C.E., 'Head Injuries Attributable to Boxing' *Lancet*, 18 September 1937.

Woodland, Les (ed.), *The Yellow Jersey Companion to the Tour de France* (London: Yellow Jersey Press, 2003).

Woods, R. Salisbury, 'Disorders and Accidents of Athletes', *Practitioner*, (September 1930).

Woods, R., 'Physician, Heal Thyself: the Health and Mortality of Victorian Doctors', *Social History of Medicine*, 9:1 (1996).

World Sports, April 1953, pp. 9–10; September 1953, pp. 5–6.

Wrynn, Alison M., 'The Athlete in the Making: The Scientific Study of American Athletic Performance, 1920–1932', *Sport in History*, 30:1 (March 2010).

Wrynn, Alison, '"Under the Showers": An Analysis of the Historical Connections between American Athletic Training and Physical Education', *Journal of Sport History*, 34:1 (Spring 2007).

Wrynn, Alison, 'The Human Factor: Science, Medicine and the International Olympic Committee, 1900–70', *Sport in Society*, 7:2 (2004).

Yesalis Charles E. and Bahrke, Michael S., 'Anabolic Steroid and Stimulant Use in North American Sport between 1850 and 1980', *Sport in History*, 25:3 (December 2005).

Zweiniger-Bargielowska, Ina, *Managing the Body: Beauty, Health and Fitness in Britain, 1880–1939* (Oxford: Oxford University Press, 2010).

Zweinigier-Bargielowska, Ina, 'Building a British Superman: Physical Culture in Interwar Britain', *Journal of Contemporary History*, 41:4 (2006).

Zweinigier-Bargielowska, Ina, 'Raising a Nation of 'Good Animals': The New Health Society and Health Education Campaigns in Interwar Britain', *Social History of Medicine*, 20:1 (2007).

Reports

Amsterdam Olympic Committee, *The Official Report of the IXth Olympiad, Amsterdam 1928* (Amsterdam: Olympic Committee of the Amsterdam Olympic Games, 1928).

Barton, Susan, Carter, Neil, Holt, Richard and Williams, John, *Learning Disability, Sport and Legacy: A Report by the Legacy Research Group on the Special Olympics GB National Summer Games Leicester 2009* (Leicester: De Montfort University, 2011).

Berlin Olympic Committee, *The Official Report of the XIth Olympiad, Berlin* (Berlin: Olympic Committee of the Berlin Olympic Games, 1936).

British Olympic Council, *The Fourth Olympiad: London* 1908 (London: British Olympic Council, 1908).

De Coubertin, Pierre, Philemon, Timoleon J., Politis, N.G. and Anninos, Charalmbos, *The Olympic Games: B.C. 776–A.D. 1896, Second Part, The Olympic Games in 1896* (London: H.G. Grevel, 1897).

Department for Culture, Media and Sport, *Coaching Task Force – Final Report* (London: Department for Culture, Media and Sport, 2002).

European Rugby Cup, Decision of Appeal Committee in Appeal by Tom Williams, held at the Radisson SAS Hotle, 301 Argyle Street, Glasgow, 17 August 2009.

House of Commons Culture, Media and Sport Committee, *Women's Football: Fourth Report of Session 2005–06* (London: Houses of Commons, 2006).

Lucas, Charles J.P., *The Olympic Games 1904* (St. Louis: Woodward and Tiernan, 1905).

Nicholls, J.P., Coleman, P. and Williams, B.T., *Injuries in sport and exercise: A national study of the epidemiology of exercise-related injury and illness, A Report to the Sports Council* (November 1991).

Recreation and Physical Fitness for Girls and Women (London: Board of Education, Physical Training Series, no. 16, 1938).

Report of the Inter-Departmental Committee on Physical Deterioration 1903–04.

Savage, Howard, Bentley, Harold W., McGovern, John T. and Smiley, Dean F., *American College Athletics, Bulletin Number 23* (New York: Carnegie Foundation for the Advancement of Teaching, 1929).

Stockholm Organising Committee, *The Olympic Games of Stockholm 1912* (Stockholm: Swedish Olympic Committee, 1912).

Wolfenden Committee on Sport, *Sport and the Community* (London: CCPR, 1960–61).

Theses

Bourne, Nicholas D., 'Fast Science: A History of Training Theory and Methods for Elite Runners Through 1975' (Unpublished PhD Thesis, University of Texas, Austin, 2008).

Day, David, 'From Barclay to Brickett: Coaching Practices and Coaching Lives in Nineteenth and Early Twentieth Century England', (Unpublished PhD: De Montfort University, Leicester 2008).

Cole, Barbara, 'The East German Sports System: Image and Reality' (Unpublished PhD Thesis: Texas Tech University, 2000).

Galligan, Frank, 'The History of Gymnastic Activity in the West Midlands, with special reference to Birmingham, from 1865 to 1918: With an analysis of military influences, secular and religious innovation and educational developments' (Unpublished PhD thesis, Coventry University, 1999).

Moon, Gregory P., 'A New Dawn Rising: An Empirical and Social Study concerning the emergence and development of English Women's athletics until 1960' (Unpublished PhD: Roehampton Institute, 1997).

Robinson, Lynne, '"Tripping Daintily into the Arena": A Social History of English Women's Athletics 1921–1960' (Unpublished PhD: University of Warwick, 1996).

Sheard, Ken, 'Boxing in the Civilizing Process' (Unpublished PhD: Anglia Polytechnic University, 1992).

Simons, David, 'The Evolution of the Endurance Athlete: Training, Diet and Performance, c.1750–1914', (Unpublished MA Dissertation: De Montfort University, Leicester, 2008).

Websites

Frederick O. Mueller and Jerry L. Diehl, 'Annual Survey of Football Injury Research, 1931–2003', National Center for Catastrophic Sport Injury Research, http://www.unc.edu/depts/nccsi/AllSport.htm [accessed 22 October 2004]

http://query.nytimes.com/gst/fullpage.html?res=990DEFDE173BF93BA1574C0A9649 C8B63&sec=health&spon=&pagewanted=3 [accessed 24 June 2011]

http://www.boxrec.com/media/index.php/USA:_New_York_Laws [accessed 15 April 2007]

http://www.boxrec.com/media/index.php/Walker_Law [accessed 15 April 2007]

http://www.guardian.co.uk/sport/2010/sep/14/steph-brennan-harlequins-bloodgate [accessed 3 August 2011]

http://www.telegraph.co.uk/sport/rugbyunion/club/8002256/Harlequins-Bloodgate-physio-Steph-Brennan-struck-off-by-Health-Professions-Council.html [accessed 3 August 2011]

Pickstone, John V., 'A brief history of medical history', http://www.history.ac.uk/makinghistory/resources/articles/history [accessed 20 June 2011]

Tony Blair's speech on healthy living, http://politics.guardian.co.uk/print/0,,329538655-1070979,00.html [accessed 26 July 2006]

http://www.acsm.org/AM/Template.cfm?Section=About_ACSM [accessed 10 August 2010]

http://www.coylehamiltonwillis.com/gaa/gaa.htm [accessed 24 September 2005]

http://www.guardian.co.uk/sport/2006/oct/06/rugbyunion.gdnsport3 [accessed 20 December 2007]

http://www.telegraph.co.uk/sport/othersports/drugsinsport [accessed 21 March 2011]

http://www.unc.edu/depts/nccsi/AllSport.htm [accessed 27 September 2007]

Index

00212981

42636550R00170

Made in the USA
Middletown, DE
17 April 2017